Planning and making crowns and bridges

Planning and making crowns and bridges

Third Edition

Bernard G N Smith

BDS, PhD, MSc, MRD, FDSRCSEng, FDSRCSEdin

Professor of Conservative Dentistry
The United Medical and Dental Schools, Guy's Hospital, London

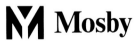 Mosby

St. Louis Baltimore Boston Carlsbad Chicago Naples New York Philadelphia Portland
London Madrid Mexico City Singapore Sydney Tokyo Toronto Wiesbaden

MARTIN DUNITZ

© **Bernard GN Smith 1986, 1990, 1998**

First published in the United Kingdom in 1986 by

Martin Dunitz Ltd
The Livery House
7–9 Pratt Street
London NW1 0AE

Second Edition 1990
Third Edition 1998

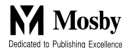

Dedicated to Publishing Excellence

A Times Mirror
Company

Distributed in the U.S.A. and Canada by
Mosby–Year Book
11830 Westline Industrial Drive
St. Louis, Missouri 63146

Times Mirror Professional Publishing Ltd.
130 Flaska Drive
Markham, Ontario L6G 1B8

A CIP catalogue record for this book is available from the British Library

ISBN 1 85317 314 2

Typeset by Scribe Design, Gillingham, Kent, UK
Printed and bound in Singapore by Toppan Printing Company (s) Pte Ltd

Contents

Preface   vii

Preface to the third edition   ix

Acknowledgements   x

Part 1 Crowns

1 Indications and contraindications for crowns   3

2 Types of crown   24

3 Designing crown preparations   41

4 Occlusal considerations   62

5 Planning and making crowns   85

6 Clinical techniques for crown construction   100

Part 2 Bridges

7 Indications for bridges compared with partial dentures and implant-retained prostheses   149

8 Types of bridge   173

9 Components of bridges: retainers, pontics and connectors   191

10 Designing and planning bridges   207

11 Clinical techniques for bridge construction   222

Part 3 Splints

12 Fixed splints   241

Part 4 Failures and repairs

13 Crown and bridge failures and repairs   255

Further reading   275

Index   279

Preface

The aim of this book is to answer at least as many of the questions beginning with 'why' as those that begin with 'how'. A textbook is not the ideal medium for teaching practical, clinical or technical procedures. These are best learnt at the chairside and in the laboratory. However, the mass of material which must be learnt, usually in a restricted timetable, in the clinic and laboratory means that there is often insufficient time to answer the questions, 'Why am I doing this?' or, 'When should I not do this?' or even, 'What on earth can I do here?'

The book is meant for clinicians, both undergraduate and postgraduate, and so although the emphasis is on treatment planning, crown and bridge design and the related theory, clinical techniques are also described in some detail. Laboratory technique is, though, almost completely omitted, both to keep the book to manageable proportions and because most clinicians no longer undertake this themselves. It is nevertheless abundantly clear that a good standard of laboratory work is as important as the other phases in the construction of crowns and bridges. The process may be divided into three stages:

Initial decision making and mouth preparation
Clinical procedures
Technical procedures.

The purpose of this book is to help quite a lot with the first stage, rather less with the second (a book cannot replace clinical experience) and hardly at all with the third.

The intention is to help solve real clinical problems. The student sitting in a technique laboratory faced with an arch of intact perfectly formed natural or artificial teeth planning to undertake 'ideal' crown preparations will find little help here. It may be good initial teaching to cut 'classic' preparations, but this is only part of the training towards solving the real problems of real patients in the real world. The opinions expressed in a textbook can only a go a little way further towards solving these problems.

Undergraduate and postgraduate students need also to take advantage of their own and others' clinical experience and learn by thinking about their clinical problems and talking about them with others. Making the right decision is as important as executing the treatment well.

There is no reference to 'case selection' or 'patient selection' for the techniques described. That is not the way things are in practice. There it is necessary to select the appropriate technique for the patient in front of you rather than select the patient for the technique. Things are different in dental schools. It often happens that in order to provide a balanced range of experience for undergraduate students in a limited period of time, patients are selected to go on to particular waiting lists to provide a flow of 'clinical material' for the students' needs. This may be necessary but the attitudes it sometimes develops are unfortunate. The essential feature of any profession is that it attempts to solve the problems of its clients before concerning itself with its own welfare.

Because this is the approach, clinical photographs or at least photographs of extracted teeth or casts, are used to illustrate the text in preference to line drawings, except where a photograph is impractical. Photographs are used even when the work shown is not 'perfect'. No apology is made for this. In reality, although we should strive for perfection (if we know what perfection is in a given case, and we often do not), we will frequently not achieve it. It is more realistic to talk about levels of acceptability. This is not to advocate unnecessary compromise, but to recognize that in many situations a compromise (from knowledge, not ignorance) is necessary. After all, the ideal would be to prevent caries, trauma and congenital deformity so that crowns and bridges were not necessary in the first place. Once they are needed there is already a situation that is less than perfect.

Some of the work photographed is mine, some is undergraduate and postgraduate student work with a greater or lesser amount of help by teachers, some of the technical work is carried out by the clinicians themselves but most by technicians or student technicians, and some illustrations have been kindly lent by colleagues. In view of the likelihood, and indeed the intention that readers will find fault with some of the illustrations and because some illustrate the work of a team rather than an individual, no acknowledgment is given for individual illustrations. I am, however, extremely grateful to all those who have allowed me to photograph their work and in particular to those who have lent me their own illustrations. Their names appear in the Acknowledgments.

Also omitted are text references. In a book of this size, which is not intended to be a reference book, it is not possible to be comprehensive, while it is impolite to use phrases such as 'there is evidence that . . .' without making proper reference to the source of the evidence. Isolated references in these cases could well lead the enthusiastic student into an unbalanced reading programme. There is also no bibliography of the major reference texts on crown and bridge work, as a more up-to-date source for this will be the catalogue in your local dental library. The further reading suggested at the end of the book is a personal selection from the literature which contains evidence to support at least some of the opinions expressed, and which will guide the reader deeper into the subject.

B.G.N.S.

Preface to the third edition

The purpose of this book and the way it is written remain as set out in the original preface.

The developments in this field continue apace and are reflected in this third edition by more than one hundred new colour photographs and revisions to the text of every chapter. Some of the earlier line drawings have also been replaced by colour photographs.

Some restorations and techniques are now used less and so the emphasis on them has been reduced or they have been dropped altogether. This applies particularly to anterior partial crowns although the importance of posterior partial crowns remains.

New sections have been added on implant retained prostheses, in particular emphasising their role in the replacement of missing teeth in comparison with bridges and partial dentures. The level of detail is sufficient to assist with the initial treatment planning process but there is no attempt to provide details of the detailed planning for implants or their construction which are subjects beyond the scope of this book.

Another change is to put greater emphasis on fixed-moveable designs for posterior minimal-preparation bridges and cantilever designs for anterior minimal-preparation bridges. Other additions include changing attitudes towards composite and porcelain veneers, methods for producing minor axial tooth movement and crown lengthening procedures in treating worn dentitions and the introduction of the automix gun simplifying the mixing and placing of many impression and other materials.

Some restorations which are no longer made are still included in relation to their maintenance and repair.

Acknowledgements

The following have lent photographs but for reasons explained in the preface, specific credit is not given to each one. I am, however, extremely grateful to them for their generosity: Chris Allen; David Bartlett; Nicholas Capp; John Cardwell; Russell Greenwood; Leslie Howe; George Kantorowicz; Bernard Keiser; Orthomax Limited, Bradford; David Parr; Ian Potter; John Richards; David Ricketts; Paul Robinson; Michael Thomas; John Walter; Katherine Warren; Tim Watson.

Other help with illustrations has been given by: Ruth Allen; Osama Atta; Dennis Bailey; Peter Chittenden; Cottrell and Co., London; Usha Desai; Terence Freeman; June Hodgkin; Orodent Limited, Windsor; Peter Pilecki; Peter Rhind; Nicholas Taylor; Leslie Wilcox. Bill Sharpling has helped considerably with the illustrations for the third edition.

Permission to reproduce Figure 4.11, which first appeared in Restorative Dentistry, has been kindly given by A E Morgan Publications Limited.

Part 1   Crowns

1 Indications and contraindications for crowns

Before the acid-etch retention system, composite resin restorative materials and efficient, simple pin retention systems were developed, crowns were the only way of restoring many teeth that can now be restored by these other means. At the same time, more patients are keeping more of their teeth for longer and are expecting faulty teeth to be repaired rather than extracted. Therefore, although there are fewer indications for crowning teeth than there were, more teeth are actually being crowned than ever before. About two million crowns per year are made in the UK National Health Service, representing 2–3 crowns per week per dentist. This figure has more than doubled between 1980 and 1990. Similar increases have occurred in most Western countries.

When the only choice for a tooth was a crown or extraction, the decision was relatively simple. Now, with more options it is more difficult. This chapter discusses the current indications for crowns and their alternatives, and guides the reader towards a decision. However, clinical decision making is the very substance of the dentist's work and cannot be done by textbook instructions: do not expect a set of clear rules to follow. Each set of clinical judgements and decisions must be unique, taken in the context of the patient's circumstances.

General indications for extra-coronal restorations

Crowns versus fillings

Most dental restorations are provided as treatment for dental caries. Once the initial lesion has penetrated the enamel, the caries spreads along the enamel–dentine junction and balloons out in dentine towards the pulp. The growth of the carious lesion is much faster in dentine than it is in enamel, so the enamel becomes undermined and then suddenly collapses into the cavity. Because of this, our forefathers thought that caries started inside the tooth and worked its way to the surface. Today, many carious lesions are detected and treated at an early stage while the enamel is still largely intact. Indeed, even more lesions are prevented from occurring at all.

Since caries produces most of its damage inside the tooth rather than on the surface, the commonest type of restoration is intra-coronal. Often, sound enamel has to be cut away to give access to the caries. Only very rarely is the surface of a tooth extensively destroyed by caries leaving a base of sound dentine, and it is therefore most unusual in the treatment of primary caries for an extra-coronal restoration (a crown) to be made on a preparation consisting of intact dentine. When secondary caries develops around existing fillings, intra-coronal restorations are still more conservative and more closely relate to the pattern of development of caries than crowns, and are therefore preferred whenever possible. Indeed, a high caries rate is a contraindication to crowns. In these cases the caries should be removed, the tooth stabilized and a preventive regime instituted before crowns are made.

With larger lesions and particularly when cusps are lost, the decision between filling and crowning a tooth becomes more difficult (see pages 17–20).

General indications for crowns

Having established that primary caries is not a common or desirable reason for making crowns, the following are the main indications for extra-coronal restorations:

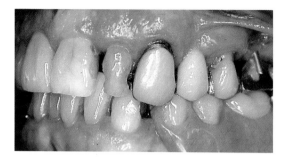

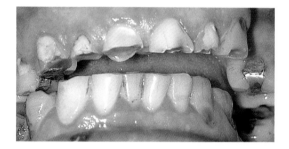

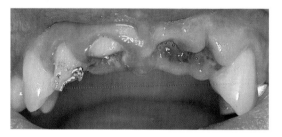

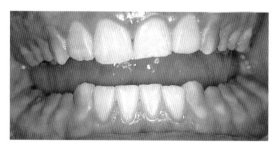

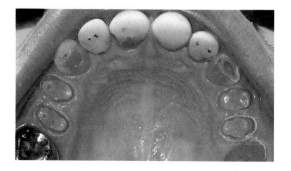

Figure 1.1

General indications for crowns.

a This mouth has been well treated in the past but the restorations are now failing. In particular the lateral incisor has lost two fillings, the pulp has died and the tooth is discoloured. It now needs a crown (see Figure 2.1*i*, page 27).

b Trauma: the result of a blow from a hockey stick. Two incisors have been lost and the upper right central incisor is fractured, exposing the pulp, the fracture line extending subgingivally on the palatal side. The lateral incisor is fractured involving enamel and dentine only. The pulp retained its vitality. Although it could be restored in other ways, a crown would be the most satisfactory solution since it would then match the other anterior restorations. If the central incisor is to be retained, it will need to be crowned, probably as a bridge abutment (see later).

c Gross tooth wear arising from a combination of erosion and attrition. This has passed the point where the patient can accept the appearance, and crowns are necessary.

d A moderate degree of amelogenesis imperfecta in a sixteen year old. The posterior teeth are affected more than the anterior teeth but the upper incisors are slightly discoloured and are chipping away at the incisal edge. Crowns were made for all the teeth except the lower incisors and these will be kept under review.

e Dentinogenesis imperfecta in a teenage patient. The incisor teeth have been protected with acid-etch-retained composite from shortly after their eruption and the first molar teeth have been protected with stainless-steel crowns. It is now time to make permanent crowns for all the remaining teeth.

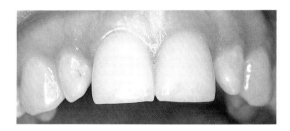

f Peg-shaped upper lateral incisors.

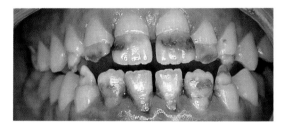

g Typical distribution of enamel hypoplasia, in this case due to typhoid in the patient's early childhood.

Badly broken-down teeth

Usually these teeth will have been restored previously, and may have suffered secondary caries or parts of the tooth or restoration may have broken off. Before crowns can be made the lost dentine will usually need to be replaced by a suitable core of restorative material (see Figure 1.1a).

Primary trauma

An otherwise-intact tooth may have a large fragment broken off without damaging the pulp and leaving sufficient dentine to support a crown (see Figure 1.1b).

Tooth wear

The processes of erosion (damage from acid other than that produced by bacteria), attrition (mechanical wear of one tooth against another) and abrasion (mechanical wear by extraneous agents) occur in all patients. What is remarkable is that teeth, which have little capacity for regeneration and which are in constant use, do not wear out long before the patient dies. Although tooth wear is normal, if it is excessive or occurs early in life, crowns or other restorations may be needed (see Figure 1.1c).

The lifelong management of excessive tooth wear is a topic of increasing interest as patients keep their teeth longer. In general the approach should be:

- Early diagnosis and prevention
- Monitoring any further progression until the patient complains of the appearance, sensitivity (which does not respond to other treatment), function is affected, or the wear reaches a point where restorations will become technically difficult
- At this point provide minimal restorations
- If the problem continues, provide crowns.

Hypoplastic conditions

These may be subdivided into hereditary and acquired defects. Examples of the former are amelogenesis imperfecta (see Figure 1.1d), dentinogenesis imperfecta (see Figure 1.1e) and hypodontia (for example peg-shaped upper lateral incisors – see Figure 1.1f). Examples of acquired defects are fluorosis, tetracycline stain and enamel hypoplasia resulting from a major metabolic disturbance (usually a childhood illness) at the age when the enamel was developing (see Figure 1.1g).

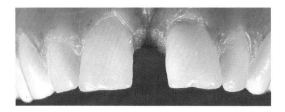

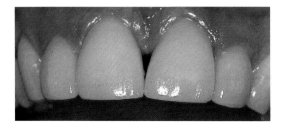

Figure 1.2

Changing the shape and size of teeth.

a A large midline diastema that the patient found aesthetically unacceptable.

b The same patient after the central incisors have been moved closer together orthodontically and all four incisors crowned. The patient must be warned of any compromise in the appearance that is anticipated – in this case the triangular space that remains at the midline. It is possible to increase the width of the incisal edges to fill the space, but the width of the crowns at the neck is determined by the width of the roots, so that only minimal enlargement is possible without creating uncleansable overhanging crown margins.

To alter the shape or size or inclination of teeth

Major changes in the position of teeth can be made only by orthodontic treatment, though minor changes in appearance can be achieved by crowns. Teeth can be made larger but not usually smaller. For example, a diastema between teeth which the patient finds unattractive can be closed by means of oversized crowns (see Figure 1.2).

To alter the occlusion

Crowns may be used to alter the angulation or occlusal relationships of anterior and posterior teeth as part of an occlusal reconstruction either to solve an occlusal problem or to improve function (see Chapter 4).

As part of another restoration

Crowns are made to support bridges and as components of fixed splints. They are also made to alter the alignment of teeth to produce guide planes for partial dentures or to carry precision attachments for precision attachment retained partial dentures (see Parts II and III).

Combined indications

More than one of these indications may be present, so that, for example, a broken-down posterior tooth that is over-erupted and tilted may be crowned as a repair and at the same time to alter its occlusal relationships and its inclination, providing a guide plane and rest seat for a partial denture.

Multiple crowns

With some of these indications, notably tooth wear and hypoplastic conditions, many or all of the teeth may need to be crowned.

Appearance

One of the principal reasons for patients seeking dental treatment is to maintain or improve their appearance. Relative prosperity, changing social attitudes and the success of modern dental materials mean that expectations of good dental appearance are rising. Fewer teeth are being extracted, and when they are it is at a later age. It is much less common now to see a mouth such as shown in Figure 1.3 than it was in the mid 1960s, when this photograph was taken.

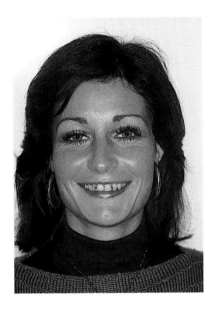

Figure 1.3

An attractive appearance spoiled by unsightly teeth.

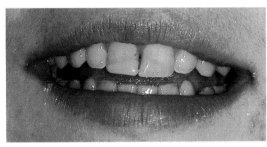

Figure 1.4

The appearance of composite restorations.

a The central incisors fractured in a riding accident eight years previously. The initial composite restorations were placed by the patient's mother, a general dentist. They were subsequently replaced, once by a specialist practitioner and once at a dental school. The composites shown had been in place for three years, and the patient was now 21 years old. She refused to consider further attempts at composite restorations, and crowns were made.

b Composite restorations to erosion lesions at the necks of the upper right central and lateral incisors, the canine and first premolar. These have been present for 18 months and are maintaining their appearance.

As standards of appearance and expectations rise, some dental defects, or types of restoration, which at one time would have been tolerated, are no longer acceptable to patients.

Composite and glass ionomer restorations, which have improved considerably, still tend, after a few years in the mouth, to wear or stain, or the margins begin to look unattractive (see Figure 1.4). In some of these cases, even though the fillings are more or less satisfactory, the patient may be justified in demanding crowns for the sake of appearance.

In several of the general indications listed above, for example, tetracycline stain and midline diastemas, the only reason for considering crowns is to change the patient's appearance. In others, for example fractured incisal edges and tooth wear, there may be other problems such as sensitive exposed dentine or functional difficulty as well as the need to restore appearance.

Appearance is important to the patient and must therefore be important to the dentist. After the relief and prevention of pain and infection it is probably the next most important reason for providing dental treatment.

Function

With modern cooked diets it is possible to masticate — and speak — without any teeth, or with complete dentures, but most patients (and probably all dentists) would not want to. As with appearance, this is again a question of the quality of life. An occluding set of natural, or second best, restored teeth is better at coping with a full varied range of diet than dentures.

Restoring function is part of the reason for several of the general indications above such as the restoration of badly broken down teeth, tooth wear, and providing support for bridges or partial dentures.

Mechanical problems

Sometimes, although it would be possible to restore a tooth by means of an intra-coronal restoration, the pattern of damage to the tooth gives rise to anxieties about the retention of the restoration, the strength of the remaining tooth tissue, or the strength of the restorative material. Fillings fail because they fall out, because of secondary caries, or because part of the tooth or part of the restoration fractures. These failures are upsetting to the patient and embarrassing to the dentist, and it is therefore tempting to prescribe crowns when there is even a faint possibility that one of these problems will arise.

However, crowns can also fail. If a filling fails, it is often possible to make a more extensive restoration or a crown. If a crown fails, a further crown may not be possible and extraction may be all that is left.

In deciding between a crown and a filling there are two considerations to be weighed up. First, how real is the risk of mechanical failure of the filling or surrounding tooth and what can be done to minimize this risk? Second, how much more destruction of sound tooth tissue is necessary to make a crown?

In general, it is better to take the more conservative approach first, even if this involves some risk of the restoration failing. The alternative is to provide far more crowns than are strictly necessary and perhaps give rise to even greater problems for the patient later on.

Indications for anterior crowns

Caries and trauma

All the general indications listed above may apply to anterior crowns. Before the days of acid-etch retained composite restorations or glass ionomer cements, anterior crowns were indicated much more frequently for the restoration of carious or fractured incisors. Today many of these teeth can be restored without crowns; these are often not needed until the pulp is involved (see Figures 1.1a, b).

Non-vital teeth

When a pulp becomes necrotic the tooth often discolours due to the haemoglobin breakdown products. This discolouration may be such that it can only satisfactorily be obscured by a crown (see Figure 1.5).

Tooth wear

The ideal approach to problems of tooth wear is to prevent the condition getting worse by identifying the cause and eliminating it as early

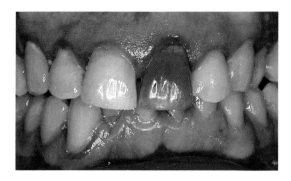

Figure 1.5

The central incisor has a necrotic pulp and is grossly discoloured. This degree of discolouration could not be resolved by bleaching or veneering the tooth. The periodontal condition must be improved before a crown can be made successfully.

as possible. Crowns should be made only when the cause of the tooth wear cannot be identified or cannot be eliminated, and the damage is serious. Sometimes the rate of tooth wear slows down or stops with no obvious explanation and the teeth remain stable for some years. Crowns are not a good preventive measure except as a last resort.

Hypoplastic conditions

In many of the hypoplastic conditions the patient (or parents) will seek treatment at an early age, often as soon as the permanent teeth erupt, and treatment may be carried out in conjunction with orthodontic treatment. In some of these cases large numbers of teeth are affected, and so the decision whether to crown them, offer some alternative form of treatment, or simply leave the condition alone, is a fairly momentous one. Figure 1.6 shows several cases of tetracycline staining affecting many teeth. Differences in the lip morphology, the depth of uniformity of the colour, and the patient's age and general attitude will all influence the decision. In the last case illustrated, 16 crowns have been provided to disguise the colour in all the visible teeth. This is a considerable undertaking and should not be embarked upon lightly by either patient or dentist. In particular with young patients, the lifelong maintenance implications must be fully understood. It should be explained that crowns are unlikely to last the whole of a natural lifetime and replacements will

be costly if they are possible at all. However, if after proper consideration crowns are made, they can dramatically improve the patient's appearance in a way that is impossible by any other form of treatment.

To alter the shape, size or inclination of teeth

Again, treatment is frequently sought at an early age and is likely to be combined with orthodontic treatment (see Figure 1.2).

As part of other restorations

Anterior crowns are often made as components of anterior bridges and splints. They are less often needed to support partial dentures. Bridges and splints are dealt with in Parts II and III.

What are the alternatives to anterior crowns?

Bleaching

Some teeth discoloured by a necrotic pulp can be bleached with hydrogen peroxide or other oxidizing agents (see Figure 1.7a,b).

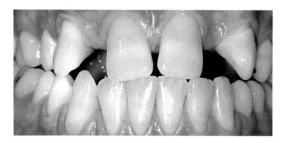

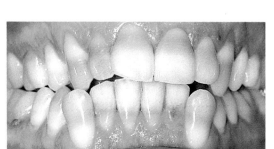

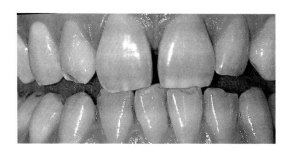

Figure 1.6

Tetracycline stain

a Mild, uniform staining. It is unlikely that treatment will be necessary other than to replace the missing lateral incisors.

b Tetracycline staining with severe banding. The extent of treatment depends on the lip line. In this case the lower lip covered the gingival half of the lower incisors, and therefore treatment for the lower teeth was not necessary.

c Darker but more uniform tetracycline staining. In this case a vital bleaching technique was used.

Restorations in composite materials or glass ionomer cements

The appearance of modern aesthetic restorative materials can be excellent (see Figure 1.4b). Although they sometimes deteriorate to give the sort of appearance also shown in Figure 1.4a, it is of course possible to replace them, usually without destroying very much more tooth tissue. It can be argued that with rapid development of anterior restorative materials, it may be preferable to replace composite restorations until such time as a more durable material is available rather than make crowns. The problem is that many of these patients are young, attractive and more concerned with their appearance now than about long-term maintenance problems with crowns.

It is clear that no absolute rules can be given on whether crowns or fillings are indicated other than to say that in general the more conservative procedures are to be preferred.

Gold or porcelain inlays

Before the advent of acid-etch retained composite materials, the conventional way to restore a fractured incisal edge was by means of a Class IV gold inlay with or without a facing (see Figure

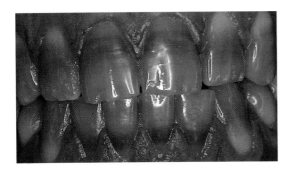

d Extreme tetracycline staining with banding.

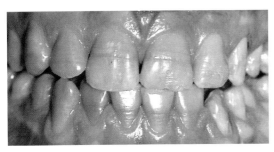

e Darkly stained teeth with four teeth prepared for crowns.

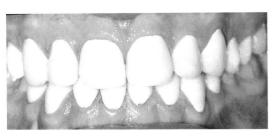

f Sixteen crowns made for the patient shown in e. The shade is too uniform and light, but this was at the insistence of the patient, who has remained happy with the appearance for several years. Today, veneers would probably be used rather than crowns.

1.7c). The alternative, if the appearance of gold or the facing material was not acceptable, was to make a crown. Today, acid-etch retained composite restorations have completely replaced Class IV gold inlays.

Similarly, porcelain inlays for Class V lesions have also almost completely disappeared. This is not because they were unsatisfactory in appearance but because laboratory costs and the time involved were much greater than for composite or glass ionomer restorations. However, there are times when a really durable restoration that will not wear or discolour or alter its surface texture may be an advantage (see Figure 1.7d).

Veneer restorations

The earliest veneer restorations were made from polyacrylic and were preformed. They provided a reasonably satisfactory and less destructive solution to many of the problems described earlier, in particular where multiple restorations of intact teeth were needed, for example in cases of tetracycline stain. These polyacrylic veneers are no longer made and have been replaced by better materials. However, some patients still have them in place, and they need to be recognized and, in most cases, replaced (see Figure 1.8a, f–l).

There is now a choice between two materials for veneer restorations: composite and porcelain.

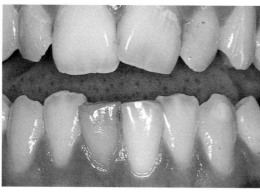

Figure 1.7

Alternatives to crowns

a A discoloured, non-vital lower central incisor.

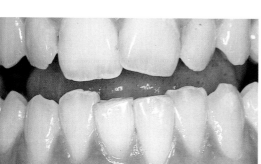

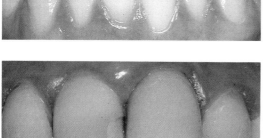

b The tooth shown in *a* bleached to produce a satis-factory appearance.

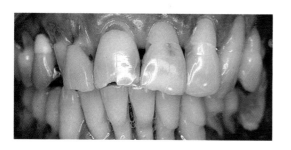

c A Class IV gold inlay and tooth-coloured facing. This is wearing and the restoration is unsightly, but it was placed many years before composites were available and has given satisfactory service. The other central incisor has a PJC.

d Porcelain inlays restoring the four upper teeth on the left. Similar restorations are to be made for the right side. Crowns would be extremely difficult in this case; consider, for example, the shape of the prepara-tion for the upper right lateral incisor. Composite or glass ionomer cement restorations could be made but would need constant maintenance and probably period-ical replacement. Porcelain inlays are likely to be more durable.

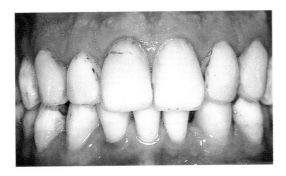

Figure 1.8

a Polyacrylic veneers that are failing after several years in the mouth. The margins are staining and chipping.

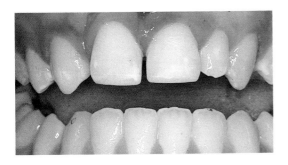

b Broken and eroded incisor teeth.

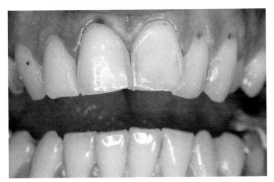

c The same patient as shown in *b* with composite veneers three years after being placed.

d Eroded upper central incisors.

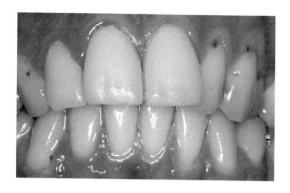

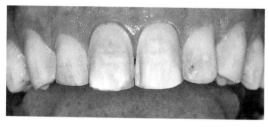

e The same patient as shown in *d* with two porcelain veneers in place.

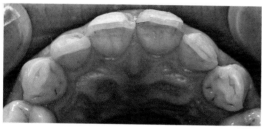

f The same patient as shown in *a* with the polyacrylic veneers removed and the teeth reprepared.

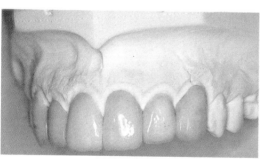

g An incisal view of the prepared teeth.

h Porcelain veneers on the model for the patient shown in *f* and *g*.

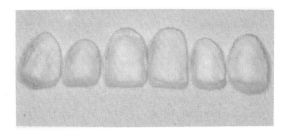

i The etched fit surface of the porcelain veneers.

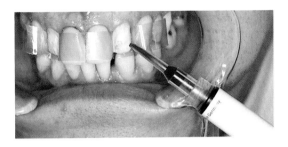

j The teeth have been isolated with acetate strip and are about to be etched with phosphoric acid gel.

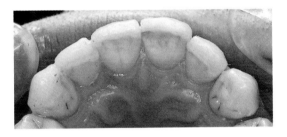

k An incisal view of the porcelain veneers in place. In this case it was necessary to carry the porcelain over the incisal edges because this had been done with the previous veneers. When possible, covering the incisal edge should be avoided since this probably produces a stronger restoration.

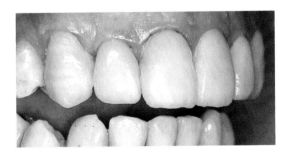

l The completed porcelain veneers.

Both systems can be used after simply acid-etching the enamel, or some preparation of the enamel may be first carried out. It is easier to produce a feather edge at the gingival margin of an unprepared tooth with composite than it is with porcelain, and this is regarded as one of the advantages of composite over porcelain if a relatively non-interventional approach is preferred. This means that composite veneers can be placed as a provisional restoration so that the patient can see how much the appearance is improved. If the enamel has not been prepared, this is a completely reversible procedure, and so, if there is any doubt about the wisdom of going ahead with porcelain veneers, trial composite veneers are to be recommended. The other advantages of composite are that the veneers are simple and quick to apply at the chairside and require no laboratory procedures. They are therefore much less expensive. They can also be repaired and adapted. On the other hand, composite materials sometimes discolour and wear and it is difficult to produce a graduated colour along the length of the tooth or to mask a deeply discoloured underlying tooth (see Figures 1.8b,c).

Porcelain veneers have become very popular in recent years and have been successful in solving some problems. However, they are nearly as expensive as crowns, and although less enamel needs to be removed than for a crown, the fit at the gingival margin is often less satisfactory than with a crown and there is anxiety about the difficulty of cleaning adequately the awkward junction between the porcelain and enamel at the approximal surfaces (see Figures 1.8e, k, l).

Some medium-term studies of porcelain veneers have now been reported and it may well be that the porcelain veneer will be increasingly used instead of crowns. Although these studies show reasonably good results for porcelain veneers, in one typical study of veneers placed by undergraduate dental students the success rate was only 73% after 4 years.

Porcelain veneers should, if possible, be bonded to enamel rather than dentine. In the case of the upper right central incisor shown in Figure 1.8d this was possible, but a large part of the labial surface of the upper left central incisor was eroded through to dentine. When this is the case the prognosis for a porcelain veneer is less good than when an intact enamel surface can be preserved after tooth preparation. However, if a rim of enamel remains, as is the case in Figure 1.8d, then either the dentine surface may be covered with a thin layer of glass ionomer cement or a dentine bonding agent may be used.

A number of different ways have been suggested for preparing teeth for veneers, the most common of these is illustrated in Figure 1.9a.

Indications for posterior crowns

Restoration of badly broken-down teeth

The most common indication for a posterior crown is a badly broken-down tooth usually resulting from repeated restorations, each of which fails in turn until finally a cusp or larger part of the tooth fractures off. In almost all cases it is necessary to build up a core of amalgam or other material, usually retained by pins, before the crown is made. Two such teeth are shown in Figures 1.10c and d.

Restoration of root-filled teeth

There is a strong clinical impression and some scientific evidence that root-filled teeth are more likely to fracture than teeth with vital pulps. It follows that some thin and undermined cusps of root-filled teeth need to be protected or removed where similar cusps in vital teeth would be left. Together with the original damage that necessitated the root filling and the access cavity, this means that many, but by no means all, root-filled posterior teeth are crowned. The fact that a posterior tooth is root-filled is not in itself sufficient justification for a crown.

As part of another restoration

In Parts II and III partial and complete crowns are discussed as retainers for bridges and fixed splints. In addition, they may be indicated in conjunction with conventional or precision-attachment retained partial dentures.

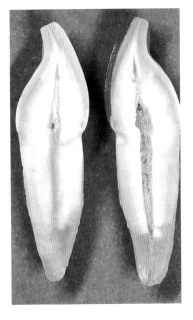
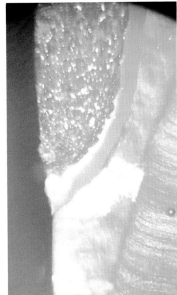
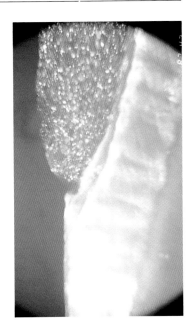

Figure 1.9

a A sectioned upper central incisor tooth. *Left* the intact tooth, *right* the tooth has been prepared for a veneer and the profile of the veneer is illustrated in wax. The features of this preparation are that the gingival margin is chamfered and is in enamel and the incisal edge preserves the bulk of the natural tooth. Had the incisal edge been more worn the veneer preparation could have been taken over it.

b A view through the confocal microscope of the margin of a porcelain veneer. From the *left* the veneer, the luting cement, enamel and dentine. This is a good fit.

c A porcelain veneer which has been sandblasted too much in its preparation leaving the margin deficient.

What are the alternatives to posterior crowns?

Gold inlays

Figure 1.11 shows a gold inlay that has been present for many years. It would clearly have been wrong to have destroyed yet more of this tooth in order to make a crown.

Pin-retained amalgam restorations

Figure 1.11 also shows an excellent amalgam restoration, which has also been present for many years. A crack is visible on the mesial palatal aspect of this tooth; this has also been present for some years. The tooth is symptomless and remains vital. It could be argued that all teeth with large lesions, such as this one, should be

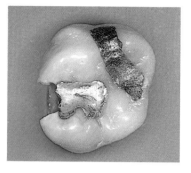
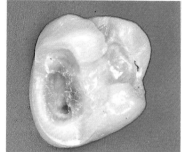

Figure 1.10

Badly broken-down teeth to be restored. *Left*: the tooth on presentation. *Right*: after removing old restorations, caries and grossly overhanging enamel. Only at this stage can a final decision be made on the most suitable restoration. These teeth would be treated with:

a a pin-retained amalgam restoration;

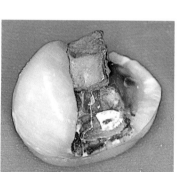
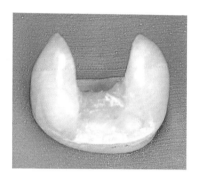

b a gold inlay with cuspal protection or a glass ionomer/composite layered restoration to strengthen the cusps;

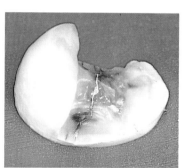

c a pin- or post-retained core and partial crown;

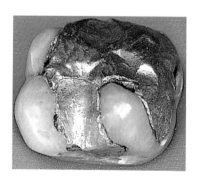
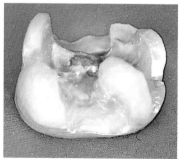

d a pin- or post-retained core and complete crown.

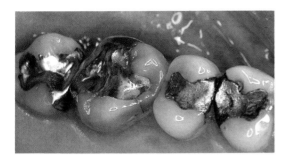

Figure 1.11

Amalgam and gold restorations. The inlay in the second molar has been present for 20 years and the amalgam in the first molar, which has just been repolished, for 15 years. The amalgam restorations in the premolar teeth are more recent, and less satisfactory.

crowned in order to prevent such cracks occurring. However, it is impossible to predict which teeth will crack and what the effects will be. It is therefore not justified to crown all teeth with large cavities just as a preventive measure. To do so is overtreatment and is not cost-effective. It is better to apply a general policy of minimum intervention, with prophylactic restorations only when there is a clear risk of failure. When occasional failures, such as broken cusps, do occur, these problems can usually be solved without the need for extraction.

Tooth-coloured posterior restorations

Composite materials suitable for posterior restorations have been developed intensively in recent times. One reason for this is increasing anxiety in some parts of the world and in some patients about the wisdom of continuing to use amalgam restorations in view of the possible risk of mercury toxicity or allergy. The subject has received much attention in the popular press and in the rest of the media. The scientific evidence is that mercury allergy does exist in a very small proportion of the population, although in some parts of the world, for example Japan, it appears to be greater, probably due to patients being sensitized by eating fish contaminated with mercury that has got into the marine food chain.

Mercury toxicity is a proper concern of dentists, and over the last 30 years or so considerable improvements have been made in mercury hygiene. Most amalgam used now is capsulated,

avoiding the need for liquid mercury to be available in bulk in the dental surgery, and other precautions are also used to protect the staff in the dental surgery. It is the staff, who are likely to be exposed over a long period to mercury vapour should mercury hygiene not be adequate, who are at risk rather than individual patients. There is no reliable scientific evidence that the mercury from amalgam restorations is a serious toxic hazard to patients, despite occasional flurries of media hype. It is also possible that the alternatives to amalgam may have equally low levels of toxic effect.

Nevertheless there are some patients who will now refuse to have amalgam restorations, and hence there has been a drive to develop satisfactory, cost-effective alternatives for the restoration of posterior teeth. The materials are improving year by year, but some dentists still feel that they are not yet comparable to amalgam for the larger posterior restoration. These dentists will therefore more commonly prescribe crowns than composite restorations in teeth that would otherwise be treated with an amalgam restoration, for example the tooth shown in Figure 1.10a. The tooth shown in Figure 1.10b still has substantial buccal and palatal cusps and a good ridge of dentine between them. However, if the tooth is subject to occlusal stress (and wear facets can be seen on the cusps) then a restoration either protecting or reinforcing the cusps is indicated with this amount of tooth loss.

There is good evidence that the layered restoration (a core of glass ionomer cement replacing the dentine, with an occlusal surface veneered with a posterior composite) is successful in binding weakened cusps together and

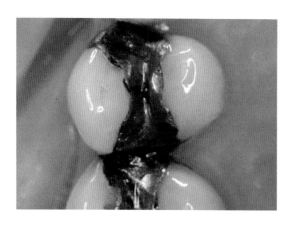

Figure 1.12

a A failed MOD amalgam restoration with secondary caries beneath both the boxes. The mesial surface of the amalgam was also unsightly.

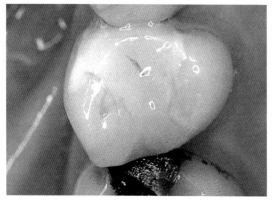

b A laboratory processed composite inlay shortly after insertion.

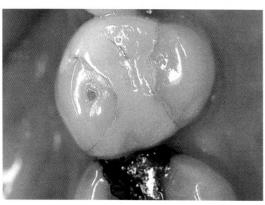

c The same composite inlay after eight years.

producing a stronger tooth than one restored with amalgam alone. This restoration is therefore being used increasingly instead of the MOD gold inlay with cuspal coverage. It is, however, not a substitute for a crown, and it is used when there is a large MOD cavity where a crown preparation would simple remove all the remaining tooth tissue.

In an attempt to increase wear resistance and to minimize the effects of polymerization contractions, systems have been developed to process composite inlays outside the mouth by a combination of heat, pressure and light. One system consists in preparing a non-undercut inlay cavity, lubricating it and filling it with a light-cured composite material. This is cured and then removed from the mouth and further processed by heat and light in a piece of equipment in the surgery. It is then cemented with more composite resin. In other cases an impression is taken of the prepared tooth and the composite inlay (or onlay) made in the laboratory (see Figure 1.12).

Ceramic inlays

Posterior ceramic inlays have many of the advantages of posterior composite restorations in that, because they are bonded by the acid-etched system, they strengthen weakened cusps, and they are tooth-coloured. However, the porcelain occlusal surface is more wear-resistant than composite and there is, of course, no polymerization contraction. As with composite inlays, there are two systems: one that includes a laboratory stage and one that does not. With laboratory-made ceramic inlays, an impression of the prepared tooth is sent to the laboratory and a porcelain inlay is made by condensing porcelain into a refractory die of the tooth (see Figure 1.13a).

The chairside system consists in milling a porcelain inlay from a design produced in a computer from a three-dimensional video image of the prepared tooth. Naturally this requires a very complex, sophisticated and expensive piece of equipment (see Figure 1.13b). It is too soon to say whether this approach to dental restorations (CAD/CAM or computer-aided design/computer aided manufacture) will be revolutionary or will stay on the fringes of dental treatment.

Choosing the right posterior restoration

In some of the teeth shown in Figure 1.10 the failure is due to the restoration fracturing or becoming lost and in others it is the tooth itself that has failed. In some the problem is secondary caries. In all these cases decisions must be made between restoring or extracting the tooth, and if it is to be restored, whether the pulp is healthy or whether endodontic treatment is necessary. Leaving these considerations to be discussed in Chapter 3, and assuming that all these teeth will be restored, the next decision is whether the appropriate restoration is:

● An amalgam, composite or glass ionomer cement
● A layered restoration of glass ionomer and composite
● An amalgam with additional retention (for example pins)
● A ceramic inlay
● A gold inlay
● A gold inlay with occlusal protection (an onlay)
● A partial crown
● A complete crown
● A core of material to replace the missing dentine followed by a partial crown
● A core and complete crown.

A further decision that must be made is whether, if a complete crown is to be used, it should be an all-metal or a metal–ceramic crown, or even in some cases an all-porcelain crown (see Chapter 2 for a description of these different types of crown).

These decisions cannot be made without further information, and some of this will be gathered from the history, examination of the rest of the mouth, radiographs, and so on (again, these matters will be discussed in Chapter 3). However, even with all this information it is usually also necessary to remove the existing restorations and caries before a final decision can be made; Figure 1.10 shows the same teeth before and after the caries and old restorations are removed.

The decision depends upon three factors:

● Appearance
● Problems of retention
● Problems of strength of the remaining tooth tissue and the restorative material.

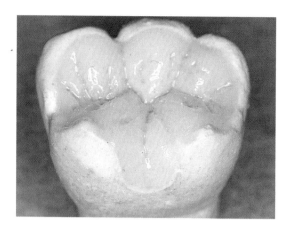

Figure 1.13

a A laboratory-made ceramic inlay. The inlay is returned from the laboratory with a contoured occlusal surface and occlusal staining. It should only require cementation.

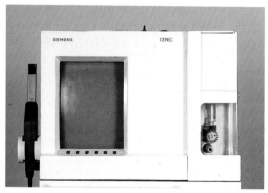

b The Cerec machine. The miniature video camera is on the left, the computer and monitor in the centre and the three-dimensional milling machine on the right.

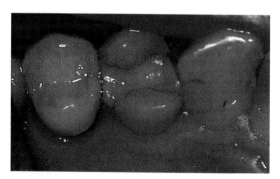

c A failed composite restoration in the first premolar tooth is to be replaced by a ceramic inlay.

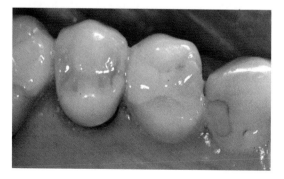

d The completed ceramic inlay milled at the chairside in the Cerec machine. The machine produces a good fit and contact points that only require minor adjustment and polishing. However, the occlusal surface is not finished, and needs to be adjusted and polished in the mouth after cementation. The main advantage of the system is that the whole procedure is carried out in one visit at the chairside and there are no laboratory stages.

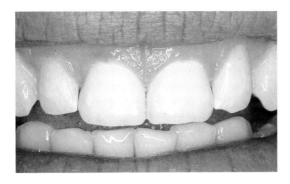

e Strengthened porcelain crowns (Hi-Ceram) on both central incisor teeth.

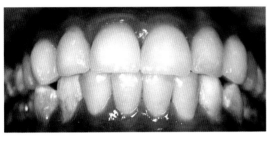

f Empress crowns on the upper and lower incisor teeth in a patient with mild amelogenesis imperfecta.

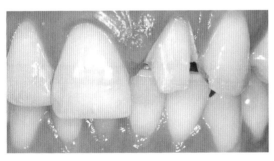

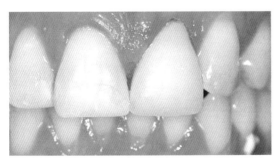

g and *h* The upper left lateral incisor tooth has been moved into the position of the central incisor and crowned with an Inceram crown (h) to resemble the missing central incisor.

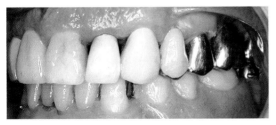

i A metal–ceramic crown on the upper lateral incisor. This is the patient shown in Figure 1.1a.

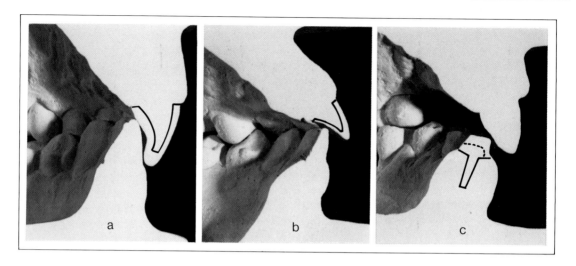

although these do not yet have quite the convenient handling properties or the precision of the high-percentage precious metal alloys.

The preparation for an anterior metal–ceramic crown differs from that for a PJC in two ways; first rather more tooth tissue needs to be removed from the buccal surface to allow for the thickness of the metal as well as porcelain, and second rather less usually needs to be removed from the palatal or lingual surface since only metal will cover at least part of this surface.

Advantages

The main advantages of metal–ceramic anterior crowns are:

Strength The metal–ceramic crown is a very strong restoration, which resists occlusal and other forces well.

Minimum palatal reduction Some teeth, particularly those severely worn by erosion and attrition that have then over-erupted back into occlusion, may not be sufficiently bulky for a porcelain jacket crown preparation with adequate palatal reduction, whereas a metal–ceramic crown preparation may be possible. Figure 2.2 illustrates this problem in comparison with a normal incisor tooth.

Adaptability The metal–ceramic crown can be adapted to any shape of tooth preparation

Figure 2.2

Sections through three sets of casts of patients in intercuspal position showing the profile of crown preparation.

a This is a Class I Division 2 incisor relationship with deep overbite and minimal overjet. It often appears, when looking at these patients from in front, that there will be insufficient clearance for porcelain jacket crown preparations. In fact, the bucco-lingual thickness of the teeth is often normal and conventional preparations are possible.

b Gross erosion of the palatal surfaces of the upper incisor teeth due to recurrent vomiting. If crowns are to be made, there will not be room to provide a palatal porcelain surface without the occlusal vertical dimension being increased. However a metal–ceramic crown preparation is possible. Because the diagnosis is erosion (chemical damage) rather than attrition (physical damage), the additional strength of the metal is not particularly important.

c Attrition has worn the lower incisors to approximately one-half their original length. A conventional crown preparation would not be possible but a one-piece metal–ceramic post-retained crown is. The dotted line shows the metal–porcelain junction.

whereas the process involved in making PJCs requires a smooth and uniform preparation. Additional retention can be gained in difficult preparations by the use of pins or grooves, which are not possible with PJCs.

Can be soldered For bridges or splints, metal–ceramic crowns can be attached to other crowns or artificial teeth by soldering or casting them together. This cannot be done with PJCs.

Disadvantages

The disadvantages of metal–ceramic crowns are:

Strength An accidental blow may result in the tooth preparation or root fracturing because the crown is stronger than the natural tissues.

Appearance Because of the metal framework, it is often more difficult to match the natural appearance of a tooth than with a PJC, particularly at the cervical margin.

Destruction of tooth tissue The metal–ceramic crown requires more tooth reduction buccally than the PJC and so is more likely to endanger the pulp. If this tooth reduction is not sufficient – as is often the case – the eventual crown either has a poor, opaque appearance or is too bulky.

Cost Even if the relatively inexpensive base metal alloys are used, the laboratory time taken to construct a metal–ceramic crown is more than for a PJC and therefore the overall cost is usually greater. When the precious metal alloys are used, the cost is naturally greater still.

Other types of anterior complete crowns

Although the majority of anterior crowns fall into one of the two previous groups, other alternatives exist:

● Cast-metal crowns with cemented porcelain facings
● Cast-metal crowns with acrylic or composite facings
● Acrylic-jacket crowns.

A number of techniques exist for making crowns with cemented-porcelain facings, but since the introduction of the metal–ceramic crown these are now obsolete. However, a number of patients still have these crowns, and so the clinician needs to be able to recognize them (see Chapter 13).

The acrylic-faced cast-metal crown was popular for a time before the general introduction of metal–ceramic crowns. It is still sometimes made, since it can be more economical than the metal–ceramic crown, although there seems little reason why this should be, since the time taken to produce it is rather similar. It is also sometimes made as a long term provisional crown as an intermediate stage in a large-scale oral reconstruction. The simple laboratory-processed acrylic facing deteriorates in the mouth by being worn away, discolouring and leaking at the margins (see Figure 13.4).

Composite faced crowns are also used as long-term provisional restorations. The laboratory-grade composite is cured by an intense light in a special light box, sometimes with the addition of heat or pressure. The cast-metal framework needs to be mechanically retentive for the facing.

Acrylic-jacket crowns discolour and wear, usually within a few years. Because acrylic has a high coefficient of thermal expansion, the constant fluctuations in temperature in the mouth produce breakdown of the margins of these crowns, and they leak, often with secondary caries formation. However, laboratory-processed acrylic-jacket crowns are useful as provisional crowns, since they are more permanent than the usual simple temporary crowns and less costly than cast-metal crowns. They are used when other forms of treatment, for example periodontal or orthodontic treatment, are necessary before the final crowns can be constructed (see Chapter 6).

Anterior crowns for root-filled teeth

Often the endodontic access cavity together with the crown preparation will leave insufficient

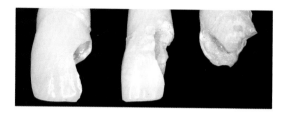

Figure 2.3

a If these three teeth had not been extracted, they would have had to be root-filled. The caries and old restorations have been removed. The left-hand tooth could be restored by a simple composite restoration, the centre tooth has sufficient dentine remaining for a glass ionomer cement or composite core followed by a crown to be satisfactory, but the right-hand tooth does not have sufficient dentine, and retention by means of a post cemented into the root canal is necessary.

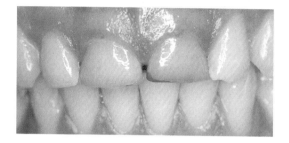

b Both central incisors are fractured and have been root-filled.

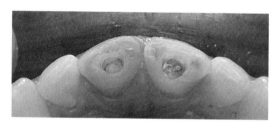

c An incisal view of the teeth shown in *b* with the restorations removed from the access cavities.

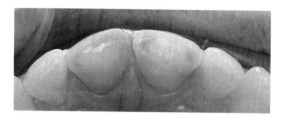

d The access cavities restored with glass ionomer cement.

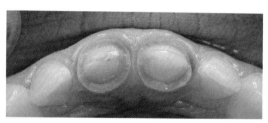

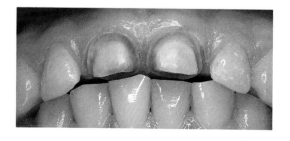

e and *f* The teeth prepared for PJCs. The completed crowns are shown in Figure 2.1e.

dentine to support a crown. In this case retention is gained by means of a post fitted into the enlarged root canal. These posts are used only for retention, and the idea that they add strength to the tooth has now been discounted. For this reason, if it is possible to obtain retention for the crown without using a post, this is nowadays regarded as preferable, even though there is some evidence that the dentine of root-filled teeth is more brittle than that of natural teeth. Figure 2.3a shows examples of teeth that would be restored by means of a simple composite restoration, a glass ionomer cement or composite core and crown or a post-retained crown. There are four groups of crowns for root-filled anterior teeth:

● Glass ionomer cement or composite core and crown
● Post and core and separate crown
● One-piece post crown
● Other types.

Glass ionomer cement or composite core and crown

When sufficient dentine remains, the endodontic access cavity can be filled and missing dentine replaced with glass ionomer cement, which bonds directly to dentine. Alternatively, dentine bonding agents may be used to adhere composite to the dentine, or the dentine may be etched (since there is no longer a pulp) and retention achieved by micromechanical interlocking of the composite bonding layer into the dentinal tubules.

Glass ionomer cement has the advantage that it does not contract on setting, and it also releases fluoride so that should the crown margin leak, there is less risk of secondary caries developing. Composite is stronger and is rather easier to prepare, since it cuts with a similar 'feel' to dentine (see Figure 2.3b–f).

Post and cores and separate crowns

The crown will be either a PJC or metal–ceramic crown as described previously. Posts and cores may either be made in the laboratory or purchased ready-made. The former have the

advantage of adaptability and can be used in very tapered root canals that have suffered caries in the coronal part of the root canal, in root canals with an oval cross section, and in two rooted teeth where the roots are parallel.

The ready-made posts have the advantage of normally being fitted at the same time as the tooth is prepared, thus avoiding the need for a temporary post crown. They are usually stronger and may be much more retentive than the laboratory-made posts and cores. Laboratory charges are lower when preformed posts are used, although any savings may be outweighed by the extra clinical time taken to fit some of them.

Post shapes

There are four shapes of post (see Figure 2.4):

● Parallel-smooth or serrated
● Tapered-smooth or serrated
● Parallel-threaded
● Tapered-threaded

Comparisons of post shapes

Parallel-smooth or serrated (see Figure 2.4b and c)

● Either preformed metal to which a composite core is added, or made with a preformed plastic post, which is incorporated into a pattern for a cast post and core
● More retentive than tapered-smooth posts, and serrations further increase retention
● Greater risk of lateral perforation of the root (see Figure 6.15b, page 121).

Tapered-smooth or serrated

● Usually laboratory-made in cast gold or other alloy
● Least retentive design, but if long enough and a good fit, the retention is sufficient in most clinical circumstances (serrations increase retention but weaken the post)
● Easy to prepare and easy to follow the root canal
● Similar to the shape of the root and therefore less likely to perforate through to the periodontal membrane

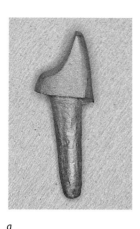
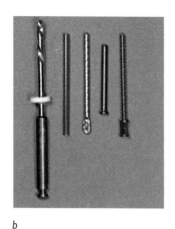
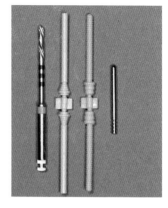
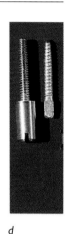

a   b   c   d

Figure 2.4

Post shapes.

a Cast gold post and core (tapered smooth shape). The surface has been sandblasted to improve retention.

b A parallel-sided, serrated post system. This manufacturer produces five diameters ranging from 0.9 to 1.75 mm. This is the middle of the range, 1.25 mm diameter. From the *left* a twist drill with a rubber disc which can be moved up and down to set the length, a smooth plastic impression post, a stainless steel serrated post which can be used in the direct technique (see Chapter 6), an aluminium post with a small head used for making temporary post crowns and a serrated plastic burn-out post used in the laboratory as part of the pattern.

c A post system from a different manufacturer with the same five diameters. This is 1.5 mm diameter. From the *left* the twist drill has three permanent marks to measure the length of the post hole, two impression posts (separated before use), serrated burn-out posts and a stainless steel post for use in the direct, chairside technique.

d Left a parallel-threaded post with attached head which will be prepared as the core after the post hole is threaded and the post cemented. *Right* a preformed tapered-threaded post which is no longer recommended (see text).

- Adaptable technique and therefore can be used with oval, irregular-shaped or multiple-root canals
- A diaphragm may be added to cover the root face and extended as a bevel around the margin. This reduces the risk of root fracture and may also replace areas of dentine lost through caries or trauma
- Cast posts are not as strong as wrought posts.

Parallel-threaded (see Figure 2.4d)

- Must be preformed and made of base metal. A thread is cut into the walls of the prepared root canal with an engineer's tap. The post is then cemented and screwed in with minimal force (like assembling a nut and bolt) so that stresses are not introduced into the dentine
- The post can be shortened
- The most retentive post design
- Post and core are made of different materials. The post may be fitted alone and the core added in composite (see Figure 2.7b, centre) or a post with a metal core already attached is fitted and the core prepared (see Figure 2.4d, left).

Tapered-threaded (see Figure 2.4d)

- Must be preformed and made of base metal
- Cuts its own thread as it is inserted (like a wood screw) and therefore introduces considerable stresses into the dentine
- Roots liable to split either as the post is being inserted or subsequently
- Because of the difficulty of inserting without root fractures, retention is unreliable

● Not recommended as the sole means of retention for a single-rooted post crown.

Making the choice

Many successful posts of all types have been made, and although each dentist has his or her own preference, and certain sets of clinical circumstances dictate that one type or another is preferable, there is no one type that is uniformly superior to the others.

However, in most cases with sufficiently long roots where the coronal part of the root canal has not been excessively tapered, the first choice is usually either a preformed or cast parallel-serrated post. A preformed post is preferable for single, uncomplicated crowns, since it avoids the need for a temporary post crown and also avoids the risk of a casting failure. A relatively common cause of such failures is porosity in the cast metal at the junction of the post and the core. As the metal cools, after being cast, it contracts and the more rapid cooling of the relatively thin post compared with the bulkier core can produce porosity at the junction between them. This porosity is within the casting and is not visible.

Cast parallel-serrated posts and cores are preferred when the core needs to be extended as a diaphragm to cover part or all of the root surface or when a stronger core is needed. Cast posts and cores are sometimes more convenient when several post-retained crowns are being made and a single impression can record all of them together.

The next best choice is usually the tapered-smooth (or serrated) cast post and core, which is used when the root canal is particularly tapered or oval or when the root is very tapered so that there is a greater risk of lateral perforation.

Parallel-threaded posts are used when the available root canal is very short due to an obstruction or when particularly robust retention is necessary. The technique for inserting them is rather precise and time-consuming, particularly if it is only used occasionally, and so it is not employed as frequently as the other types.

The tapered-threaded type should not be used for single-rooted post-retained crowns. The post material is relatively weak and the technique often introduces excessive stress into the dentine, which may then fracture. If the self-threading

characteristics of the post are not used in order to avoid these stresses then the post is not as retentive as other systems.

One-piece post crown

In some cases, for example with very short clinical crowns or with lower incisors, there is insufficient space within the crown of the tooth to make both a retentive core and a separate crown. Then, a crown made of metal–ceramic material with the post cast as part of the crown is often the solution (see Figure 2.2c).

Other types of crown for root-filled teeth

Occasionally the root canal is obliterated by a fractured post that cannot be dislodged, or the root canal is completely closed with secondary dentine. A crown can still be made by building up a core, usually in composite retained by pins (see Figure 5.5, page 93): alternatively a metal–ceramic crown retained by pins cast together with the base of the crown can be used.

Neither of these two techniques is likely to be as retentive as a post crown, and particular attention must be paid to avoiding excessive occlusal forces.

Anterior partial crowns

Before the days of metal–ceramic crowns when there was no satisfactory facing material for a metal crown, partial crowns of one sort or another were commonly used to restore individual teeth and as retainers for bridges and splints. Today, with acid-etch retained composite restorations and with metal–ceramic crowns, partial anterior crowns are much less common. However, there are occasions when there are advantages in maintaining the natural buccal surface and where it would be difficult to prepare the tooth for a full crown. Figure 12.9, page 248 shows such a case.

The restoration shown in Figure 12.9 would not be made today. Instead the first choice would be a splint made with minimum-preparation retainers (see Chapter 12). However, patients still have restorations like this and also individual anterior partial crowns, and so it is necessary to recognize them and understand how they were constructed in case they need to be removed or maintained in some way.

The traditional 'three-quarter' anterior crown was retained by mesial and distal grooves and usually a cingulum pin. It covered the palatal surface and part of the mesial and distal surfaces, but usually showed through on the labial side. The incisal edge was also usually covered.

Posterior complete crowns

Cast-metal crowns

Although traditionally a gold alloy is used for complete metal posterior crowns, the cost of gold and the considerable improvements that have been made in the alternative alloys have resulted in a rapid increase in the number of crowns made with alloys containing less gold, and in some cases none. The term 'metal' is therefore used as more accurate than 'gold' in most cases.

The American Dental Association (ADA) classification of dental gold alloys is more useful than the British Standard (BS 4425). The ADA classification refers to the proportion of noble metals (gold, platinum and palladium) in the alloy. The classification is:

High noble   At least 60% noble metals, including at least 40% gold.
Noble   At least 25% noble metals
Base metals   Less than 25% noble metals

However, some of the low-gold alloys are produced in a gold colour, which can be confusing.

High noble metals are still considered better than the others because of their great resistance to tarnish and corrosion and the easy way in which they can be worked. However, they are substantially more expensive than the other metals and so are now used less often.

Metal crowns are used either when the patient does not mind the appearance of metal or when the tooth does not show during the normal movements of the patient's mouth. When a complete crown is necessary, it is the restoration of choice since it requires the minimum reduction of tooth tissue, the margins are uncomplicated by the presence of facing material, the occlusal surface is readily adjusted and polished, and the time taken to produce the restoration in the laboratory is less than other types of crown so the cost should be less. It is the most convenient restoration for providing rest seats, guide planes, reciprocal ledges and undercuts in conjunction with partial dentures.

It can be soldered to other structures to make bridges and splints, and solder can be added to it to reshape its surface. The only significant disadvantage of the cast-metal posterior crown is its appearance (see Figure 2.5).

Metal–ceramic crowns

The principal advantage of metal–ceramic crowns over metal crowns is their appearance (see Figure 2.5). Porcelain can be used on the most commonly seen buccal and occlusal surfaces. It is often more important to produce a tooth-coloured occlusal surface than a buccal surface with lower teeth, but usually only the buccal surface shows with upper teeth. Any or all of the other surfaces may also be covered with porcelain.

The disadvantages of the metal–ceramic crown for posterior teeth are that more tooth tissue needs to be removed in order to allow for the thickness of porcelain, and when this is on the occlusal surface of a tooth with a short clinical crown, there may be difficulty with retention because of the reduced length of the preparation. When this is the case, additional retention by means of pins or grooves is necessary.

With an amalgam core retained by pins, a preparation for a metal–ceramic crown is more likely to give rise to trouble than one for a metal crown, because the greater reduction of the core material may expose the pins and thus jeopardize the retention of the core (see pages 36–38).

Ceramic crowns

Occasionally it is reasonable to use a porcelain jacket crown on a posterior tooth, for example in conjunction with a post and core on a single-rooted

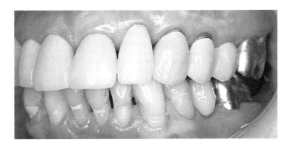

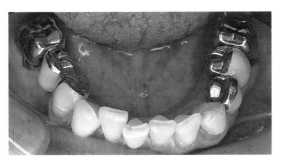

Figure 2.5

a and *b* Gold crowns on the first molar teeth which, with this patient's lip morphology, were aesthetically acceptable. There are metal–ceramic crowns on the upper canine and premolar teeth and PJCs on the upper incisor teeth.

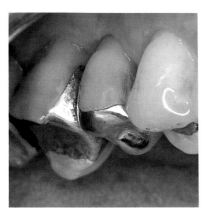

c A partial crown (three-quarter crown). The tooth is vital: the grey colour comes from the amalgam core. A composite core would have been better.

premolar tooth. Care needs to be taken in assessing the occlusion, but if this is favourable a castable or high-strength ceramic crown often has a better appearance than a metal–ceramic crown.

Posterior partial crowns

'Three-quarter' crowns

'Three-quarter' posterior crowns actually cover four-fifths of the tooth's surface – mesial, distal, occlusal, lingual or palatal.

They are retained by grooves on the mesial, distal and occlusal surfaces that effectively perform the same function as the buccal surface of a complete crown (see Chapter 5). They are always made of cast metal, and are used when the buccal surface of a tooth is intact and reducing it as part of a complete crown preparation would either produce an unsightly and unnecessary display of metal or where reducing the buccal cusp would weaken it, reducing the strength of the preparation. An example of a tooth where a three-quarter crown is needed is shown in Figure 1.10c (page 18). Clinical examples are shown in Figure 2.5c and 2.6e, f and g.

The advantages of posterior 'three-quarter' crowns are that they are more conservative of tooth tissue than complete crowns, and the margin of the crown does not approach the gingival margin buccally. It is still possible to test the vitality of the tooth via the buccal surface, and the appearance is preferable to a complete metal crown, without there being the need for the extra tooth destruction.

Some operators find the preparation difficult, but they would do well to learn the skill involved since the posterior 'three-quarter' crown is still a useful part of the dentist's repertoire.

Other types of posterior partial crowns

There are a variety of alternative posterior crowns. The 'seven-eighths' crown covers all but the mesial buccal cusp of an upper molar tooth, the 'half' crown covers the mesial half and occlusal surface of a lower posterior tooth where the distal wall is very short, and other variations leaving various odd bits of the tooth surface exposed are also made. Principles governing the design of all these partial restorations are the same and are covered in Chapter 5. It is for the dentist to use these principles to plan the detailed design of each restoration to solve its particular problems. It is not good practice to follow classic cookery-book-type preparation designs, none of which may be suitable.

A further variation of the posterior partial crown is the occlusal onlay, made to alter the shape of the occlusal surface or the occlusal vertical dimension but without necessarily covering any of the axial walls. It is retained by intra-coronal features, adhesive techniques or pins, and sometimes whole quadrants of opposing teeth are restored by these means.

Cores for posterior crowns

Badly broken-down posterior teeth are rebuilt to the general shape of the tooth using amalgam, composite, glass ionomer cement or cast metal before preparing them for crowns. These cores are usually retained by pins or posts.

Cores of amalgam, glass ionomer cement or composite

The commonest type of posterior core is made of amalgam retained either by pins or by posts in the root canals. The pins are usually threaded self-tapping pins screwed into dentine. Pin-retained cores are used in vital teeth, but it is preferable to use post-retained cores when the tooth has been root-filled. The dentine of root-filled teeth is thought to be more brittle than vital teeth, and so the stress introduced by self-tapping pins may produce a greater risk of the tooth fracturing. In any case it seems commonsense to use the relatively large holes that already exist down the root canals rather than drill yet more holes into the tooth for pins.

When pins are used in a vital tooth, it is important to choose the correct number of pins and to site them properly. In deciding the number and location of pins, the final design of the preparation must be anticipated. For example, pins should not be placed in the middle of the mesial or distal surfaces of a core when the tooth is going to be restored by means of a partial crown. If they are, the grooves in the mesial and distal surfaces of the preparation may expose the pins (see Figure 2.6a). If a substantial cusp remains, the pins should be set at an angle relative to the inner surface of this cusp so that there is a retentive undercut between the pins and the cusp.

When the final restoration is to be a metal–ceramic crown, the pins must be kept well clear of the buccal shoulder area so that they are not exposed during the preparation of the tooth. Also when a metal–ceramic crown is planned, any remaining buccal cusp will usually be severely weakened by the preparation, and cannot be relied upon to retain the core. Sufficient pins must therefore be placed to retain the core without this cusp, and it is sometimes good practice to remove the cusp completely before the core is placed (see Figure 2.6b, c).

A conventional amalgam matrix may be used to retain the amalgam while it is being condensed,

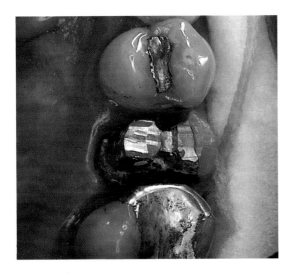

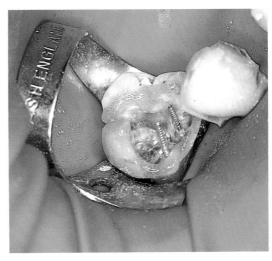

a The amalgam core for the partial crown shown in Figure 2.5c. Pins must be sited with a view to the eventual preparation design – in this case avoiding the mesial and distal surfaces, where grooves are to be prepared. The alternative, a complete metal–ceramic crown, would have relied entirely on pin retention, the remaining cusp having been removed during preparation. Elective endodontic therapy and a post-retained crown would have been less conservative.

b Tooth prepared with pins for a pin-retained composite core. The enamel margin is being etched with gel, taking care to avoid the gel making contact with the dentine. Once the gel is washed off, the deep part of the cavity will be lined.

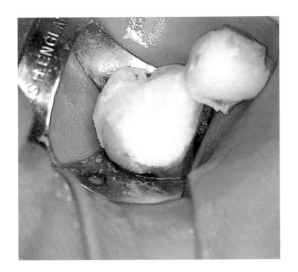

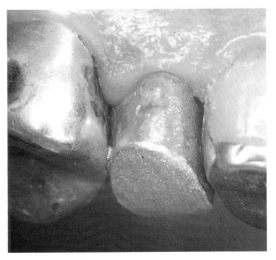

c The composite core in place, having been built up in several increments of light-cured posterior composite.

Figure 2.6

Cores for posterior crowns.

d An amalgam core retained by a copper ring. The patient was unable to return for the crown preparation until eight months after the core was placed. There is some gingival inflammation distally, but apart from this the gingival irritation has been minimal.

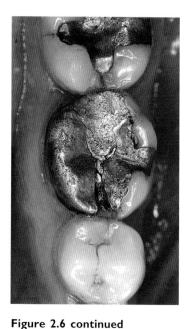

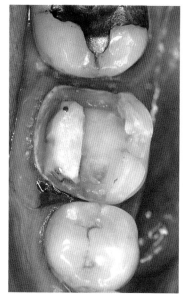

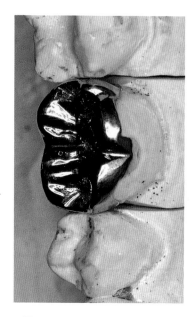

Figure 2.6 continued

e A large failed amalgam restoration.

f The amalgam removed and a composite core placed, retained by two pins. The heads of the pins can be seen. They are sited within the composite core, away from the periodontal membrane and pulp and will resist lingual displacement of the core.

g The partial (three quarter) crown on the die.

but when considerable tooth tissue loss has occurred it is often better to use a copper or orthodontic band that can be left in situ until the crown preparation is started. This supports the amalgam while it is setting, and reduces the risk of the amalgam core fracturing before preparation (see Figure 2.6d).

Composite cores can be used in the same way as amalgam cores, and they have the advantage that they can be prepared at the same visits as they are inserted (see Figures 2.6e, f and g). They should be built up in increments, light-curing each increment to reduce the effects of polymerization contraction. Despite this precaution, there is some concern about the risks of microleakage between the composite core and the dentine surface. In some cases pin retention is not necessary. Glass ionomer cement may be used as a core material provided there is sufficient dentine

to retain it. Pin retention is not usually used. It does not contract on setting and so has an advantage over composite, although it is less strong.

Cermets (glass ionomer cements containing metal powder sintered into the glass) are sometimes used as core materials. They have the advantages of glass ionomer cement, they are easier to distinguish from enamel and dentine while preparing the tooth, and they are radio-opaque. When posts are used to retain posterior amalgam or composite cores, the commonest type is the parallel-serrated preformed metal post (see Figures 2.4b and c and Figure 2.7). If a substantial cusp remains and the post is placed in one of the root canals at an angle to the inner surface of the cusp, this will produce an under-cut and therefore retention for the core. In other situations where more of the enamel and dentine have been lost or will be removed in the crown

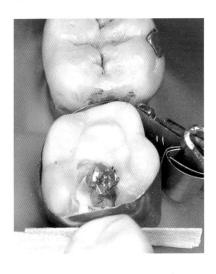

Figure 2.7

a A root filled tooth which is to be restored by a post-retained amalgam restoration and in due course by a partial crown. Two parallel-serrated posts have been placed, one in the distal canal and one in one of the mesial canals.

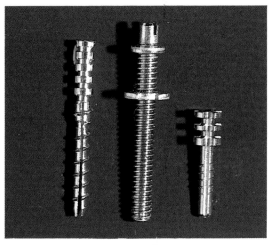

b Three threaded posts used to retain composite or amalgam cores on anterior or posterior teeth. *Left* has a split post that collapses towards itself as it is inserted so that excess force is not applied to the walls of the root canal. *Centre*: a thread is cut into the walls of the post hole first, and the post is then screwed in with light pressure, together with cement. *Right* has a very fine thread that cuts into the walls of the post hole without causing undue strain.

preparation, two, or even three posts should be used.

A cemented post may be sufficient for some single-rooted posterior teeth, but in other cases it is not sufficiently retentive in view of the greater occlusal force usually applied to posterior compared with anterior teeth. A number of post systems have therefore been designed to overcome this problem (see Figure 2.4d and Figure 2.7b). These are usually threaded posts, tapered or parallel-sided posts, either self-tapping or requiring a thread to be cut in the root canal walls. They are very retentive, and, provided they can be inserted without putting undue strain on

the root of the tooth, they provide an excellent way of retaining a core.

Cast posterior cores

With currently available posts and pins used to retain amalgam and composite posterior cores, there is less need for cast-metal posts and cores in multi-rooted posterior teeth than there once was. However, cast posts and cores are still useful for single-rooted premolars, and two-part posts and cores are occasionally used for posterior teeth with divergent roots.

Practical points

- Porcelain jacket crowns are preferred for anterior teeth when possible.

- Metal–ceramic crowns are stronger but may not give such a good cosmetic result, and require more labial tooth reduction.

- Vital posterior teeth commonly need pin-retained cores.

- Root-filled anterior teeth may need post-retained cores, and root-filled posterior teeth need post-retained cores.

- Posterior partial crowns are less destructive of tooth tissue, but often show gold.

- Partial crown designs vary considerably, but are all based on a common set of principles.

- When making pin-retained cores, the number and siting of the pins must be planned with the final crown preparation in mind.

3

Designing crown preparations

Teeth vary so much in their general shape and in the effects upon them of caries, trauma, tooth wear and previous restorations that it is less helpful to describe classical 'ideal' preparation designs than it is to give the principles determining the design and then show how these should be applied.

The principles of crown preparation design

The following factors need to be considered:

● Materials
● Function
● Appearance
● Adjacent teeth
● Periodontal tissues
● Pulp.

Related to materials

Metal crowns

Dental casting metal is strong in thin sections and can be used to overlay and protect weakened cusps against the occlusal forces. It is, however, ductile, and can be distorted if it is too thin or if it is subjected to excessive forces. Normally no metal surface should be less than 0.5 mm thick and occlusal surfaces should be more. This usually means that an equivalent amount of tooth tissue has to be removed. When distorting forces are anticipated, the design can be modified either by reducing the tooth more, and producing a thicker metal layer, or by introducing grooves or boxes into the preparation to stiffen the metal by producing ridges on the fit surface. If high noble metals are used, their ductility allows finely

bevelled margins to be burnished against the tooth surface. This means that the tooth preparation for high-noble-metal restorations is usually finished with an oblique cavosurface angle (see Figure 3.1).

Noble and base metals

Some of the alternatives to high noble metals that are increasingly being used in dentistry, particularly the nickel–chromium-based alloys, are less prone to distortion than the older conventional dental casting golds. It is therefore possible to remove rather less tooth tissue in preparing teeth for these materials. However, because of their greater stiffness and reduced ductility, it is not possible to burnish the margins of these metals.

Porcelain

Porcelain is brittle when subjected to impact forces, and must be in sufficiently thick sections to withstand normal occlusal and other forces. When a high-alumina core is used to strengthen the restoration, this is opaque, and so it is necessary to provide a sufficient thickness of more translucent porcelain on the buccal surface of the crown to simulate the appearance of a natural tooth. It follows that the minimum reduction for a porcelain jacket crown (PJC), made by any of the techniques, is much greater than for a metal crown. A thickness of 1.5–2 mm of porcelain is ideal, particularly on the labial or buccal side. However, with vital teeth this can only seldom be achieved, and the minimum is 1 mm of porcelain. This is acceptable only on the lingual (occluding) surfaces of upper incisor crowns, where the occlusal forces are minimal. With normal occlusal forces this thickness is inadequate, and either the preparation should be deepened or a metal–ceramic crown used.

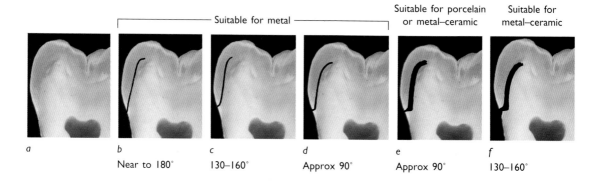

Suitable for metal   Suitable for porcelain or metal–ceramic   Suitable for metal–ceramic

a   *b*   *c*   *d*   *e*   *f*

Near to 180°   130–160°   Approx 90°   Approx 90°   130–160°

The edge strength of porcelain is low, and therefore the compromise at the cavosurface angle between brittle enamel and brittle porcelain is a 90° butt joint (see Figure 3.1e).

Metal–ceramic materials

Even greater reduction of tooth tissue is necessary for metal–ceramic crowns on the visible surfaces, because the metal layer will need to be covered by an opaque layer of porcelain, and this in turn will need to be covered by translucent porcelain. A thickness of 2 mm is ideal, but in many situations, for example lower incisor crowns, this is impossible because of the smallness of the tooth. Where part of the crown is all metal, for example on the lingual side, the preparation is as it would be for a metal crown.

The margin of the crown may be constructed in porcelain or metal, or the two materials may join at the periphery. The cavosurface angle will depend upon this decision (see Figures 3.1e, f).

Figure 3.1

Margin configurations for crown preparations.

a A section of a molar tooth

b A knife-edge margin with a cavosurface angle approaching 180°.

c A chamfer margin with a cavosurface angle of 130°–160°.

d A finishing line with minimal tooth reduction but with a sharp step, prepared with a square-ended instrument producing a cavosurface angle of approximately 90°.

e A full shoulder with a 90° cavosurface angle. When used for a metal–ceramic crown, the metal is either brought to the margin or finished short, leaving a porcelain margin.

f A full shoulder with bevelled margin.

Related to function

Occlusion

The occlusal relationships of the tooth to be crowned will influence the design of the preparation. Those areas of the crown subjected to heavy occlusal loading in the intercuspal position (see Chapter 4) or in one of the excursions of the mandible should be sufficiently thick to withstand these forces without distortion if the crown is metal, and without fracture if the crown is porcelain or metal–ceramic. This means that in

an Angles Class I occlusion there should be adequate reduction of the occlusal surfaces of the posterior teeth, the palatal surfaces of upper incisor teeth and the incisal edges of lower incisal teeth. Other surfaces may also be involved in different occlusal relationships.

When there is posterior group function, that is, several pairs of posterior teeth slide against each other as the jaw moves to the working side (see Chapter 4), the result of applying this principle is that the cusps that function against each other in

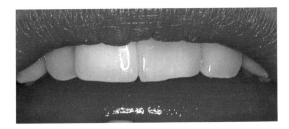

Figure 3.2

Inadequate reduction of the labial incisal area of the preparation so that the core shows through the PJC on the upper right central incisor.

this way should be reduced more than other parts of the preparation. This is often referred to as 'bevelling the functional cusp'. Before this is done, the actual relationships of the cusps in question should be studied during the full range of movements. In the majority of patients the posterior teeth are discluded in lateral excursion by the canine teeth. These 'functional' cusps therefore only function in the intercuspal position and are less vulnerable to wear and to lateral forces. There is therefore less need to bevel them excessively.

In some cases the crown is being made to alter the occlusal relationship, and it may be necessary to reduce the occlusal surface less than usual if the intention is to increase the occlusal vertical dimension.

Future wear

All restorative materials wear in use, and the rate is determined by the occlusion, the diet and parafunctional (bruxing) habits. Where the tooth surface is intact before crown preparation is started, careful note should be made of any wear facets, and these areas of the tooth surface should be prepared sufficiently to allow for an adequate thickness of crown material so that future wear will not produce a perforation of the crown.

Related to appearance

Buccal, incisal and proximal reduction

Adequate reduction of the tooth surface must be carried out on those surfaces where the appearance of the crown will be important.

Insufficient buccal or incisal reductions for PJCs results in the core material showing through (see Figure 3.2) or the crown being too prominent. Proximal reduction is important to achieve translucency at the mesial and distal surfaces of the crown. Further back in the mouth it is more important to reduce the preparation mesio-bucally than disto-bucally since this is the more important surface aesthetically.

Occlusal reduction of posterior teeth

In most patients the occlusal surfaces of the lower premolar and molar teeth are more visible than the buccal surfaces in normal speech and laughter. If metal–ceramic crowns are made for lower posterior teeth, it is usually necessary to reduce the occlusal surface sufficiently for porcelain to be carried over it.

In the upper jaw the occlusal surfaces are far less visible, the buccal surfaces being more important aesthetically. It follows that it may be necessary only to reduce the occlusal surfaces of upper posterior teeth sufficiently for a thickness of metal.

Crown margins

The position of the crown margin in relation to the gingival margin affects the appearance. Subgingival margins may have a better appearance initially but will often produce a degree of gingival inflammation that, apart from possibly leading to more serious periodontal disease, is itself unattractive. Crown margins at the gingival margin or slightly supragingival need not be obvious and will be less likely to produce gingival inflammation

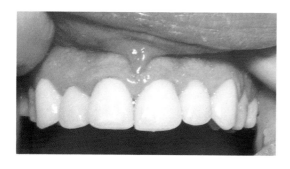

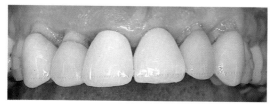

Figure 3.3

Crown margins.

a Six crowns made in 1969 with subgingival margins.

b The same crowns, except for the central incisors, which have been replaced, photographed in 1978. There has been extensive periodontal disease and surgery throughout the mouth. The crowns were replaced with slightly supragingival margins, and the gingival tissues have remained stable.

(see Figures 2.5a and 3.3). It is also easier to take impressions of supragingival margins, to assess the fit and to maintain them. The intention to make visible margins supragingival should be discussed with the patient, explaining the reasons, before the teeth are prepared.

Related to adjacent teeth

Clearance to avoid damage to adjacent teeth

If only one tooth is being prepared for a crown, it is clearly important to avoid damage to the adjacent teeth. This is much easier said than done, and a number of studies have shown that slight damage to adjacent teeth during crown preparation is extremely common. In preparing the approximal surface of a tooth with burs, the tooth surface must be reduced sufficiently to allow the full thickness of the bur to pass across the contact area within the contour of the tooth being prepared, leaving a tiny fragment of enamel or amalgam core in contact with the adjacent tooth. This falls away once the bur emerges at the other side of the tooth. This means that extensive reduction is often inevitable at the approximal surface (see Figures 3.10 and 6.10b, pages 52 and 112).

Path of insertion

When teeth are unevenly aligned, although a crown preparation can be made and an impression taken, the finished crown sometimes cannot be seated because the overlapping adjacent teeth prevent its insertion. The solution is either to reshape the adjacent teeth or to design the preparation at an angle that permits the insertion of the crown.

Technical considerations

Proximal reduction should preferably be continued to allow clearance between the gingival margins and the adjacent tooth sufficient for a fine saw blade to be passed between the dies, so that they may be separated in the laboratory. This also facilitates cleaning the margins once the crown is fitted (see Figure 3.14k, page 59). With convergent roots of adjacent teeth this may not be possible.

Related to periodontal tissues

The importance of supra- or subgingival crown margins to periodontal health has already been discussed. The shape of the crown margin (the cavosurface angle) should be designed so that the

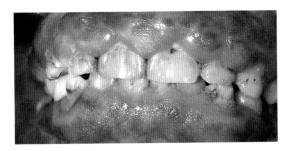

Figure 3.4

a Gross gingival hyperplasia and enamel hypoplasia.

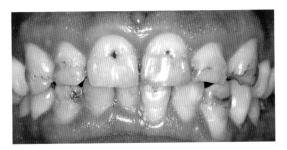

b The hyperplastic gingival tissue has been removed surgically.

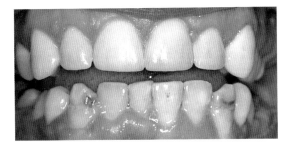

c Crowns on the upper incisor teeth for the same patient.

crown surface can conveniently be made in line with the tooth surface. Insufficient reduction at the margin can result in an overbuilt crown, which in turn produces a plaque retention area at the margin (see Figure 3.1b).

It is not always possible to keep crown margins supragingival at the proximal surface. Where the gingival tissues are normal and healthy when crown preparation starts, the interdental papilla fills the space beneath the contact point. Therefore if the crown margin is to include the contact point, it will usually be necessary to make the crown margin subgingival or to remove healthy gingival tissue surgically.

When the gingival tissues are inflamed, as they often are around teeth to be crowned, because of plaque retention around existing unsatisfactory restorations, it may be necessary to modify the restoration and encourage better cleaning, or to make a well-fitting provisional crown, provide periodontal treatment and then adjust the margins of the preparation.

When periodontal pockets are present that are so deep that they cannot be maintained by improved oral hygiene, periodontal surgery may be necessary, and this will usually have the effect of moving the gingival margin apically so that more of the clinical crown (and root) is visible. This makes crown preparation with supragingival margins easier, but the appearance may be poor, with large triangular spaces between the necks of the teeth (see Figure 7.5, page 155).

This surgical procedure is certainly justified where there has been alveolar bone loss through periodontal disease or in other periodontal conditions (see Figure 3.4).

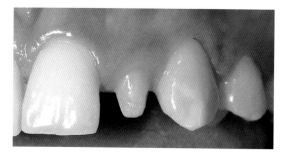

Figure 3.5

a A peg shaped lateral incisor with a low gingival margin.

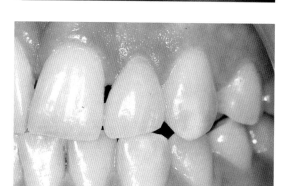

b Elective crown lengthening. This photograph was taken a week after the surgery and the sutures are about to be removed.

c The upper lateral incisor crowned.

A similar procedure known as 'crown lengthening' is also sometimes carried out where there is a normal level of alveolar bone and healthy gingival tissues but where the clinical crown height is reduced and it is perceived that there is a problem with retention. Crown lengthening usually involves the removal of healthy alveolar bone, and is therefore destructive, and is quite uncomfortable for the patient. Alternative means of improving retention should therefore be used whenever possible, and crown lengthening should be reserved for those cases where part of the purpose is to move the gingival margin apically for aesthetic reasons or where alternative means of retention are considered to have a poor prognosis.

Figure 3.5 shows a patient who has had elective crown lengthening.

Related to the pulp

When a vital pulp is to be retained within the crown preparation, a minimal thickness of dentine must be preserved to protect it. The thickness of this layer will depend upon the age of the patient, the condition of the dentine (i.e. the amount of peritubular and secondary dentine) and the type of preparation. Only an approximate estimate can be made of the size of the pulp in a given case, even with good radiographs. So, confusingly, the design of the crown preparation is partly determined by the need to preserve the pulp undamaged without really knowing in detail where it is within the tooth.

The size of the pulp will also be determined by the condition that has necessitated the crown preparation. If this has been a slowly progressing condition such as caries or toothwear then the probability is that the pulp will have laid down a substantial amount of secondary dentine and will therefore be much less vulnerable than if the tooth has been fractured in an accident. If the natural crown of the tooth is small (microdontia) and the purpose of making a crown is to increase the size then very little tooth preparation is necessary and the pulp is not significantly jeopardized even with young patients (see Figure 3.5).

This need to protect the pulp often conflicts with the need for an adequate thickness of crown material, particularly in extreme cases such as metal–ceramic crown preparations on lower incisor teeth. Here the ideal thickness of crown material commonly has to be compromised in favour of the need to protect the pulp.

A good way to gain experience that should help avoid too many dead pulps or failed crowns is to make preparations on a variety of extracted teeth and then section them to see how much dentine is in fact remaining.

Retention

There are two principal systems used to retain restorations in crown and bridge work. The conventional method, which has been used for many years, involves preparing the tooth to a retentive shape and then cementing the crown or bridge retainer with a luting cement, which is not usually chemically adhesive to either the tooth surface or the fit surface of the crown. The crown is retained by a combination of the design features to be discussed shortly.

The second system is to use an adhesive luting cement that bonds either chemically or micromechanically to both the tooth surface and the restoration. Restorations cemented in this way therefore do not need to be made in the conventional manner. Examples of these restorations are porcelain veneers (see Figure 1.8, pages 13–15) and minimal preparation bridges and splints (see Chapter 8). At present there are three such adhesive luting cements:

- Glass ionomer luting cements, which adhere chemically to both enamel and dentine but not to cast-metal surfaces or other restorative materials
- Chemically adhesive resin-based cements, which adhere to a freshly sandblasted cast-metal surface and which lock micromechanically into an etched enamel surface
- Composite luting cement consisting of a lightly filled resin that retains restorations by physically locking into micromechanical retentive features on both the tooth surface (etched enamel) and the restoration.

These adhesive cements have produced significant changes in the practice of crown and bridge work in recent years but have not replaced conventional techniques in the majority of cases. This is because with all these adhesive materials there must be sufficient sound enamel or dentine left for the cement to adhere to. In many of the situations described so far, this is not so, and in others there is a need to remove substantial amounts of tooth tissue in order to replace it with crown material for aesthetic reasons.

These adhesive systems are still in the process of development, and it is likely that they will have an influence over the principles of retention used in conventional crown and bridge work. Glass ionomer and resin-based luting cements are already commonly used with conventional crowns and bridges, and time will tell whether this will allow modifications of the conventional preparation designs. In the meantime it is wise to continue to apply the general principles of retention that have been shown to be effective over many years. The following paragraphs all relate to conventional crowns and bridges rather than those retained by adhesive cements.

Retention against vertical loss

A crown is inserted from an occlusal or incisal direction and can be lost in the reverse direction.

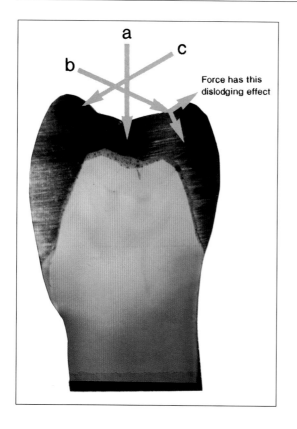

a

c

b

Force has this
dislodging effect

Figure 3.6

This extracted molar tooth has been prepared with a taper of 35°. This is more than the recommended figure (page 49). An occlusal force, a, will not dislodge a crown, however unretentive the preparation. A force directed at an inclined cusp plane, b, occurring in lateral excursions of the mandible will, though, have a dislodging effect if the crown preparation is unretentive as in this case. Loss of retention is unlikely to occur as a result of a single contact of this sort. It is more likely to result from small repeated forces in alternate directions, b and c.

Forces unseating crowns in this direction fall into three categories. First, there can be a direct pull on the crown such as that exerted by biting into a sticky toffee and the jaw then being opened sharply. Other direct unseating forces are the removal of partial dentures and leverage in some bridge designs. Second, there are forces arising as a component of lateral force against an inclined plane (see Figure 3.6), and third, there are forces exerted by the dentist in a deliberate attempt to remove the crown. Apart from the force exerted by the dentist, these vertical unseating forces are less than the forces applied in normal function, which are in directions that seat the crown onto the preparation.

The path of insertion may be inclined away from the long axis if an anterior crown is being constructed to give the appearance of proclination or retroclination, or if a large amount of tooth tissue has been lost on one or other side of the tooth due to caries or trauma so that inclining the path of insertion would allow more of the remaining tooth tissue to be preserved.

Interlocking minor undercuts

Figure 3.7 shows a section through a dentine/cement/crown interface. The surface irregularities of the dentine are typical of those produced by fine diamond or tungsten carbide burs. The irregularities of the cast-metal surface are typical of a surface that has been cleaned by light sandblasting. Even without an adhesive cement, it would not be possible to detach the crown from the tooth by sliding it away parallel to the tooth surface or at an angle from the tooth surface, until an angle of more than 30° were reached, without crushing and shearing the cement within the minor undercuts on the two surfaces.

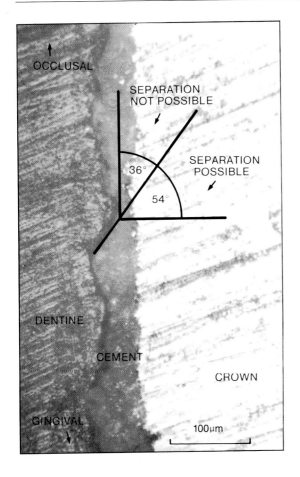

OCCLUSAL

SEPARATION
NOT POSSIBLE

SEPARATION
POSSIBLE

36°

54°

DENTINE

CEMENT

CROWN

GINGIVAL   100µm

Figure 3.7

A section through a typical dentine/cement/crown interface showing the irregularity of the two surfaces and the angle at which separation must occur unless the cement is to be crushed.

Taper of the preparation

Depending upon the size of these minor undercuts and the compressive strength of the cement used, the taper of the preparation (the angle between opposing walls) and its length determine the degree of retention against axial unseating forces. A parallel preparation is impractical, since cement cannot be extruded from the crown during cementation leaving an excessive thickness of cement occlusally and at the margin. Once the taper of the preparation exceeds 30 or so, failure through loss of retention becomes common. Under 'ideal', artificial, laboratory conditions and using artificial materials rather than natural teeth, a taper of 7 has been shown to be the optimum with minimum cement film thickness and maximum retention. However, in the mouth it is impossible to achieve consistently a uniform 7 taper without producing some undercut preparations and damaging many adjacent teeth. The human eye cannot, in the clinical situation, detect the difference between a parallel preparation and one of 10 or so. Several studies have shown that the average taper for posterior crown preparations that have been clinically successful in a large number of cases is approximately 20 (see Figure 3.8).

Most clinicians do not have a protractor amongst their instruments and so rather than aiming to achieve a taper of x – which cannot be conveniently measured and which will vary around the tooth – the object should be to produce a preparation that is as conservative of tooth tissue as possible (including adjacent teeth), but where an absence of undercut can clearly be

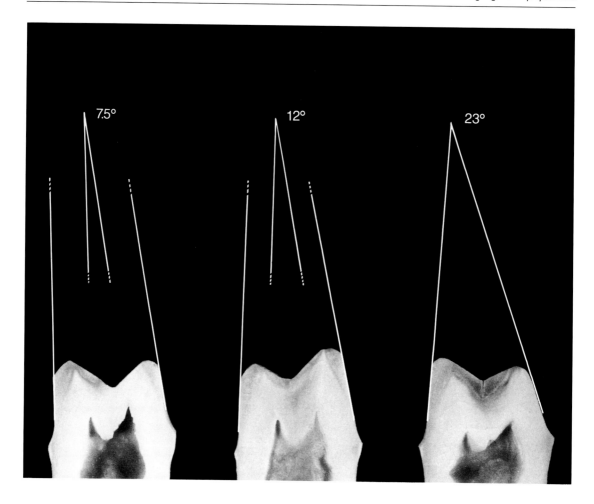

7.5°   12°   23°

seen. In most cases this will produce an accept-able taper of between 10 and 20 .

Length of the preparation

The greater the length of the preparation, the more retentive the crown will be. The minimum acceptable length will depend on other circumstances, including the nature of the occlusal forces, the number of other teeth and whether the crown will be subjected to withdrawing forces from a partial denture or bridge.

The relationship between length and taper is important. The shorter the clinical crown, the more parallel should be the taper attempted.

Figure 3.8

Bucco-lingual sections through crown preparations on three premolar teeth. The taper of the preparations is shown. The 7.5 and 12 preparations would be suffi-ciently retentive in virtually any clinical situation. The 23 preparation would probably be satisfactory in most clinical situations unless subjected to undue lateral or axial withdrawing forces. Note that in the 7.5 prepa-ration both buccal and lingual enamel is hardly reduced at all towards the occlusal surface. This is also true of the 12 preparation. This would result in an overbuilt, bulbous crown in this region.

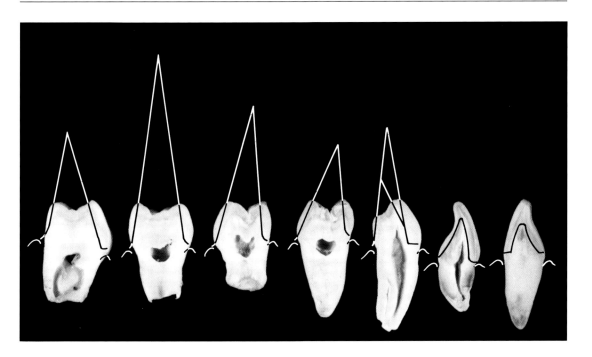

When the clinical crown is assessed as being too short for adequate retention it must be built up with a core (if there is sufficient occlusal clearance), or a surgical crown lengthening procedure may be carried out (see Figure 3.5, page 46), or additional retention may be achieved by means of pins or grooves.

Retention against other displacing forces

Provided the taper of a complete crown preparation is uniform between all the opposing surfaces, the only way the crown can be lost is along the path of insertion. However, some crowns cannot be made with uniform taper. Incisor teeth, for example, can be prepared with a small angle of taper between the mesial and distal surfaces, but it is impossible to produce a narrow angle of taper bucco-lingually – similarly with some molar teeth (see Figure 3.9). Partial crowns must also be designed to prevent loss in directions other than axial (see page 61).

Figure 3.9

Sections through several teeth showing the difficulty of preparing opposing walls nearly parallel.

In all these cases it is helpful to envisage the crown as potentially being dislodged from the preparation in one of five directions:

● Occlusally
● Buccally
● Lingually
● Mesially
● Distally

or at any angle between these directions. The preparation needs features that prevent loss in all these directions. These features also need to be distributed around the preparation so that the complex (and not fully understood) forces applied to the crown do not dislodge it. All crown materials, and certainly dentine, have a degree of flexibility, and unless the crown preparation has

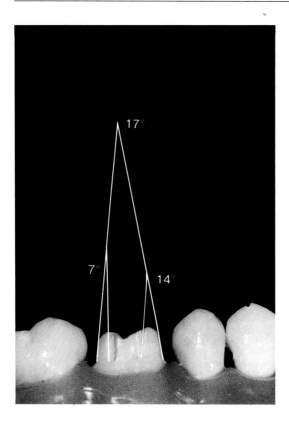

Figure 3.10

A complete crown preparation that is inevitably over-tapered mesio-distally because of the relationship with the adjacent teeth. This overtaper has been compensated by buccal and lingual grooves.

these retentive features, this flexibility may eventually lead to a breakdown in the cement lute, leakage and either caries or loss of retention.

These additional retentive features are usually either grooves or pinholes. Both have the potential not only to resist loss of the crown in a direction other than in the long axis, but also to reduce the angle of the path of insertion. For example, a crown preparation with an excessive mesio-distal taper may be improved with buccal and lingual grooves (see Figure 3.10).

Avoiding failure from other causes

Fracture or distortion of tooth tissue

The remaining tooth tissue, once the crown preparation is completed, must be sufficiently robust to withstand not only the forces to which it is subjected when the crown is completed and cemented, but also the forces that it will encounter during impression taking, while a temporary crown is in place, and during try-in and cementation of the final crown. This may be a problem in preparation for anterior post crowns where a rim of tooth tissue is left around the post hole and with partial crowns.

Fracture of porcelain jacket crowns

Stresses are developed within PJCs as a result of contraction on cooling after the firing cycle. These stresses produce minute cracks, some of which originate at the fit surface and propagate to produce failure if the crown is subjected to sufficient force. These stresses are concentrated around sharp internal angles of the fit surface, so

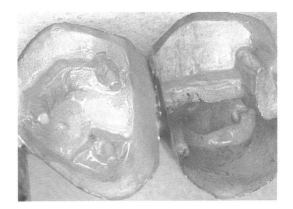

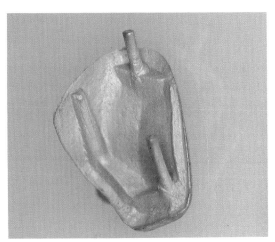

Figure 3.11

Rigidity in partial crowns.

a The fit surface of a premolar partial crown showing the ridge of metal running across the occlusal surfaces. The partial crown for the canine is retained by three pins rather than grooves. This is reasonably rigid except for the proximal surfaces, which would have been stiffer if grooves had been used instead of pins. Although the premolar preparation is still used, the canine preparation would now be uncommon, although many patients still have successful bridges retained by this type of partial crown.

b The fit surface of an anterior partial crown showing mesial and cingulum pins and a distal groove. Only the palatal and distal surfaces of the tooth are prepared. Note the ridge of metal running around the periphery of the restoration and stiffening it. Although uncommon, this type of preparation (with a larger distal box) is still used for a minor retainer for a fixed–movable bridge (see Chapter 8).

the external angles of PJC preparations should be rounded to reduce them (see Chapter 6).

Rounded angles have other advantages: it is easier to lay down a platinum foil matrix without tearing it, sharp corners on a refractory die might be damaged, and during cementation the flow is improved, producing a thinner film of cement.

Distortion of metal

A common cause of failure of anterior partial crowns is leakage producing discolouration and caries behind the incisal tip, and caries starting at the approximal gingival margin. Both types of failure result from inadequate attention to the need to stiffen the casting against distorting forces. The internal mesial and distal ridges of a classical partial crown provide both stiffening and retention. The internal occlusal ridge, which should connect the other two ridges, produces a stiff U-shaped bar (see Figure 3.11a). In less classic preparations the principle should be for a ridge of metal to run all the way round the periphery of the preparation to prevent distortion (see Figure 3.11b).

Casting difficulties

The external angles of crown preparations for metal castings should also be rounded to prevent one of the faults that may occur in the following chain of events:

● Stone die material may not flow into the impression adequately, trapping air bubbles in the sharp angles of the impression
● The sharp edges may be damaged at the wax-up stage
● Investment material may not flow adequately into the wax pattern to produce rounded internal angles on the casting, preventing the casting from seating fully
● It may be difficult to remove the investment material entirely from sharp internal angles without damaging the casting
● Cement will flow less readily around sharp angles, increasing the likelihood of an unnecessary thick cement layer at the margins.

Designing specific crown preparations

The principles outlined above are common to all preparations. Some are more important than others, however, with different types of crown.

Posterior complete crown preparations

All-metal crowns

Whether the preparation is on a natural tooth or an artificial core, application of the principles will usually result in preparations as shown in Figure 3.12.

Variations include additional axial grooves or pinholes to limit the path of insertion when a pair of opposing walls are more tapered than is desirable.

Metal–ceramic crowns

Posterior metal–ceramic crown preparations will usually have an all-metal lingual surface and a porcelain buccal surface, and may have a porcelain occlusal surface. The decision where to finish the porcelain will influence the preparation. The

margin may well be a bevelled shoulder to allow a small line of metal to show, simplifying the finishing of the crown margin (see Figures 2.5a and 3.1f). In the posterior part of the mouth this appearance is usually acceptable. Figure 3.13 shows typical posterior metal–ceramic preparations.

Anterior crown preparations: crowns for vital teeth

Porcelain jacket crowns (PJCs)

A series of PJC preparations is shown in Figure 3.14, demonstrating the application of the principles in a variety of cases, including lower incisor teeth. In all but Figures 3.14d and g, the crowns will be retentive and there is sufficient tooth reduction to enable a crown to be made of adequate thickness for strength and appearance.

Metal–ceramic crowns

Figure 3.14 also shows preparations for metal–ceramic crowns. Compared with PJC preparations, the buccal reduction is greater and lingual reduction less where possible.

Post-retained crowns

The shapes of post holes were described in Chapter 2. The margin of the crown preparation will be similar to that for a vital crown of the same material, the difference being that in the case of a post crown there is no pulp to protect, and therefore the shoulders can be wider and the core thinner than for an equivalent vital tooth preparation. This is possible not only because of the absence of a pulp but also because the core material is often cast metal or reinforced with a metal post (see Figure 3.15a) and therefore stronger than dentine. Besides, a laboratory-produced core can be made more parallel-sided and retentive than a clinical preparation.

The dentine remaining between the post hole and the shoulder, or other margin, may be retained or removed, depending upon its thickness. With a preformed post and composite core,

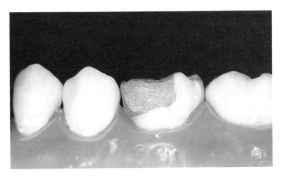

Figure 3.12

Full metal crown preparation on a molar tooth with an amalgam core.

a Preoperative

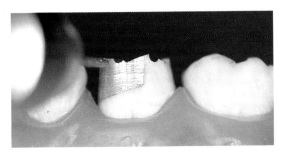

b Mesial and distal preparation with a thin diamond instrument with pointed tip to produce a chamfer finishing line.

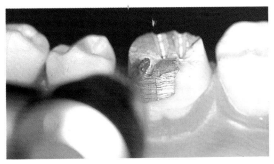

c The axial preparation has been carried round the buccal and lingual surfaces, and grooves are now being placed in the occlusal surface to ensure uniform reduction.

d Reduction of the occlusal surface.

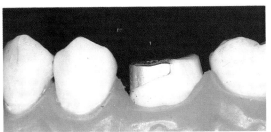

e The axial walls of the preparation finished with plain-cut tungsten carbide burs. The axial–occlusal angle will now be rounded.

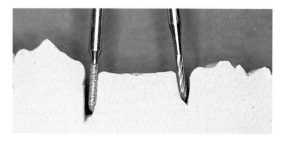

f A mesio-distal section of a cast of the finished preparation with the diamond and tungsten carbide burs used to prepare the tooth. The relationship between these burs and the adjacent teeth can be seen, and it is clear that this is the minimum achievable taper avoiding damage to the adjacent teeth and an excessive shoulder preparation mesially and distally. The mesio-distal taper is 14°.

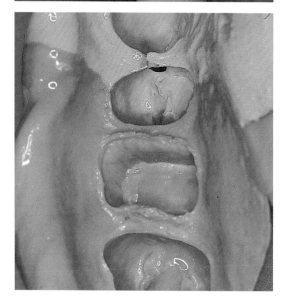

g Occlusal view of typical complete gold crown preparation on an upper first molar tooth with an amalgam core.

h Impression of the preparation in *g* showing the chamfer finishing line.

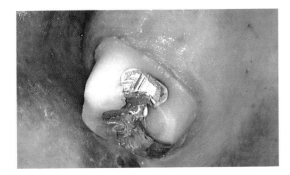

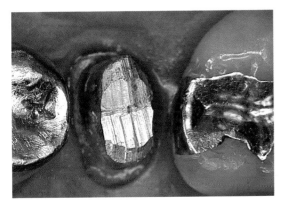

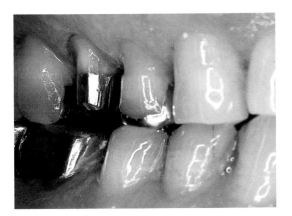

Figure 3.13

Posterior metal–ceramic crown preparations.

a A tooth prepared as a bridge abutment. Only a small amalgam restoration was present. The buccal margin is a bevelled shoulder, the palatal margin is a chamfer finishing line and the entire margin is supragingival.

b and *c* A typical metal–ceramic crown preparation on a root-filled tooth with a post-retained amalgam core. Note the amount of occlusal clearance. The axial wall has been finished smooth but the occlusal surface has not. This is of little significance, except that the mesial and distal corners of the occlusal surface should have been rounded.

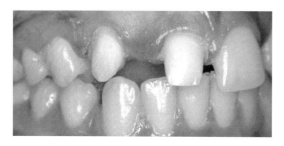

Figure 3.14

Anterior crown preparations.

a Sufficient sound dentine remains for conventional PJC preparations. These preparations were made for an all-porcelain bridge before the days of minimal-preparation bridges.

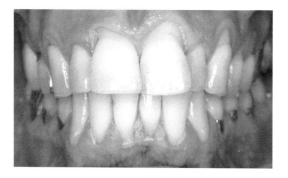

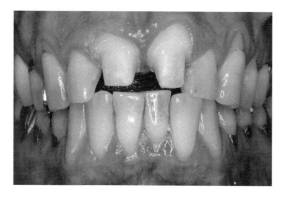

b and *c* The objective is to reduce the size of the upper central incisors. Preparations in *c* are as extensive as possible, allowing PJCs to be constructed that are narrower and less prominent than the natural teeth, except at the neck.

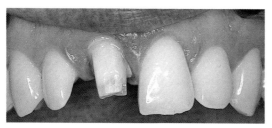

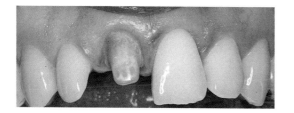

d An inadequate PJC preparation. The previous crown had broken. The angles of the preparation are too sharp and there is insufficient reduction for an adequate thickness of porcelain for strength and appearance.

e The preparation shown in *d* modified for a cast ceramic (Dicor) crown. Note the rounded external and internal angles and the greater reduction.

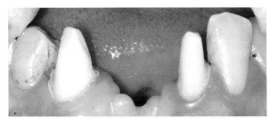

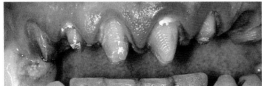

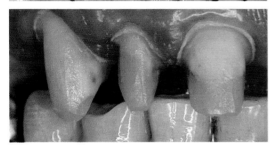

f Metal–ceramic crown preparations to retain a bridge on the lower incisor and lower canine teeth.

g Totally inadequate preparations on a number of upper anterior teeth. The preparations are over-tapered, all except the central incisors are far too short, and the surfaces are too rough. All these restorations failed with disastrous consequences.

h Metal–ceramic crown preparations on badly worn incisors that have been built up with composite cores (the same patient as in Figure 5.5, page 93). The temporary composite restorations shown in Figure 5.5 are retained by acid etching to the enamel. These were replaced by pin-retained permanent cores, since the crown preparations removed all the enamel.

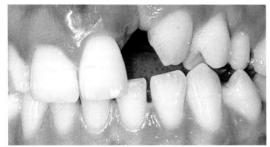

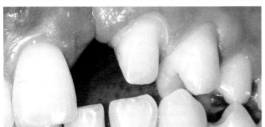

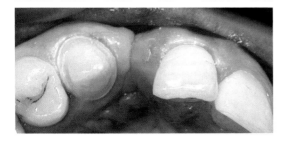

i, j and *k* PJC preparation on an incompletely erupted tilted upper canine tooth in a patient with a repaired cleft palate. The final crown will have a very different alignment and appearance to the unprepared tooth. There has been almost no enamel removed from the incisal edge and the adjacent buccal surface. A trial preparation on a study cast is essential with this type of problem (see later).

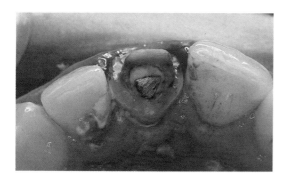

Figure 3.15

Posts and cores.

a A preformed stainless-steel post has been cemented, preserving as much dentine as possible. The tooth was root-filled at age 9, before the apex was closed, so that a large access cavity was necessary. Therefore only a thin shell of dentine remains, and this needs to be reinforced by a post.

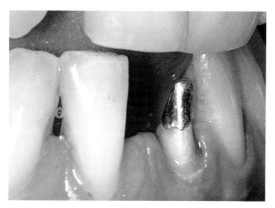

b A cast post and core with a substantial amount of dentine remaining as part of the preparation.

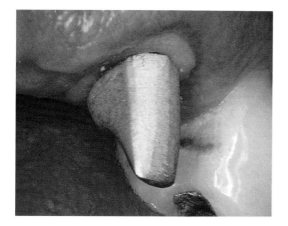

c A cast post and core with no coronal dentine.

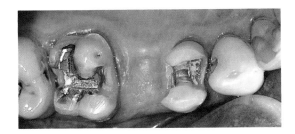

Figure 3.16

A posterior partial crown preparation for an upper first molar tooth. Mesial and distal boxes have been prepared rather than grooves, since there was a previous MOD amalgam. The occlusal groove has been prepared through the remaining amalgam. The stained dentine is firm, and further removal is unnecessary. The tooth has been prepared as an abutment tooth for a bridge, which will be fixed–movable with an MOD inlay with cuspal coverage in the premolar tooth (see Chapter 8).

virtually all the dentine can be saved (see Figure 3.15a). The advantage in retaining a collar of dentine around the post hole when a cast post and a core is to be made is to guide the technician in the dimensions of the core required. The rim of dentine also slightly lengthens the post and improves the retention of the whole restoration (see Figure 3.15b).

Partial crown preparations: posterior teeth

A typical posterior partial crown is much like a complete gold crown except that the buccal wall of the tooth is left unprepared. This means that the crown can be inserted or lost not only from the occlusal direction but also lingually. A posterior partial crown must therefore incorporate features that will prevent lingual loss, usually

mesial and distal grooves connected by an occlusal groove, the important area being the lingual wall of the groove (see Figure 2.6, page 38 and Figure 3.16). With other types of posterior partial crowns, similar grooves or pins are used.

Anterior teeth

Both the design and the preparation of teeth for anterior partial crowns are difficult. Retention is achieved by at least three pinholes or grooves, one each mesially, distally and in the cingulum. The surfaces prepared will depend upon the type of partial crown, which in turn will depend upon its purpose, the occlusion and the importance of appearance. This difficulty, and the availability of less destructive, adhesive restorations have contributed to the decline in the use of individual anterior partial crowns.

Practical points

- There is no ideal crown preparation.

- Preparation and design should follow general principles suitably adapted to the particular case.

- Adequate reduction is necessary where appearance is important.

- Retention still depends in many cases on conventional methods.

- Remaining tooth tissue and adjacent teeth must be preserved.

4

Occlusal considerations

There are excellent textbooks on occlusion, and the reader who has studied these will be forgiven for skimming this chapter. For those who are not yet conversant with the principles of occlusion, this short explanation together with the practical techniques for recording and reproducing occlusal relationships is intended as an introduction to the subject. It will be sufficient for making crowns and bridges for patients with no functional disturbances or pathological changes in the temporomandibular joint or the oro-facial musculature and no major occlusal abnormalities, i.e. most patients. For more difficult occlusal problems the reader is referred to the comprehensive texts.

In recent years there has been considerable interest in normal and abnormal occlusions and in the effects of abnormality. There is a rapidly expanding literature, both research-based and empirical. An unfortunate side-effect of this enthusiasm is that the whole subject seems to be confused in some dentists' minds with the use of complex articulators, recording devices and expensive full mouth 'rehabilitations'. The all or nothing law seems to apply, with some dentists apparently blaming most of the human race's ills, and all of its dental ones, on the odd aberrant cusp, while some others remain unconvinced, throwing the baby out with the bath water − paying little or no attention to occlusal relationships other than when a filling or crown is 'high in the bite'.

An understanding of a few simple principles of occlusion related to natural teeth and in particular how to examine occlusions encourages a middle course between these extremes and will be of great value in preventing some of the failures that occur with restorations that replace occlusal surfaces.

Elaborate equipment is unnecessary for the application of these principles to the restoration of small groups of teeth; equipment should be seen simply as a means to an end. In fact, the principles determining the design of articulators and recording devices are fairly simple, but their conversion into three-dimensional reality leads to the complexity of the equipment.

A functional approach to occlusion

The most useful way for a restorative dentist to look at occlusion is from the functional point of view; the morphological details of the occlusion are less important. The fact that an occlusion is Angles Class I, II or III is less important than the way the teeth move across each other in various movements of the mandible. For example, in lateral excursions in some patients, the canines are the only teeth in occlusion, and in others several of the teeth are in occlusion (see Figure 4.1).

The restorative dentist should also recognize that crowns, bridges or any restorations involving the occlusal surface will often affect the way the occlusion functions. This effect should be deliberately planned rather than be allowed to influence the occlusal movements by accident.

The functional compared with the orthodontic approach

Orthodontic treatment is aimed primarily at improving the patient's appearance and producing a stable posterior occlusion in a single static position. Some forms of orthodontic treatment go further and establish deliberate patterns of contact between the teeth in various movements of the mandible.

Most orthodontic treatment is carried out on young people who have not yet developed rigid patterns of involuntary neuromuscular control of

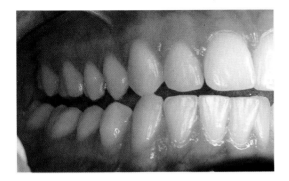

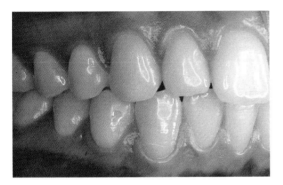

Figure 4.1

Lateral guidance

a Canine guidance in lateral excursion with the posterior and incisor teeth completely discluding. Contact in this position is sometimes shared between the canine, lateral and central incisor teeth.

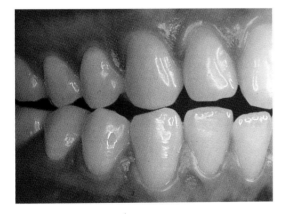

b and c Group function. The patient is shown, *b*, in intercuspal position, and when she moves to the working side, *c*, contact is shared between the posterior teeth. The lateral and central incisors disclude.

their mandibular movements. They are therefore capable of adaptation to fairly drastic changes in their occlusal relationships in a way that some older patients find difficult.

From the functional point of view there should be no difference in the objectives of the orthodontist and restorative dentist – only different means of achieving them.

Fixed compared with removable prosthetic approaches

The main purpose of designing the occlusion for complete dentures is to produce stability of the denture bases. This is an entirely different concept from the restoration of natural teeth with intact roots and periodontal membranes. Occlusal considerations for partial dentures fall somewhere between these two positions. In complete denture construction, consideration of where the occlusal surfaces of the artificial teeth should be in relation to the ridge, the presence of balancing contacts on the non-working side, and the angulation of cusps or absence of cusps altogether, are important. None of these applies in the same way to the construction of fixed restorations.

The methods of recording and reproducing mandibular movement are similar whether fixed or removable appliances are being made. However, the principles governing the design of the occlusal relationships, although similar in some respects, are different in others.

Mandibular movements and definition of terms

The movements that the mandible can make and the names of the important positions within this range of movements are shown in Figure 4.2.

Inter-cuspal position (ICP)

This is the position of maximum contact and maximum intercuspation between the teeth. It is therefore the most cranial position that the mandible can reach. The term 'centric occlusion' has been used to describe this position, but this is confused with 'centric relation' (see below) and may also imply centricity of the condyles in their fossae, centricity of the midline of the mandible with the midline of the face, or centricity of the cusps within the fossae of the opposing teeth, none of which may be the case. The term 'centric occlusion' is therefore better not used.

Retruded contact position (RCP)

This is the most retruded position of the mandible with the teeth together. It is a clinically reproducible position in the normal conscious patient. Patients with conditioned patterns of muscle activity may not be able to manipulate the jaw into it, even with assistance by the dentist. In

less than 10% of the dentate population the RCP coincides with the ICP. In the remainder RCP is up to 2 mm or more posterior to ICP. The term 'centric relation' has been used to describe this position, but it has the same disadvantages as the term 'centric occlusion' and will not be used.

Mandibular movements

Those patients who have a discrepancy between RCP and ICP usually close straight into ICP from the postural or rest position. However, contact occurs in the range between ICP and RCP during empty swallowing (particularly nocturnal swallowing), during the mastication of a tough bolus and during parafunctional activity. Thus the mandible can slide from ICP in four main directions with the teeth in contact, or in an infinite number of directions at angles between these main pathways. The four excursions are:

● Retrusive
● Protrusive
● Left lateral
● Right lateral

Retrusive movements

Movements between ICP and RCP are usually guided by a limited number of pairs of cusps of posterior teeth. Figures 4.3a, b and c illustrate the occlusal contacts produced in RCP and other excursions in a typical natural dentition. The angle of the slide between RCP and ICP, its length and the individual pairs of teeth that produce it are important and should be examined. Of even greater importance is any unevenness of the movement producing bulges or lumps in the path of movement. These disturbances to the smooth movement of the mandible are one form of occlusal interference (see page 65).

Protrusive excursion

In forward movement of the mandible with the teeth together it is usually the incisor teeth that guide the movement. This will not be the case in anterior open bites or in Class III incisor relationships.

The angle and length of movements will be determined by the incisor relationship so that, for example, in a Class II Division II incisor relationship with an increased overbite and reduced overjet, the movement of the mandible has to be almost vertically downwards before it can move forwards. Anterior guidance is important when making anterior crowns or bridges. Sometimes, when the teeth are a normal shape, it is helpful to reproduce the patient's existing guidance as accurately as possible; on other occasions, for example, with worn teeth, it is unnecessary or undesirable to do so, and in fact the purpose of the treatment may be partly to alter the incisor guidance.

Left and right lateral excursions

In lateral excursions the side that the mandible is moving to is known as the working side and the opposite side the non-working side. The term 'balancing side' has been used to refer to the non-working side, but since it implies a balanced occlusion, balancing or stabilizing a complete denture base, it should not be used in reference to natural teeth.

The contacts on the working side are either between the canine teeth only (canine-guided occlusion – see Figure 4.1a) or between groups of teeth on the working side (group function – see Figures 4.1b, c). Occasionally, individual pairs of posterior teeth will guide the occlusion in lateral excursion, but this is not regarded as ideal.

Contact on the non-working side in lateral excursions should not normally occur. It does sometimes after extractions and over-eruption and occasionally following orthodontic treatment, particularly when this treatment has been carried out with removable appliances that have allowed the posterior teeth to tilt (see Figures 4.3d, e). Contact may also occur in cases of posterior crossbite where the lower teeth are placed buccally to the upper teeth.

Occlusal interferences and occlusal harmony

An occlusal interference may be defined either as a contact between teeth in one of the excursions of the mandible so that the free sliding movement of the mandible is interrupted or uneven, or as the guidance of the mandible being carried on teeth that are unsuitable for the purposes. In many cases occlusal interferences develop some time after the eruption of the permanent dentition and are the result of dental treatment.

Figure 4.4 illustrates an alteration to the movement between ICP and RCP resulting from the over-eruption of a tooth. This constitutes an occlusal interference in this excursion. Figures 4.3d and e illustrate an interference in lateral excursion.

These interferences are often difficult to detect because the sensory mechanism within the periodontal membranes of the teeth involved detects the interference and triggers a conditioned pattern of mandibular movement to avoid it. This accounts for the difficulty many patients have in permitting their mandible to be manoeuvred into the RCP and also the difficulty they have in voluntarily making lateral excursions with the teeth together.

An interference in the intercuspal position resulting from a 'high' restoration involving the occlusal surface will be readily detected by the patient, who will usually comment on an occlusal change as soon as the restoration is inserted. These instant, entirely artificial interferences are obviously easier to deal with than occlusal interferences in the various excursions of the mandible – which may be artificial but can also develop slowly and naturally following extractions, tooth movements, occlusal wear and over-eruption.

Interferences should be suspected if the patient has difficulty in making voluntary protrusive and lateral excursions with the teeth in contact or there is difficulty in manoeuvring the mandible into a reproducible RCP. Interferences can also be detected by the dentist resting a finger gently under the patient's chin while the various excursions are performed. Irregular movements, which the finger will feel, indicate interferences that need fuller investigation.

Occlusal harmony – the absence of occlusal interferences – allows comprehensive movements of the mandible in all excursions with the teeth together without strain or discomfort, the movements not causing harmful effects to the teeth (for example tooth mobility, fractured cusps or excessive wear). A harmoniously functioning occlusion will usually also involve fairly shallow angles of movement in the guidance from ICP in all four directions. Patients who do not have free sliding movements may not have symptoms. They have adapted to their occlusal interferences. However, if the occlusion is altered to produce new and different occlusal interferences (for example by unsatisfactory crowns or bridges), the patient's neuromuscular mechanism may well experience difficulty in adapting to these, resulting in damage to the restorations or teeth, or a dysfunctional disorder leading to temporomandibular joint pain, muscle pain and spasm, or postural and

functional problems. These disorders arising from occlusal disharmony are fully described in specialist textbooks.

'Premature contact'

The term 'premature contact' should not be used in relation to the natural dentition. With complete dentures there is no natural ICP, and ICP and RCP are made to coincide, i.e. the artificial teeth interdigitate on the retruded path of closure. The patient learns, subconsciously, to close on this reproducible path of closure and closes into intercuspation. When, as

Figure 4.2

Border movements of the mandible.

a The maximum possible movement of the tip of a lower central incisor. The teeth are in occlusion from RCP to the fully protruded position (P). In opening from RCP to X, the mandible rotates in a pure arc of a circle around an axis (the terminal hinge axis, THA), which passes through the condyles. X is the maximum opening that can be made without the condyles moving forwards and O is the maximum opening with the condyles fully protruded.

b The view from above, showing RCP and ICP. The movements are not pure arcs of circles, because when the mandible moves to the side the condyle on the working side shifts laterally (Bennett movement) and the condyle on the non-working side moves forwards and medially (Bennett angle).

c The border movements viewed from in front. The movement from ICP to the cusp-to-cusp contact (C) is guided either by canines, all the anterior teeth or a group of posterior teeth (see Figure 4.1). From C to the maximum lateral position, L, the guidance is irregular and usually controlled by the anterior teeth or teeth on the non-working side. This is a non-functional range not usually involved in parafunctional activity, and is therefore of little importance.

d Changes in the lateral guidance will either expand the original border movements, Y, or encroach upon it, Z.

Both changes constitute occlusal interferences. The change, Y, would result, for example, from the fracture or extraction of a canine tooth that previously governed lateral guidance. The change, Z, might result from overbuilding the cusps of a posterior crown in a group function occlusion or from the development of non-working-side contacts.

e This occlusal interference, an irregularity developing in the smooth movement from ICP to RCP, may also result from crowns. An example of extraction and over-eruption causing this change is shown in Figure 4.4.

f An expansion of the border movement is often an objective of occlusal adjustment in the range from ICP to RCP. For example, if the original movement was from ICP to RCP1, with large vertical and horizontal components to the movement, an adjustment could be carried out to produce a 'long centric', so that the movement was flat from ICP to RCP2. This would not change the horizontal component of the movement, but would reduce the vertical component to zero. The alternative of making ICP and RCP coincident (RCP3) usually involves multiple crowns or other restorations as well as occlusal adjustment. This is because either the border movement space needs to be encroached upon (the dashed line) or a substantial amount of tooth tissue must be removed. When this is done the process is known as 'reorganizing' the occlusion. If ICP is left undisturbed, the occlusal plan is known as 'conformative'.

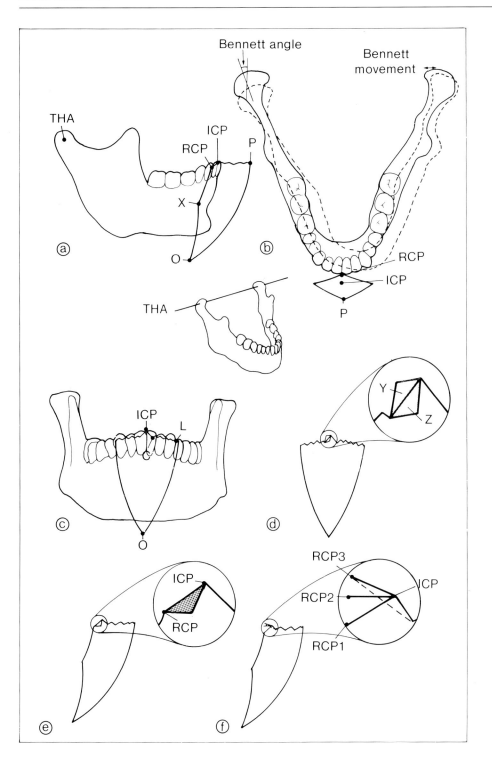

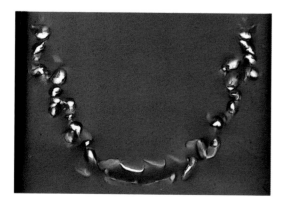

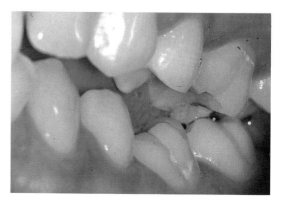

Figure 4.3

Occlusal contacts.

a Perforations in a 0.5-mm-thick sheet of soft wax produced by the patient closing in ICP.

d A different patient making a right lateral excursion. The left (non-working) side is shown, and there is contact between the lower second molar and the first upper molar. This is a non-working-side occlusal interference.

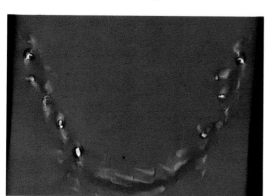

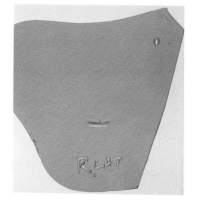

b The same patient contacting in RCP. There are of course fewer contacts, but they are evenly distributed, both anterio-posteriorly and between left and right.

e A wax occlusal record of the patient shown in *d* in the same right lateral excursion, showing this interference to be the only contact at this point.

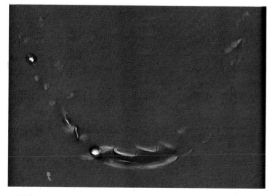

c The same patient making contact in right lateral excursion, mainly on the canine teeth, although a contact is also present posteriorly.

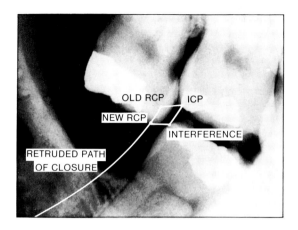

Figure 4.4

Since the lower third molar has been extracted, the upper third molar has over-erupted, changing the RCP. Previously the mandible could slide smoothly back from ICP to RCP, but it now has to make a detour to the new RCP to circumnavigate the mesial surface of the upper third molar. This is an occlusal interference. This patient presented with pain diagnosed as mandibular dysfunction, which disappeared once the upper third molar had been extracted. Caries, although present in the mesial surface of the upper third molar well below the original contact point, was not the cause of the pain.

a result of inaccurate occlusal records, the ICP and RCP of the complete dentures do not coincide, the patient may close on the retruded path of closure, and then may slide into maximum intercuspation or alternatively the dentures may move. This is known as premature contact and is clearly unsatisfactory. The artificial teeth do not have a periodontal proprioceptive system, and so the position of an artificial ICP cannot readily be detected. With a natural dentition the ICP is well recognized by the neuromuscular mechanism and the mandible closes directly into ICP in the great majority of involuntary closing movements. It may not do so in the artificial environment of the dental chair when the mandible is brought under voluntary rather than involuntary control. In these circumstances, even if the first contact appears to be a premature contact, this should not be assumed to be the normal pattern of closure, but only the result of the patient concentrating on a movement that is usually entirely automatic.

For these reasons the term occlusal interference as defined and described above is preferred to the term premature contact for the dentate patient.

Occlusal stability

A stable occlusion is one in which over-eruption, tilting and drifting of teeth cannot occur and

therefore cause new occlusal interferences. For an occlusion to be stable, there must also be sufficient posterior contacts to prevent a general collapse of the posterior occlusion resulting in a loss of occlusal vertical dimension. Figure 4.5 shows a disordered but stable occlusion, a disordered and unstable occlusion, and an occlusion that has lost posterior support to the point where collapse and loss of occlusal vertical dimension has occurred.

In a stable occlusion all the teeth should have occlusal contact with either another tooth or a prosthesis (occlusal stops). Mesial drifting should be prevented by the presence of contact points, either with other teeth or a prosthesis, or by adequate cuspal locking with the opposing teeth in intercuspal position.

Not all partially edentulous occlusions are unstable. For example, if all the molar teeth are extracted, the remaining teeth may still be in stable occlusion. Therefore extracted teeth are not always replaced (see Chapter 7). In any case, a degree of instability is sometimes acceptable.

Occlusal vertical dimension (OVD)

The occlusal vertical dimension is the relationship between the mandible and the maxilla with the teeth in ICP, that is, the face height with the

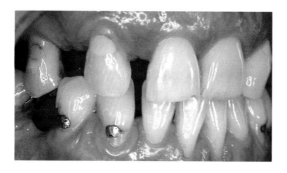

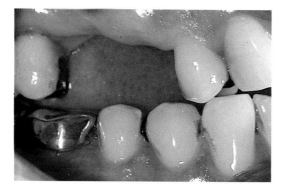

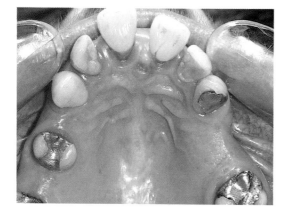

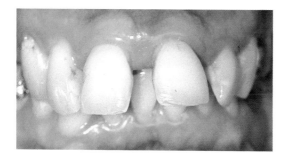

Figure 4.5

Occlusal stability.

a A disordered but stable occlusion. Several teeth are missing and there have been a number of tooth movements, some producing aesthetic problems and potential occlusal interferences. However, the occlusion is now stable and study casts taken five years before this photograph show that no change has occurred in that period. There are no symptoms of mandibular dysfunction and no other complaints by the patient, even of the appearance of the missing upper teeth. Treatment of this occlusion is therefore not justified.

b There have been recent extractions in the upper arch and undesirable tooth movements, including over-eruption of the lower teeth, can be anticipated.

c and *d* A 'collapsed bite' with loss of a number of posterior teeth, periodontal disease, drifting upper incisors, an increase in overbite and a reduction in occlusal vertical dimension.

teeth in occlusion. It is usual to measure the difference between rest position and ICP (the freeway space) to give an indication as to whether the OVD is within the normal range. However, rest position is difficult to measure with any precision, particularly in dentate patients, and the normal freeway space may be 2–5 mm or more. OVD is therefore judged as much as it is measured by the patient's general facial appearance with the teeth together and apart. In most cases requiring crowns or bridges the OVD is satisfactory. In some it has been reduced by the extraction of teeth, by tilting, drifting and collapse of the posterior occlusion or by rapid wear of the teeth (see Figures 4.5c, d and 5.5a). In these it is necessary to restore the original occlusal level for both aesthetic and technical reasons. In other cases gradual wear of the dentition has resulted in very short teeth so that making aesthetic and retentive crowns is a problem, yet there is no loss of facial height because the tooth wear has been compensated by over-eruption. In these cases a decision must be made between:

● Artificially increasing the OVD by restoring or replacing all the occlusal surfaces in one jaw
● Accepting that the crowns will have a short appearance
● Artificially lengthening the clinical crowns by gingival surgery and sometimes alveolar surgery (crown lengthening)
● Creating inter-occlusal space between the teeth to be crowned without altering the other occlusal relationships
● A combination of these approaches.

When a change in OVD is planned, whether or not it is to restore lost facial height, it is usual to assess the tolerance of the patient's neuromuscular mechanism to the change. A removable acrylic plate covering all the occlusal surfaces of one arch and increasing the OVD by at least the same amount as is proposed for the final restorations may be fitted. Alternatively the teeth may be temporarily built up using acid-etch composite restorations (when sufficient enamel remains), amalgams or temporary crowns. The temporary adjustment to the OVD should be left for at least six weeks and preferably three months or more to ensure that problems do not arise with the neuromuscular mechanism or the teeth before

the change is made permanent (see Figure 5.5, page 93).

Creating interocclusal space for teeth to be crowned

In certain circumstances, particularly extreme wear of anterior teeth, it is helpful to carry out minor orthodontic treatment to enable crown preparations to be carried out without further preparation of the worn surfaces. Often the wear has been sufficiently slow that over-eruption has kept pace with it, carrying the gingival margin along with the over-eruption. Conventional orthodontic treatment can be used, but a simple, reliable and rapid technique is to use either a removable or fixed appliance commonly known as a 'Dahl' appliance. Dahl originally described a removable anterior bite plane made of cast cobalt–chromium but modern adhesive technology has enabled a simpler fixed appliance to be made that is well tolerated by most patients and that usually achieves the required result in about three months. Figure 4.6 shows the appliance in use.

Mandibular dysfunction

Many terms are used to describe this condition, for example temporomandibular joint dysfunction, myofascial pain dysfunction syndrome and muscle hyperactivity disorder. This illustrates the fact that the condition is poorly understood and that there are many suggested explanations for it. Some explanations blame the joint itself for the symptoms, some the muscles of mastication and their control systems, and some the occlusion, which in turn affects the control system and again in turn the muscles and the joints, and some clinicians believe that the symptoms arise entirely from psychological stress and anxiety.

The least pejorative term is therefore 'mandibular dysfunction', which is simply used to label a common combination of symptoms often including tenderness, pain and tension in the muscles of mastication and pain, clicking and limitation of movements of the temporomandibular joints.

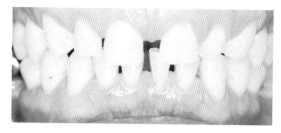

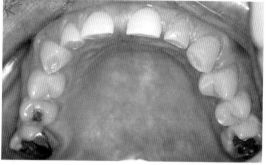

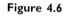

Figure 4.6

a and *b* Palatal erosion affecting the upper incisor teeth. The lower teeth have over-erupted and are making contact with the worn palatal surface.

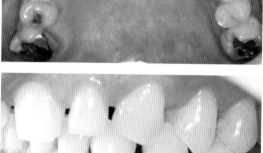

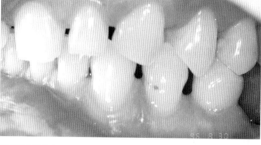

c The posterior teeth in occlusion.

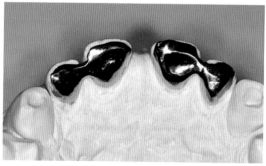

d The cast Dahl appliances. They are left separate at the midline because of the diastema.

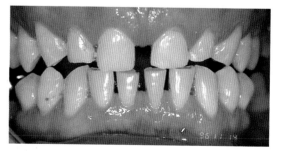

e The Dahl appliances in place propping the occlusion open on the anterior teeth.

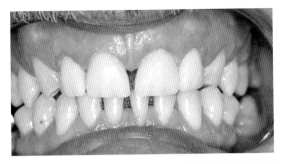

f The appliances have worked in depressing the lower incisors and the four upper incisor teeth have been crowned without any further reduction of their palatal surfaces.

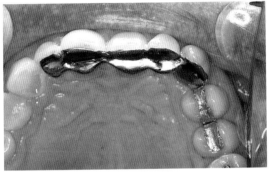

g Another typical Dahl appliance, this time in one piece and with a more pronounced shelf palatally to produce axial tooth movement.

In many cases the symptoms resolve spontaneously with or without treatment. The incidence is higher in young adult dentate female patients than in other groups. These two facts suggest that the condition is more commonly of functional and psychogenic origin than it is to do with irreversible physical changes in the joints themselves.

Changes do occur in the joints, and these can be demonstrated by conventional radiography or by special, and sometimes invasive, techniques such as arthrography, in which radio-opaque material is injected into the joint space, or arthroscopy, in which a tiny fibre-optic instrument is inserted into the joint space, which can then be viewed directly. However, the least invasive investigation is by magnetic resonance imaging (MRI), which does not involve ionizing radiation or physical invasion of the joint. When MRI is available (it is a very expensive technique) it is the best way to investigate the possibility of internal joint derangements. Confusingly, MRI surveys of normal patients with no symptoms of mandibular dysfunction have shown that a significant proportion of them have displaced discs within the temporomandibular joints, which, when such displacements were discovered by the invasive techniques (which could only ethically be used on patients with symptoms) were considered to be the cause of the symptoms. Undoubtedly some of these internal joint derangements, or more frank pathology of the joints, do cause symptoms similar to those arising from the purely functional disorder: mandibular dysfunction.

There are clearly cases in which the cause of the symptoms is dysfunction, others in which there is some organic, physical explanation and many where the cause is less clear. Sadly some dentists align themselves with one or other of the rather narrow and exclusive regimes for the management of mandibular dysfunction. This is unfortunate and unscientific. With different schools of thought about the aetiology and management of mandibular dysfunction, each supported by some, but incomplete, research evidence, the sensible dentist will keep an open mind. However, some lines of treatment are more interventive than others and so it is wiser to take a conservative approach to the management of mandibular dysfunction and assume that, in the absence of firm evidence to the contrary, most cases of mandibular dysfunction are functional rather than organic in nature.

An attractive hypothesis is that occlusal interferences (described on page 65) produce conditioned patterns of muscle activity that avoid these interferences. This increases the basic level of muscle activity, which, when it is further increased by anxiety or stress, brings the level of muscle tension above a threshold and symptoms develop. Therefore treatment aimed at removing the occlusal interferences is aimed at the cause of the problem rather than the symptoms. Similarly, treatment aimed at reducing anxiety and stress is also aimed at the cause, but this should be limited to sympathy and explanation of the cause together with a caring approach to treatment rather than, in the hands of the general dental practitioner, the use of drugs.

Occlusal interferences are not always easy to detect clinically because of the set of conditioned reflexes that avoid contact on the occlusal interference. A simple way to detect whether alteration of the occlusion is likely to reduce the symptoms of mandibular dysfunction is to provide a hard acrylic biteplane covering all the surfaces of one (usually the upper) jaw. If the symptoms improve after a few weeks of wearing the appliance at nights (or all day if it is tolerated) then this is a clear indication that the occlusion has something to do with the symptoms and justifies the expenditure of further time and effort on identifying and dealing with the occlusal interferences.

The acrylic biteplane should be used in this diagnostic way rather than as a long-term treatment of the condition. However, some patients, despite advice given to them, continue to wear the plate because it has reduced their symptoms, and for this reason plates making contact with only a limited number of anterior or posterior teeth should not be used. If they are, they will act as orthodontic appliances and produce depression or over-eruption of teeth.

The treatment of occlusal interferences in the management of mandibular dysfunction is usually fairly simple once the interference has been identified. It usually involves occlusal adjustment by grinding selected parts of the occlusal surfaces.

This is not the same as occlusal 'equilibration', which suggests recontouring the entire occlusion to fit some preconceived, idealized concept of what the occlusion should be. Similarly the treatment of mandibular dysfunction only *very seldom indeed* justifies the construction of multiple crowns or bridges. Crowns and bridges may be necessary for other reasons, and if the patient has mandibular dysfunction then this will complicate the treatment and definitive restorations should not be provided until the symptoms have resolved.

The detailed management of mandibular dysfunction is beyond the scope of this book, and the remainder of this chapter deals with practical aspects of dealing with the occlusion in a patient without symptoms of mandibular dysfunction.

Examination and analysis of the occlusion

In most cases it is sufficient to examine the occlusion clinically, but in more extensive occlusal reconstructions or where there are conditioned patterns of movement preventing clinical examination, study casts should be articulated. Provided the clinician understands what he is looking for, there is no need to articulate study casts for the majority of crowns and bridges.

Clinical examination of the occlusion

The following points should be noted:

- Any complaints the patient may have of temporomandibular joint pain, muscle spasm or unexplained chronic dental pain
- The ease or difficulty with which the various excursions can be made voluntarily by the patient
- Any occlusal interferences and whether the proposed restorations will influence these
- Mobility of teeth during excursions of the mandible with the teeth in contact
- The presence, angle and smoothness of any slide from RCP to ICP
- The type of lateral guidance and particularly the degree of contact in lateral excursion of any

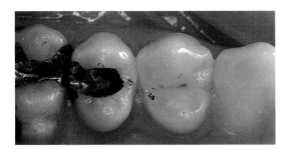

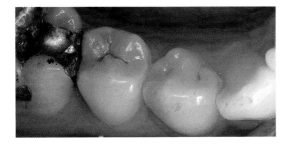

Figure 4.7

a and *b* Occlusal contacts marked in two different colours of articulating paper. The black marks on the marginal ridges of the upper premolars, *a*, and on the buccal cusp of the lower first premolar, *b*, were made with the patient in ICP. Movement to RCP produced the contacts marked in red.

teeth that are to be restored, or the likely degree of contact for any teeth to be replaced
● The presence of any contact on the non-working side
● The location, extent and cause of any faceting of the teeth to be restored
● The degree of stability of the occlusion and whether the proposed restorations will influence stability
● Over-erupted and tilted teeth, particularly if they are the teeth to be restored or if they oppose the teeth to be restored.

Clinical aids

Articulating paper

Flexible articulating paper or plastic foil of different colours may be used to mark occlusal contacts in different excursions. For example, ICP may be recorded in one colour and RCP in a second (see Figure 4.7). Articulating paper is rather difficult to use, having a tendency to mark the tips of cusps whether or not they are in occlusion, and often it does not register contacts on polished gold and glazed porcelain.

Wax

Thin, fairly soft wax with an adhesive on one side is marketed as a material for registering occlusal contacts. This is useful but rather expensive. An alternative is to use 0.5-mm-thick, dark-coloured sheet wax. Occlusal registrations in this material are shown in Figure 4.3. It has the advantage that it can be removed from the teeth and placed over the study casts for the occlusal contacts to be studied more closely. It can also be used in full arch-sized pieces. Areas of contact in the mouth may be marked through the perforations with a chinagraph pencil.

Plastic strips

Plastic strips may be used to test whether teeth are making contact in various excursions. The thinnest of these materials (shimstock) is opaque and silver-coloured and is only 8 μm thick. The strip is placed between opposing teeth and pulled aside once occlusal contact has been made. Often two pieces are used on opposite sides of the jaw to test the symmetry of the occlusion, or between the crowned tooth and its opponent, and the adjacent tooth and its opponent to test that the crown is in contact but is not 'high'.

Less accurate (40 μm thick) but more manageable mylar matrix strips, used for composite resins, is an acceptable alternative.

Study casts

Unarticulated study casts are useful for assessing the stability of the occlusion in ICP and for examining wear facets, which are often easier to see on the cast than in the mouth. They are of little value in assessing contacts in the excursions of the mandible.

Articulated study casts

When sufficient information cannot be obtained by clinical examination or examination of hand-held study casts, it is unlikely that study casts mounted on a simple hinge articulator will give adequate additional information; a semi-adjustable or fully adjustable articulator is necessary.

Figure 4.8 shows a set of study casts being mounted on a semi-adjustable articulator. For registration of the occlusion the following are required:

● A facebow record: set to an average terminal hinge axis of 10 mm in front of the superior border of the tragus of the ear on a line to the ala of the nose
● A record of RCP in one of the materials described more fully in Chapter 6
● Protrusive excursion record, usually in wax, but sometimes in one of the other materials described in Chapter 6, or
● Lateral excursion records taken in wax or one of the other materials.

The semi-adjustable articulator has a number of limitations and produces only an approximation to the tooth movements in the mouth. For the normal purposes of analysis it is quite sufficient.

Occlusal adjustments prior to tooth preparation

Once the occlusion has been assessed, adjustment prior to tooth preparation must be considered.

This will be necessary in cases where the teeth opposing a proposed bridge have over-erupted or where the occlusal plane is going to be altered by means of crowns. Sometimes the incisal plane of the lower incisors is adjusted and levelled out before making upper incisor crowns.

Occlusal adjustment is also indicated in many cases of mandibular dysfunction (see page 71).

There is no justification for prophylactic adjustments unless there is evidence of damage or pathology arising from the occlusion; our level of understanding of occlusal problems is not yet sufficient to warrant arbitrary prophylactic alterations in an established, comfortable, functioning occlusion.

Occlusal objectives in making crowns and bridges

There are two main objectives:

● To leave the occlusion with no additional occlusal interferences
● To leave the occlusion stable.

In addition, there may be secondary objectives, for example:

● To distribute the guidance in one of the excursions more evenly between a number of teeth, for example, by modifying the anterior guidance so that a number of anterior teeth share the occlusal forces in protrusive excursion.
● When a canine tooth that previously guided the occlusion is extracted, lateral forces should be distributed as evenly and as widely as possible between the remaining posterior teeth.

These latter objectives may be described as occlusal engineering, planned to produce occlusal relationships that achieve the first two major objectives of occlusal harmony and occlusal stability.

Most crowns and small bridges are made in mouths with an established ICP and RCP. These should be left unaltered by the restorations (i.e. a 'conformative' approach) unless:

● So many of the occluding surfaces are being restored that ICP will inevitably be altered

● ICP is unsatisfactory for some reason
● OVD is being altered, or
● There are symptoms of mandibular dysfunction.

In all these cases the occlusion is usually restored with ICP made to coincide with RCP (i.e. a 'reorganized' approach). This is mostly for practical reasons and does not imply that RCP is preferable to an established, comfortable, functional ICP.

Clinical and laboratory management of the occlusion

Avoiding loss of occlusal relationships

When sufficient occluding teeth will remain to register the ICP and other occlusal relationships after tooth preparation, there is no need to take any precautions to record the occlusal relationships beforehand. However, when the occlusal surfaces are being removed from a number of teeth, or when one or more of these teeth are crucial to the guidance of mandibular movements, the occlusal relationships should be registered before the tooth preparations are begun.

When large numbers of posterior teeth are being prepared or when several teeth are missing there is a risk of losing any record of the original OVD. A pair of opposing teeth on either side may be left unprepared, the remaining teeth prepared and then the opposing teeth adjusted so that ICP is the same as RCP. Impressions and occlusal records are taken with these teeth stabilizing the jaws during the occlusal registration. They are then prepared and further impressions taken. Alternatively, one pair of opposing crowns can be made for each side of the arch before the other teeth are prepared and these pairs of crowns serve the same purpose.

Maintaining occlusal relationships with temporary restorations

Prepared teeth and their opponents will over-erupt unless occlusion is re-established by means of adequate temporary restorations; and the prepared tooth and the teeth either side of it can drift together unless contact points are maintained in this way. The longer the period between the impression and fitting of the restorations, the more important are temporary restorations. They are probably also more important in younger patients, where tooth movement may occur more quickly. For this reason, individually made temporary restorations in plastic are preferred to preformed types unless the preformed temporary restoration happens to be an excellent fit at the contact points and in the occlusion.

Recording and occlusion

A decision must be made on the type of articulator to use for the working casts. Once this is done, the appropriate occlusal records will be obvious. The choice is as follows:

Hand-held models

Unless enormous care is taken, these are not satisfactory. The most common problem is that restorations are made high and are not detected because it is very difficult to see the tiny spaces between pairs of opposing teeth adjacent to the restoration. It is possible to check whether these teeth are in occlusion in intercuspal position using shimstock or other material but this can be difficult and time consuming – it is quicker to mount the models on an articulator in the first place, when a high restoration is easier to see.

Simple-hinge articulator (see Figure 4.9)

This is adequate when there are sufficient unprepared intercuspating teeth and the restoration is to be made occluding in ICP and adjusted at the chairside. For example, in a straightforward single upper anterior crown, the palatal surface can be contoured to match the adjacent palatal surfaces so that the incisal guidance will need very little adjustment. Similarly, for a single posterior crown when the occlusion is canine-guided, it is necessary only to reproduce contact in ICP. The crown will disocclude in lateral excursions, and adjustment at the chairside for protrusive and retrusive movements will be straightforward.

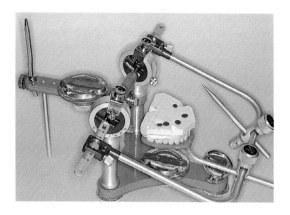

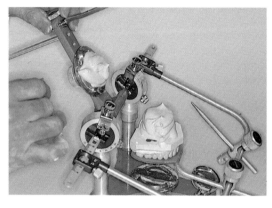

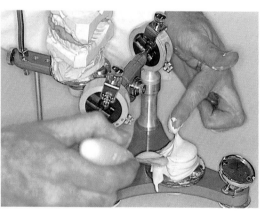

Figure 4.8

Articulating casts on a semi-adjustable articulator.

a The facebow in position and the upper cast seated in the wax impression of the upper teeth. This cast has been prepared with removable dies, and the blobs of red wax cover the ends of dowel pins. The cast has also been notched so that it can be removed from its mounting and relocated (a split cast). The facebow records the relationship of the upper teeth with the THA or an approximation of it.

b Quick-set, low-expansion impression plaster being used to mount the upper cast. When the upper arm is swung into position, the bite fork of the facebow and upper cast are supported with the other hand.

c The lower model is seated into the RCP record, in this case silicone, and plaster is applied to the lower mounting plate.

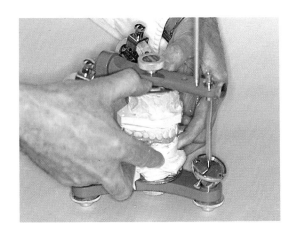

d The casts are swung over with the upper member and held in place with the fingers until the plaster sets. Alternatives are to attach the casts together with elastic bands or wax.

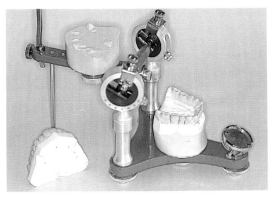

e The mounted casts showing the upper cast removed from its base.

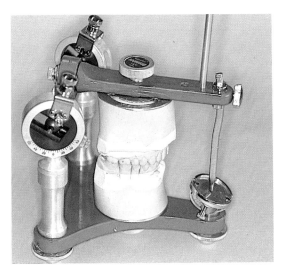

f The casts in RCP. The condylar guidance is now adjusted using protrusive or lateral excursion inter-occlusal records. The record is placed between the teeth and the condylar guidance angle adjusted until the casts are fully seated in the record.

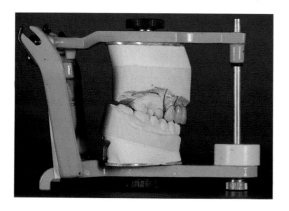

Figure 4.9

A simple articulator that is adequate for many single crowns and small bridges.

The advantage of a hinge articulator over hand-held models is that if the restoration is made high, all the other teeth will be out of occlusion, and this effect can be magnified by arranging the casts so that the restoration is nearest to the hinge.

There is often no need for any occlusal record. It is usually possible to place the models together entirely satisfactorily by hand in ICP. When there may be some doubt about ICP an occlusal record is made in wax or one of the other materials discussed in Chapter 6.

Semi-adjustable articulator (see Figures 4.8 and 4.10)

These have the following features:

● The maxillary cast is related to an arbitrary axis through the condyles

● Condylar guidance is variable, but only in straight lines
● Some adjustment of incisal guidance is usually possible.

When occlusal relationships are important in positions other than ICP a semi-adjustable articulator may be used. The maxillary cast is mounted using the facebow, and the mandibular cast is related to it by hand in ICP, by an ICP record, or by a record in the RCP, whichever is appropriate. The articulator is then adjusted using intra-occlusal records taken in either protrusive or lateral excursions. The records taken will be selected according to the circumstances. For example, if crowns on the right side are being made in a case with group function but where there is no risk of non-working side contacts occurring in left lateral excursion, only a record of right lateral excursion is necessary.

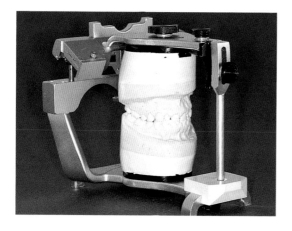

Figure 4.10

An 'arcon' type of semi-adjustable articulator. This is now the most popular design of articulator for crowns and bridges.

With this arrangement a good approximation to group function should be possible, with only minor adjustment being necessary at the chairside because of the compromises inherent with semi-adjustable articulators.

There are two broad categories of semi-adjustable articulator. The type shown in Figure 4.8 is a non-arcon type. That is, the balls representing the condyles are attached to the upper member of the articulator and the condylar guidance to the lower. This is, of course, upside down with respect to the anatomy of the joint. The articulator shown in Figure 4.9 is also non-arcon. The articulator shown in Figure 4.10 is a semi-adjustable arcon articulator, and the fully adjustable articulator shown in Figure 4.11 is also an arcon design.

In practical terms the difference between the arcon and non-arcon designs is not particularly relevant, providing that the occlusal records can be taken with the teeth in contact or nearly so. However, if the OVD is being increased or if the occlusal records have to be taken at a degree of opening of the mandible then this affects the relationship between the condylar guidance angle and the upper member of the articulator. It follows that in these circumstances an arcon design should be used.

Fully adjustable articulator

A full description of the use of these articulators is beyond the scope of this book. Suffice it to say that they are used when more accurate and comprehensive records of mandibular movements are required. The records used to mount casts on them are the facebow set to a terminal hinge axis determined specifically for the patient, a record of mandibular movement recorded by mechanical or electronic devices (pantographs), and usually several records of RCP that are checked against each other to ensure that the recorded position is reproducible (see Figure 4.11).

Fully adjustable articulators vary, but they usually have some if not all of the following features:

● The condyles are on the lower member of the articulator and the condylar guidance element on the upper membrane, i.e. an arcon design

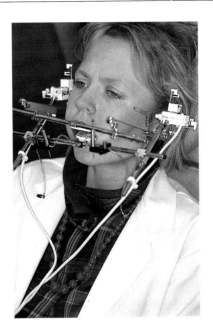

Figure 4.11

a An electronic mandibular movement recording device. The upper and lower members are attached to acrylic clutches firmly seated on the teeth. Movements of the mandible are recorded by the sensors sited over the condyles, and the information is passed to a control box (not shown), which produces a printout of information from which the fully adjustable articulator can be set directly.

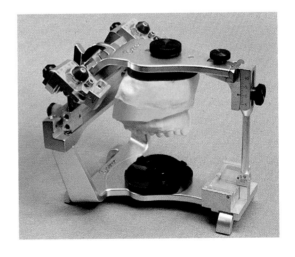

b A fully adjustable articulator.

- The inter-condylar distance is infinitely variable
- The immediate side shift (Bennett movement) and progressive side shift (Bennett angle) are adjustable
- The Fischer angle (the angle of the superior wall of the glenoid fossa to the horizontal lateral plane) is adjustable
- The superior wall of the glenoid fossa (the anterior-posterior condylar guidance) is fully adjustable and in some cases can be contoured to a curved pathway using individually made inserts
- Individually contoured anterior guidance tables can also be made.

These adjustments all allow for fine tuning of the articulator so that movements of the casts in it more closely represent the physiological movements of the patient.

Even when this costly and time-consuming equipment is used by experienced operators, there is often still a need for some occlusal adjustment at the chairside.

Laboratory stages

Trimming the casts

One of the commonest causes of restorations being high when tried in the mouth is distortion of the casts, particularly the opposing casts, which may be made from an alginate impression. Commonly, small air bubbles trapped in the occlusal fissures will prop the models apart slightly, so that if the restoration is made to touch the opposing model, it will be high in the mouth. Impression techniques for crowns and bridges should concentrate on the crowns of the teeth, injecting impression material into the occlusal fissures or rubbing alginate into them with the fingers. If air bubbles do occur, great care should be taken to trim occlusal defects from the models, and if individual teeth are suspect, they should be cut right away from the model unless they are opposing or adjacent to the teeth being restored.

Articulating the casts

As small an amount of plaster as possible should be used since the expansion of the plaster distorts the relationship of the articulator with the casts. Ideally, impression plaster or plaster containing an anti-expansion agent should be used; alternatively, there are plasterless designs of articulator.

Shaping the occlusal surfaces

The technique of shaping the occlusal surface will depend upon whether the surface is to be gold or porcelain:

Wax carving With this technique wax is built up to excess on the occlusal surface and then carved to the required occlusal contour. Small increments of wax are added when necessary to repair over-carving. When completed, occlusal contact should be checked using shimstock, both between the carved tooth and its opponent and between adjacent teeth and their opponents (see Figure 4.12).

The wax-added technique Small increments of molten wax are flowed from the tip of an instrument to build up cones, each one forming the tip of a cusp. The other features of the occlusal surface are then added, often with different coloured waxes to identify each feature. Using this technique, the occlusal relationships in all excursions can be checked from the beginning and adjusted as the process continues (see Figure 4.12).

Occlusal shaping with porcelain Although there are cones of high alumina available that can be used in techniques similar to the wax-added technique, there is often not sufficient room for them and they are difficult to use.

Usually porcelain surfaces are built up slightly to excess and then ground to shape, stained and glazed. Again shimstock or similar material is useful in checking the occlusal relationships in the articulator.

An alternative approach: the functionally generated wax record

The principle of this technique is that the prepared teeth are coated in wax contained in a suitable matrix that allows free movements of the mandible. The patient then makes excursions of the mandible with the teeth in contact, effectively

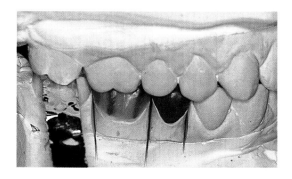

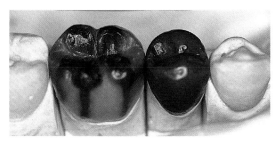

Figure 4.12

a and *b* Two crowns waxed up on the lower second premolar and first molar teeth. The lower second premolar has been waxed using a carving technique, starting with an excess of wax on the occlusal surface. The first molar has been carved by a wax-added technique, cones of wax being built up to the required contact with the opposing teeth and the gaps between filled in with a different-coloured wax. Shimstock is being used to check that contact just occurs between the unprepared second molar teeth, and will be used between the wax patterns and the opposing teeth.

carving the wax with the opposing teeth. A cast is made against this occlusal record and set up against the working cast. This ensures that no occlusal interferences are introduced as the full range of movements of the opposing teeth are recorded in the functionally generated cast. It is, however, sometimes difficult to achieve occlusal stability, and so a normal anatomical model of the opposing jaw is also set up, so that not only is the occlusion made stable but the appearance of the restoration is made to harmonize with the opposing teeth. To allow these alternative opposing casts to be used with the working cast, special designs of articulator are available. One type has two upper arms: one carrying the functionally generated cast and the other the anatomical cast. They can be hinged over alternately to occlude with the lower cast.

Adjusting the occlusion of restorations in the mouth

Occlusal marking materials

Articulating paper and 0.5-mm-thick darkly coloured wax have already been described. An alternative technique for metal occlusal surfaces is to sandblast them lightly with a mild abrasive which gives the surface a matt appearance. Burnish marks will then appear in areas of contact with the opposing teeth.

Adjusting in intercuspal position

A patient who does not have a local anaesthetic will be immediately conscious of a high restoration in ICP. Even with a local anaesthetic the opposing teeth will normally sense a high restoration. The patient will not of course be aware of a restoration that is short of the occlusion, and so occlusal contact should be checked with shimstock or mylar matrix strip. If occlusal contact is not present (i.e., the restoration is not occlusally stable), the tooth or its opponent will over-erupt and occlusal interferences may be introduced.

High restorations should be ground. With crowns short of the occlusion, additions may be made, if this is possible, or the crowns cemented and the occlusion adjusted when over-eruption has occurred.

Adjustments in lateral, protrusive and retrusive excursions

The occlusion of the restoration is examined for interferences in these excursions of the mandible and adjusted if necessary.

Stability

Following these adjustments, a final check of the stability of the occlusion is made by confirmation of the presence of centric stops on the restoration and the adjacent teeth. The adequacy of the contact points is checked with dental floss.

Adjustment techniques

ICP is adjusted first and the centric stops marked with articulating paper or wax. Interferences are marked with a different colour and adjusted.

Gold and porcelain can be adjusted with mounted stones or diamond burs. Gold can be finished with finishing burs and polished with mounted rubber wheels or points. Porcelain can be finished with the mounted points or discs used to finish composite and with specially produced kits of instruments. With these instruments, the finished surface is as smooth as the glazed surface, and re-glazing is unnecessary.

Practical points

● In restorative dentistry a functional rather than orthodontic or complete denture approach to occlusion is necessary.

● Clinical examination of the occlusion and simple records are often sufficient for straight-forward crowns and bridges.

● In cases of more complicated occlusal movements, a semi or fully adjustable articulator will be needed.

● Occlusal adjustment should be considered only where the restoration will interfere with a harmonious or stable function.

● The occlusion of the restoration itself will have to be checked and if necessary adjusted, using recording and clinical techniques similar to those for the preliminary occlusal examination.

5 Planning and making crowns

There is a natural sequence by which the history and examination of the patient lead to a decision on the advisability or otherwise of crowns in the context of the overall treatment. This general decision leads to a further series of stages in the detailed planning of treatment. This sequence is:

History and examination:

- Of the whole patient
- Of the mouth in general
- Of the individual tooth

Decisions to be made:

- Keep the tooth or extract
- If the tooth is to be kept – crown or other restoration
- If the tooth is to be crowned – preparatory treatment necessary

Detailed planning of the crown:

- Appearance
- The remaining structure of the tooth and its environment, including any necessary core
- Choice of type of crown, including material
- Detailed design of the preparation

Planning and executing the clinical and laboratory stages:

- Appointment sequence – agreement with patient and laboratory, including agreements on fees and laboratory charges
- First clinical stage
- Laboratory stage
- Second clinical stage
- Maintenance.

It would be very nice if life were as simple as this. It is convenient to have such a sequence of events in mind but it is not often possible to follow the pattern precisely. For example, if endodontic treatment is necessary as part of the preparatory treatment then a temporary crown may well have to be made at an early stage before the preparation can be finally planned. This outline sequence may have various repeat loops arising within it. The dentist must be prepared to rethink the options as new circumstances arise and allow full freedom to his or her professional judgement.

History and examination

Considering the whole patient

Patient attitude and informed consent

Complex and time-consuming procedures such as crowns should not be contemplated unless the patient is enthusiastic and cooperative about the treatment. There is always some other way of treating the tooth, even if it means extracting it. The patient's attitude is particularly important when crowns are being considered for purely cosmetic reasons. The dentist must be satisfied that the patient fully understands the limitations of what can be achieved. Techniques for demonstrating cosmetic changes to patients before the teeth are prepared are described later.

Patients generally appreciate having the reasons for treatment explained to them together with some of the details of treatment. A common source of dento-legal problems is the patient who claims an inadequate understanding of what was being proposed and that had it been fully understood, he or she would not have gone ahead with the treatment. Again this applies particularly to treatment provided mainly for cosmetic reasons.

Age

There is no upper age limit for crowns provided the patient is fit enough to undergo the treatment

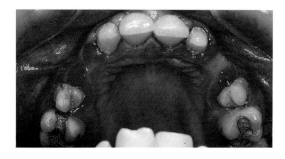

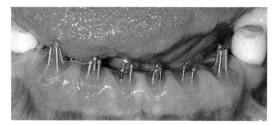

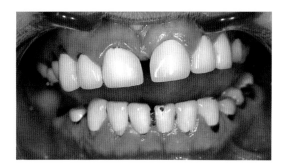

Figure 5.1

Crowns and bridges for young patients.

a Bridge preparations for a patient aged 13 with oligodontia. The teeth prepared are the canines and second premolars: the diminutive and unattractive canines are in the position of the missing lateral incisors. At this stage, minimal preparations are carried out and metal–acrylic provisional restorations placed for a period of six months to a year. This encourages secondary dentine formation so that the definitive preparations can be made with less risk to the pulp (see the text for an explanation of the poor gingival condition).

b Threaded-pin retention for composite cores in a patient aged 12 with dentinogenesis imperfecta. In this condition the pulps recede rapidly, and this procedure was carried out without the need for local analgesia.

c These are the crowns made for the patient in b eighteen years after they were fitted. The porcelain at the incisal edge of the lower left central incisor has chipped and there has been some gingival recession and repairs with glass ionomer cement, otherwise the pin retained composite cores have been successful and none of the crowns have been lost.

and is in other ways suitable for crowns. There are some practical problems in extensive treatment for elderly patients; for example, the teeth tend to become more brittle with age and this affects the design of crown preparations.

Neither is there a lower age limit for crowns. It is unusual to make crowns for teeth shortly after they have erupted, and crowns are commonly delayed until the patient is 16 or so. However, this decision has traditionally been based upon three main factors:

● The size of the pulp
● The degree of eruption of the tooth
● The cooperativeness of the patients.

These will vary considerably among patients. For example, an upper incisor tooth that is fractured at the age of 7 or 8 and restored with composite, will usually develop extensive secondary dentine so that the pulp will be smaller by the age of 10 than the pulp of an undamaged tooth at the age of 16. In patients with good oral hygiene, the position of the gingival margin of the incisor does not alter much after this age, and today's children are far less anxious about dental treatment than they were a generation ago. In a case like this, therefore, there may be no contraindication to providing a permanent crown at the age of 10.

Similarly, when a successful root canal treatment has been carried out so that there is no need to worry about the pulp, post-crowns can be made for children in their early teens and even younger.

Even when the pulp has not been damaged or affected by secondary dentine, there is now evidence that the size of the pulp does not vary significantly with age in the great majority of young patients. The ratio of the size of the pulp to the size of the tooth is very varied, and certainly the pulp does not suddenly shrivel to a significantly smaller size on the patient's 16th birthday or at any other age. It is much more important to assess pulp size from a good, clear periapical radiograph than it is to adopt an arbitrary rule about the age at which teeth can be prepared for crowns.

Of course, there are far fewer indications for anterior crowns in young patients than there were a few years ago, with the introduction of a variety of new ways to restore anterior teeth and make bridges, as described elsewhere in this book.

Figure 5.1 shows bridges being made for a 13-year-old boy and a set of full mouth crowns for a girl of 12 with severe dentinogenesis imperfecta. Both patients were particularly cooperative and enthusiastic about treatment. Figure 5.1c shows the crowns for the second patient still in place at age 30.

It is argued that boisterous children and sports players who suffer damage to their teeth should not have the teeth permanently restored until they are over this energetic period. However, many of them continue to play vigorous contact sports well into their twenties or thirties or later, and, if crowns are indicated, it is quite unacceptable that patients should be deprived of them until they have become docile and sedentary. It is very much better to provide the crowns, and with them a mouth protector, not only for the crowns but also more importantly for the remaining natural teeth.

Sex

Many male patients are just as concerned with their appearance as females. They may, however, be less willing to admit to this. It is more important to determine patients' real attitudes to their appearance than to make assumptions based upon their gender.

Social history

The patient's occupation may be important. Wind instrument players, for example, are particularly anxious to retain their incisor teeth in order to support their embouchure (the particular contraction of the lips needed to form the contact with the mouthpiece).

Habits such as pipe smoking, where the stem of the pipe is clenched between the teeth, may affect the design or type of crown selected.

When extensive treatment is planned, it is important to establish that the patient will be available for appointments of sufficient length and frequency to complete the treatment. Crowns should not be started just before a patient is due to sit important examinations; and people who plan to marry usually like to have their crowns completed in time for the wedding photographs.

Cost

There is no satisfactory way of mass producing crowns, and so they will always be labour-intensive and therefore costly. Whichever way the cost is borne – by the patient, or by a private or public insurance scheme – the cost is important and must be taken into account in any treatment plan. Because crowns are expensive, they should not be made unless they will really contribute significantly to the patient's well-being and can be expected to last for a reasonable period of time.

Considering the whole mouth

Oral hygiene

There is obviously no point in embarking upon a complex course of treatment involving crowns (or bridges) in a mouth with rapidly progressing caries or periodontal disease resulting from poor oral hygiene. The first priority must be to arrest the disease process and improve the oral hygiene.

That being said, however, it is impossible for any mouth to be kept absolutely plaque-free. It is almost always possible to find some in the mouth of even the most meticulous patient. Most, despite good intentions, achieve only a moderately good level of plaque control. The problem for the dentist is therefore one of degree. He or

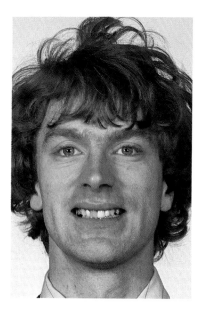
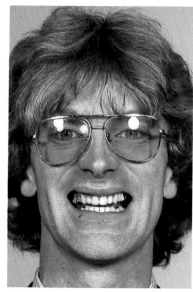

Figure 5.2

a and *b* The same patient before and after a six-month course of extensive dental treatment involving periodontal treatment and the construction of upper anterior crowns. During this period, the patient's dental awareness and motivation improved considerably and his oral hygiene became markedly better once he had more attractive teeth.

she must decide whether the patient, after instruction in oral hygiene, can achieve a level or oral cleanliness that warrants treatment which is time consuming and costly. It is also necessary to decide how to treat those patients who are assessed as having a level of oral hygiene falling below this standard but who nevertheless have teeth that can only be treated satisfactorily by means of crowns.

There is no simple guidance on these difficult decisions. Perhaps the best advice is to assess not only the level of oral hygiene, but the effect that this is having on periodontal disease and caries. Yet there is no single direct relationship between oral hygiene and disease – many other factors

influence the disease processes. The decision whether to crown a tooth or not should therefore be made on an assessment of the prognosis of the tooth without the crown or with it. If, in an otherwise-intact arch, a single badly broken-down anterior tooth is ugly, does not function well and is difficult to restore by any means other than a crown then, provided that the prognosis of the alveolar support is such that the tooth is not likely to be lost for at least a few years, it is almost certainly better to make a crown than to extract it and provide a partial denture, even if the oral hygiene is poor and cannot be improved. It would be quite wrong not to offer any form of treatment, and morally dubious to attempt to blackmail the patient to maintain a better standard of oral hygiene by refusing the crown unless the oral hygiene improves. In any case, this crude psychological approach seldom produces a permanent improvement in oral hygiene.

Although every effort should be made by both dentist and patient to improve oral hygiene when it is poor, there are those who are simply not able to improve, but who are nevertheless fortunate in having a slow rate of progress of periodontal disease and a low caries incidence, and for these patients crowns are often justified.

Figure 5.1a shows a typical 13-year-old boy who has entered puberty. This hormonal change affects the gingival response to plaque, but it also – as many parents of teenagers know – sometimes leads to expressions of independence and even rebellion. This may show as lapses in cleanliness, including oral hygiene. Fortunately most recover. This patient had several missing or misshapen teeth through no fault of his own. He had cooperated with a course of fixed orthodontic treatment. How cruel now to prescribe a removable denture, which he desperately wished to avoid, at this difficult stage in his life, just because, for the time being, his standard of oral hygiene has lapsed.

When crowns or other complex forms of treatment that improve the patient's appearance are provided, this and the general increase in dental awareness that comes with extended courses of dental treatment themselves often improve the patient's motivation and, in turn, oral hygiene (see Figure 5.2).

Condition of the remaining teeth

The state of health and repair of the whole mouth must be taken into account. When there have been no previous extractions and the prognosis of the remaining teeth is good, it is usually worth the patient and dentist putting a considerable amount of effort into saving an individual tooth. Conversely, when the patient has already lost a number of teeth and is wearing a partial denture that will need replacing fairly soon, it would be foolish to struggle to save an individual tooth unless it is a crucial abutment for the denture, or of particular importance to the patient's appearance. It is usually better to extract the tooth and remake the denture.

The periodontal condition of the remaining teeth is one of the factors in assessing their prognosis, but it is more important to determine whether any periodontal disease is progressing or whether treatment of it has produced a stable state. The effects of periodontal disease, particularly when there has been gingival recession, can affect the choice and design of the crowns. An example is given in Figure 12.9, where partial crowns are selected in preference to complete crowns partly because of the length of the clinical crowns.

Assessment of the occlusion is important (see Chapter 4). In particular, the adequacy of posterior support should be considered when anterior crowns are planned. Insufficient occluding natural posterior teeth usually means that anterior crowns should be metal–ceramic rather than porcelain, and in some cases where there has also been periodontal disease and drifting of the incisor teeth, crowns joined together may be necessary (splinting is described in Chapter 12).

Considering the individual tooth

The value of the tooth

Not all teeth are of equal value. Third molars are commonly extracted with no harmful effects on appearance or function. To crown third molars in an intact dentition would probably be no more than a display of clinical virtuosity. However, if a number of other teeth are missing, a broken-down third molar tooth that can be crowned may provide an invaluable abutment tooth for a denture or a bridge. There is a similar range of possibilities for most other teeth.

Appearance

The presence of failed restorations may suggest that crowns are advisable, but since anterior filling materials are continually improving, the possibility of replacing the restoration rather than crowning the teeth should normally be considered first. Whether the problem is one of failed restorations, intrinsic staining or the shape or angulation of the teeth, a realistic appraisal of the cosmetic advantages of crowns must be made. Sometimes patients expect more of crowns than can be achieved, and are disappointed with the end result. This should be avoided by explaining the problems, complications and compromises associated with crowns (see Chapter 1).

Condition of the crown of the tooth, the pulp and periodontium

The presence of caries, previous restorations or pulp pathology are not contraindications to making crowns, but they may well determine the type of crown and the design of the preparation. Caries or fractures extending deep below the gingival margin will make crown preparation difficult, and it may sometimes be better to extract the tooth. Alternatively, periodontal surgery may be used to expose the margin of the fracture.

Unless the tooth has been root-treated, the vitality of the pulp must always be tested and when necessary endodontic treatment carried out. The prognosis and acceptability of crowning a recently root-filled tooth will depend on the absence of signs or symptoms and its radiographic appearance.

If there is any anxiety about the success of a root filling then a choice must be made between a number of options:

1 Leave the tooth temporarily restored until the symptoms settle and a good prognosis can be given
2 Repeat the root filling, with either an ortho-grade or a retrograde approach
3 Proceed with the amalgam core (for a posterior tooth) or the post and core (for an anterior tooth), but delay the final crown until the symptoms have settled or the radiographic appearance has improved, or the tooth has been apicected.

In many cases the third option is best. If a tooth is left with a temporary restoration for too long, there is a risk of further caries and periodontal disease. With anterior teeth, if the post and core are inserted immediately, there will be no risk of disturbing the root filling later, and with most well-condensed anterior root fillings, the treatment for further endodontic problems is often

an apicectomy. It is better to cement the post and core before the apicectomy rather than afterwards, to avoid the risk of disturbing the apical seal.

A more liberal attitude should be taken to minor radiographic defects in the root filling when it has been present for some years and is symptomless. Further details of the criteria for assessing root canal fillings are left to the endodontic textbooks.

Any local periodontal problems should be assessed and treated.

Occlusion

The occlusal contacts on the surface of the tooth may be important in determining the type of crown to be used. For example, an upper canine tooth that is the only tooth in contact in lateral excursion (canine guidance, see Chapter 4) will usually need a metal–ceramic crown rather than a PJC. However, if the tooth is only one of a number that make contact in lateral excursion (group function), it may be possible to restore the canine with a PJC.

The point of contact between the tooth to be crowned and the opposing tooth is also important in determining the position of the crown margin. It is wise to design the preparation so that the opposing tooth contacts either tooth tissue or the crown but not the junction between the two. In the case of partial crowns, when occlusal protection is required, the *occluding* surfaces of the tooth to be crowned should be determined. These are not always the same as the *occlusal* surface. *Occlusal* is an anatomical term, and an extracted tooth still has an occlusal surface. The *occluding* surfaces are those that really do make contact with opposing teeth in one or other excursion of the mandible.

Root length

The length of the root should be assessed from radiographs in two ways. First, this should be done from the point of view of periodontal support, i.e. the ratio of the length of the root supported by alveolar bone to the length of the remainder of the tooth. Second, the length of the

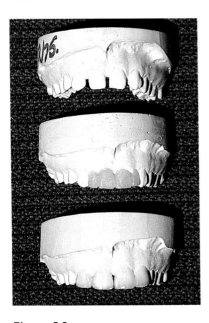

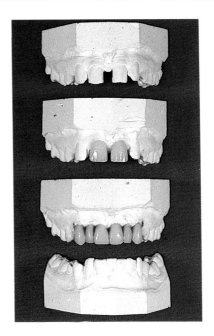

Figure 5.3

Trial or diagnostic wax-ups.

a Missing upper lateral incisors and a midline diastema. *Centre*: closing the diastema orthodontically and providing bridges to replace the lateral incisors. *Lower*: the alternative is to make four oversized crowns or veneers on the central incisors and canines to resemble four incisors. Neither solution will produce an ideal appearance.

b A similar case, but with denture teeth set on the model. This technique is less accurate and gives unrealistic results.

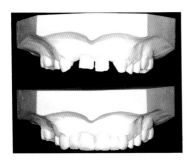

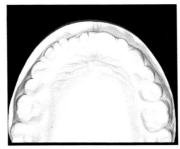

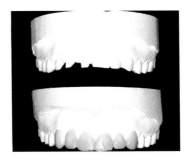

c A better diagnostic wax-up for a similar case. The lateral incisor teeth will be replaced by two 3-unit conventional bridges (see Part 2) increasing the size of the central incisor crowns and reducing the size of the canines.

d This patient has extensive palatal erosion as a result of an eating disorder. The teeth are already short and so diagnostic preparations have been made on three of them to see whether sufficient dentine remains for retentive preparations or whether some other solution is necessary.

e The preparations are judged as being sufficiently retentive and this figure also shows how short the unprepared incisor teeth have become. The diagnostic wax-up shows the appearance of the planned restorations and also provides a starting point for more detailed planning of the preparations and for making temporary crowns.

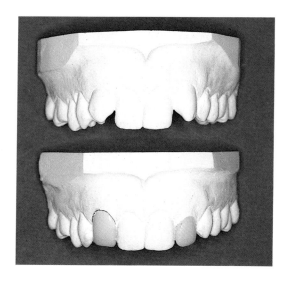

Figure 5.4

Trial wax-up 'cheating'. The upper cast shows a patient with ugly prominent canine teeth and missing lateral incisors with no residual space. The lower cast shows two trial wax-ups: *left*, with the contour of the gingival margin carefully marked in pencil before the preparation and wax-up are made; *right*, the position of the gingival margin has been lost and a more natural looking wax-up made. However, it will not be possible to achieve this result in the mouth and a decision whether to proceed with crowns must be made on the appearance of the 'honest' trial wax-up.

root is important in providing retention for a post crown. A working rule for the length of smooth tapered posts is for the length of the post to be not less than the length of the artificial crown. Variations are possible: for example, a shorter post is acceptable in the case of reduced occlusal forces (such as incisor teeth with an anterior open bite); and a longer post is necessary where there are excessive forces applied to the tooth, for example when the tooth is used as a partial denture abutment. When this length is not available, a post with improved retention, such as a threaded parallel post, should be used. An alternative is to include a full diaphragm of gold over the root face together with a collar around the periphery. This improves retention and also reduces the likelihood of root fracture.

Decisions to be made

Is the tooth to be kept or extracted?

Usually the result of the history and examination will determine this question. Sometimes,

however, it is necessary to proceed to further stages and then return to a decision to extract the tooth if further endodontic, periodontal or other treatment is not successful.

If the tooth is to be kept, is it to be restored by a crown or a filling?

In Chapter 1 the alternatives to crowns are listed, and the findings of the history and non-interventive examination will sometimes settle this question. However, it is often necessary to proceed to a further stage, actually starting the treatment by removing previous restorations and caries, before a properly informed decision can be made (see Figure 1.10, page 18).

If the tooth is to be crowned, is any preparatory treatment necessary?

Preparatory orthodontic treatment may be necessary to move the tooth into a suitable position

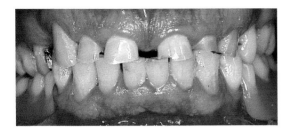

Figure 5.5

Temporary and permanent changes to occlusal vertical dimension.

a Gross erosion of the upper incisor teeth following a period of chronic vomiting. The patient had a peptic ulcer that had been successfully treated surgically two years before this photograph. The OVD is reduced because of this wear and because the lower posterior teeth are replaced only by a tissue-supported partial denture. The gingival condition at this early stage of treatment is poor.

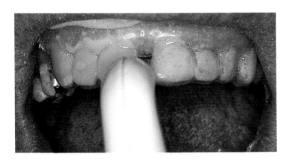

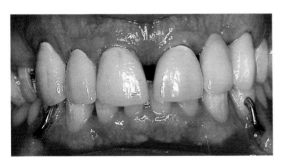

b and *c* Increasing the length of the upper incisors temporarily by means of light-cured composite placed in a vacuum-formed PVC matrix. Acrylic was added to the lower partial denture to increase its occlusal height temporarily.

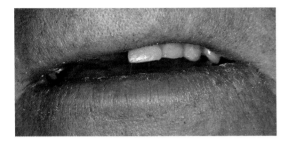

d After a period during which the patient became accustomed to the new OVD, the upper incisors were crowned and a tooth-supported partial lower denture fitted. The gingival condition has improved. Note the supragingival crown margins, which help the patient to maintain good oral hygiene. The left lateral incisor has been extracted and replaced by a bridge.

for crowning. Combinations of orthodontic treatment and crowns can often produce results that cannot be achieved by either form of treatment alone. Periodontal and endodontic treatment may also be necessary.

Detailed planning of the crown

Appearance

When a significant change in appearance is proposed, it is most important that the patient is

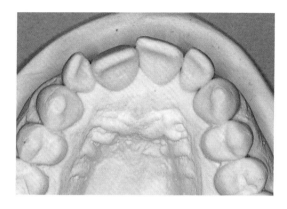

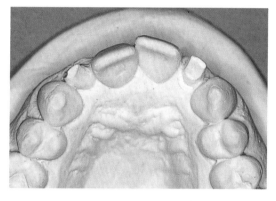

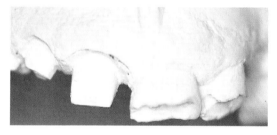

Figure 5.6

Trial preparations on study casts.

a The patient is unhappy about the appearance of the rotated lateral incisors and would like them crowned.

b *Right*: the maximum labial reduction, while preserving the vitality of the pulp would result in this preparation, allowing some reduction in the prominence of this tooth. *Left*: however, initial preparation quickly shows that devitalization would be necessary if a crown is to be made.

c The upper right central and lateral incisors were almost identical to the unprepared worn teeth left. Trial preparations show that it will be possible to achieve a retentive crown preparation for the central incisor but not for the lateral incisor.

fully informed of what can be achieved and what cannot. This can best be done by a modification of the patient's own study casts, usually in wax. Figure 5.3 shows examples of missing upper lateral incisors that could be treated by moving the central incisors mesially closing the diastema and replacing the lateral incisors by means of bridges. If this were done, all the teeth would be rather small. The alternative of not moving the teeth and enlarging the central incisors by means

of crowns and crowning the canines to resemble lateral incisors is also shown. Figures 5.3c, d and e show satisfactory trial wax-ups demonstrating retentive preparations and aesthetically pleasing crowns and bridges.

Trial or planning wax-ups are extremely valuable in predicting the final appearance, and should be used routinely.

Because the teeth and soft tissues are all reproduced in plaster or artificial stone in the cast, it

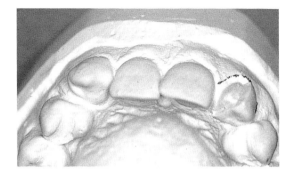

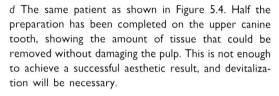

d The same patient as shown in Figure 5.4. Half the preparation has been completed on the upper canine tooth, showing the amount of tissue that could be removed without damaging the pulp. This is not enough to achieve a successful aesthetic result, and devitalization will be necessary.

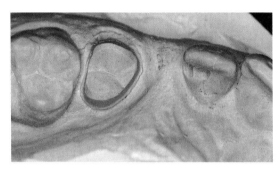

e Trial preparations for a bridge (see Part 2). These show that this design (fixed–movable) would not work in this case.

is possible to 'cheat' by making the trial wax-up in a way that would be impossible in the mouth by reshaping the gingival margin or by changing the dimensions of the root as it emerges from the gum. When the teeth are not to be moved orthodontically, it is useful to draw a pencil line around the gingival crevice on the study cast and to ensure that this is still visible after the wax-up has been completed. When the tooth is to be moved orthodontically, the mesio-distal width at the gingival margin should be measured and this width reproduced in the new position of the tooth on the study cast. Figure 5.4 shows an example of study cast 'cheating'. The plan is to crown the upper canines to resemble upper lateral incisors. This is always difficult and often disappointing. One of the distinctive features of an upper canine is the sharply curving gingival margin. This will be retained once the crown is in place, and will detract from the impression that the tooth is a lateral incisor.

These trial wax-ups serve a number of other purposes as well as informing the patient of

what can be achieved. However experienced the clinician, each case is different and modified study casts will help in planning details of the eventual appearance. The technician will know what is wanted and will have models to copy rather than have to design the patient's new appearance in porcelain.

The modified study cast, agreed by the patient, forms part of the contract between the dentist and patient. If the final outcome is an appearance similar to that of the study cast, it can be used as evidence that the contract has been fulfilled, and so dento-legal problems can be avoided. The modified study cast may also be used to produce temporary crowns (see Chapter 6).

Shade

It is wise to select the shade at this early stage, since some shades are more difficult to match than others. It is better to know about any difficulty before the teeth are prepared, both from the point of view of warning the patient and because it may be helpful to modify the preparation. For example, if there is an extensive amount of incisal translucency, the preparation may need to be shorter to allow additional incisal porcelain than if the tooth were more opaque.

Clinical modifications

In some cases it may be helpful to adjust the shape of teeth in the mouth by adding composite material – particularly when alterations in occlusal vertical dimensions are planned. Figure 5.5 shows a patient with gross erosion treated by upper anterior crowns and a new partial lower denture with an increase in occlusal vertical dimension. The patient's tolerance of an increase in OVD is assessed by means of the temporary additions of acrylic to the occlusal surfaces of the old partial lower denture and of composite material to the upper incisor teeth. Temporarily reshaping incisor teeth with composite to close diastemas and produce other changes are further examples.

Assessing the remaining tooth structure and its environment

Existing restorations and caries, especially in badly broken-down posterior teeth, should be removed, together with any completely unsupported enamel, so that the shape of the remaining tooth structure is not guesswork. Only at this point should the final restoration be planned. This preliminary cleaning away was necessary in all the examples shown in Chapter I (see Figure 1.10, page 18) for a properly informed decision to be made.

At this stage it may also be necessary to return to a decision on further preparatory treatment. For example, although the pulp may be vital in an anterior tooth, it may be decided that because of the weakness of the remaining coronal tissue, an elective root canal treatment and post crown is the preferred restoration. Similarly, where caries extends below the gingival margin, it may be decided to carry out a gingivoplasty or apically repositioned flap procedure to alter the gingival contour.

The need for a core

At this stage, when the full extent of the damage to a broken-down tooth is known, a decision is made on whether sufficient tooth substance remains for a crown preparation or whether it needs to be built up by means of a pin-retained or post-retained core, and, if so, whether the core should be of amalgam, composite or cast metal.

At the same time, the position of the crown margin should be settled. Usually the crown will extend beyond the core and completely cover it. However, when part of an amalgam core is subgingival but is well condensed and polished, it is often better to make the crown margin supragingival, leaving part of the core exposed.

The choice of the type of crown and the material

At this stage too the decision is taken between making a complete or partial crown, and what the material for the crown will be.

Detailed design of the preparation

Chapter 3 described the principles of crown preparation design. This is the point where they are applied to the particular tooth. In cases of doubt, for example where there are questions on the likely retentive qualities of the final preparation or on the likelihood of exposing the pulp in removing sufficient tooth tissue for a crown that is planned to change the shape of a tooth, a trial preparation on the study cast is of considerable value (see Figures 5.3d and e and 5.6).

Planning and executing the clinical and laboratory stages

Appointments

The treatment plan and fee having been agreed with the patient, a series of appointments is made and agreement reached with the laboratory that the technical work can be undertaken in the time. Very few dentists now carry out their own technical work and most laboratories appreciate being notified in advance when their services will be required, as least for extensive cases. This avoids the problem of promising the patient delivery of the crown by a specified date only to find when the impression is taken that your favourite technician is on holiday.

Clinical and laboratory stages

Details of clinical techniques are given in Chapter 6; at this point only the sequence of events is listed (see pages 98–99). Depending on the number of crowns involved, the experience and speed of the operator and other factors, each clinical stage may be accomplished in a single appointment or in several. The patient should be advised on oral hygiene techniques appropriate to the new crown, and he or she will need to be seen at regular intervals for the crown to be inspected and, if necessary, maintenance carried out.

It may be necessary to abort the procedure shown on pages 98–99 and return to an earlier stage, either in the construction sequence or even the planning stages. For example, a damaged working model in the laboratory stage means returning to the first clinical stage for a new impression, or a cusp fracturing after a tooth has been prepared for a partial crown means returning to the planning stage.

Practical points

● The logical sequence of history-taking, examination and decision-making, planning and execution in practice often has to be altered or adapted to particular circumstances.

● In planning always first consider the patient as a whole, the mouth next and the tooth last.

● The cooperation of the patient is essential from the start.

● The value of the tooth when crowned is an important central consideration.

● Even with imperfect oral hygiene, a crown can be the best solution, provided the prognosis for the tooth is adequate.

● Only after initial preparation of the tooth can a firm decision on the type of restoration be made.

Clinical and laboratory stages of making crowns

First clinical stage

All crowns (after making any necessary core)
- Select temporary crown technique and prepare for temporary crown
- Recheck shade
- Prepare the tooth to be crowned
- Make temporary crown (which helps to detect faults in the preparation)
- Impression of the prepared tooth and other teeth in the same arch with extremely accurate material (the working impression)
- Impression of the opposing arch, usually in alginate (unless the study cast is adequate for the opposing arch)
- Occlusal record (if necessary)
- Cement temporary crown
- Advise patient on maintenance of temporary crown

First laboratory stage

All crowns
- Make working cast and articulate with opposing cast
- The laboratory procedure will then be different, depending upon the type of crown being made

Metal crown
- Prepare wax pattern
- Cast
- Polish

Porcelain jacket crown (PJC)
- Adapt platinum foil
- Apply high-alumina core
- Apply dentine and enamel porcelain
- Glaze

or

- Make refractory die
- Apply core, dentine and enamel porcelain
- Remove die by sandblasting

or

- Follow instructions in making a crown in one of the alternative glass–ceramic materials. *Note*: These materials should only be used by people who have been specifically instructed in their use.

Metal–ceramic (MC)
- Prepare wax pattern
- Cast
- Either add porcelain or return to clinic for try-in of the metal

Cast post and core
- Prepare wax pattern (or combination of wax and plastic or metal)
- Cast
- Either make PJC or MC crown or return to the clinic for try-in or post and core only

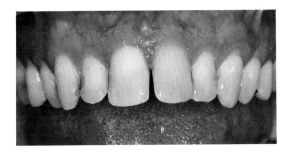

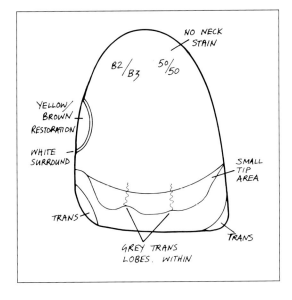

Figure 6.3

a and *b* A shade map of this patient's upper right central incisor.

Making a special tray (Figure 6.4)

When a special tray is to be used it can be made from self-curing acrylic or light-curing acrylic. Shellac and vacuum-formed materials are not sufficiently rigid or stable and so they should not be used. A spacer of wax or asbestos substitute tape approximately 3 mm thick is laid down over the study cast. This is perforated through to the occlusal surface of three or four teeth that are not to be prepared for crowns. The purpose of these perforations is to allow tray material to form stops on the occlusal surfaces of the teeth. This will localize the tray in the mouth and prevent it making contact with the prepared teeth. The tray is then formed by moulding acrylic dough or a sheet of light-curing acrylic over the study cast. Figure 6.4 shows the stages in making special trays in the two materials. Self-curing acrylic is convenient and inexpensive and does not require special equipment. Self-curing acrylic special trays can be made in the dental surgery. Light-curing acrylic special trays are quicker and easier to produce and give more consistent results. However, it is necessary to have a light-curing box in which to cure the tray, and the cost of this would not normally be justified for surgery use. The trays are therefore made in the laboratory. There is usually little difference in cost between the two types of tray if they are laboratory-produced.

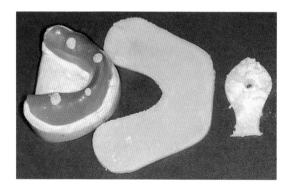

Figure 6.4

a and *b* Making a self-curing acrylic special tray.
a shows a study cast with a wax spacer with holes made in it. The holes have been filled with self curing acrylic. Self curing acrylic has been rolled out and shaped together with a handle.

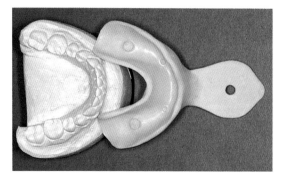

b The tray has been moulded over the study cast and spacer and the handle attached. The stops, located over teeth which are not to be prepared prevent the tray from seating too closely onto the prepared teeth.

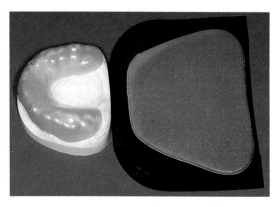

c–g The construction of a light-cured acrylic special tray.

c The study cast and wax spacer together with a preformed blank of light curing acrylic material.

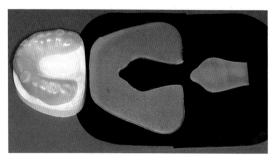

d The blank is roughly shaped, producing a handle.

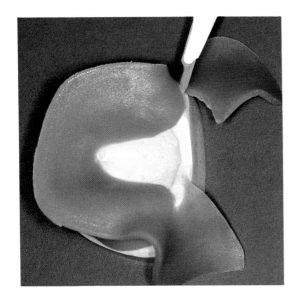

e It is moulded over the study cast and trimmed with a scalpel.

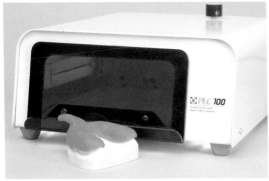

f The light curing box with the bright blue light turned on.

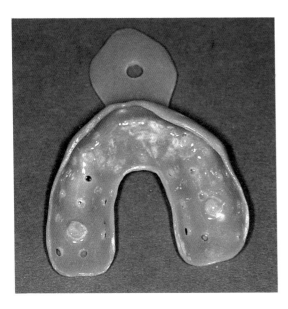

g The finished tray with stops.

Planning the temporary crown

Temporary crowns may be either purchased as preformed units or made at the chairside in a suitable mould.

Preformed temporary crowns

The following types of preformed temporary crown are available:

1 Polycarbonate, tooth-coloured temporary crowns for anterior and some posterior teeth
2 Stainless-steel posterior temporary crowns
3 Aluminium posterior temporary crowns.

When one of these is to be used the appropriate size can be selected before the tooth is prepared using the study cast as a guide.

Chairside temporary crowns

Temporary crowns can be made in the mouth, preferably using one of the higher acrylics, usually consisting of a mixture of poly(ethyl methacrylate) and poly(isobutyl methacrylate), sometimes with a nylon fibre filler. Alternatively acrylic–poly-(methyl methacrylate), epimine resin or amalgam may be used. The mould that is used to form the temporary crown may be one of the following:

● A preformed celluloid crown form
● A vacuum-formed PVC crown form made on a study cast or a modified study cast of the patient's mouth
● A silicone putty impression of the study cast
● An alginate impression of the mouth taken before the tooth is prepared
● A copper band or matrix band.

The use of these materials and moulds is described on page 122.

Building up the core

As described in Chapter 2, cores may be made of cast metal retained by a post, or of amalgam or composite retained by pins or posts or by glass ionomer cement when pins are not usually used. Techniques for constructing pin- and post-retained amalgam cores are illustrated in Figure 6.5. Other pin-retained cores are shown in Figure 2.6 (pages 37–8). With a composite or glass ionomer core the tooth can be prepared at the same visit. The site and angulation of pins is crucial (see Chapter 2). The detailed design of the preparation must be decided *before* the pins are placed; otherwise, if the pins are in the wrong place, they may be cut off during the preparation of the core for the crown.

Managing worn, short teeth

Figure 6.6a shows some very worn and short upper anterior teeth. They have continued to erupt as they have worn, and so remain in contact with the lower incisor teeth. The gingival margins have migrated incisally, following the further eruption of the teeth. The upper and lower posterior teeth remain in contact. The upper incisor teeth are to be crowned to improve their appearance and prevent further wear (other preventive measures having been unsuccessful), but the length of the crowns is not sufficient to produce satisfactory preparations and crowns with a good appearance. There are a number of ways to overcome this problem:

● Increase the whole occlusal vertical dimension by crowning all the teeth in the upper arch. This is sometimes necessary if the occlusal vertical dimension (OVD) is reduced and if the posterior teeth need crowning in any case. However, it is unjustifiably destructive if the posterior teeth do not need crowning and is likely to fail if a normal OVD is encroached upon artificially.
● Crown-lengthen the teeth by means of a periodontal surgical procedure to remove gingival tissue and usually bone. This is destructive if the gingival tissues are healthy and is usually quite painful for the patient. It can produce sufficient length for retentive crown preparations, but the worn incisal surface has to be prepared and so there is a risk to the pulp. The neck of the preparation is placed part way up the tapering root, and so is of a smaller diameter than if it were at the cement–enamel junction. This means that the interdental spaces are usually greater, and this can spoil the appearance.

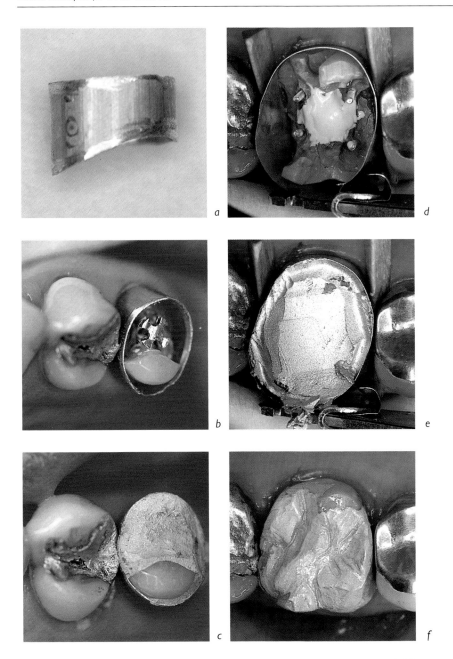

Figure 6.5

Post- and pin-retained cores.

a A copper band trimmed to shape and the margins smoothed.

b Cooper band in place ready to receive amalgam. Retention in this root-filled tooth is provided by a preformed post (see Figure 2.7, page 39).

c The amalgam core placed. Note that the palatal gap between the cusp and copper ring has been filled with amalgam. This will fall away when the copper ring is removed at the next visit. As the copper band will be left in place, the amalgam can be left in occlusion – note the marks from articulating paper.

d Pins, lining, matrix and wedges placed. Pins are used when the pulp remains vital.

e Amalgam placed.

f Matrix removed and amalgam roughly carved. The amalgam is left out of occlusion to avoid undue stresses before the crown is placed.

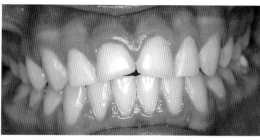

Figure 6.6

a A patient who has suffered from bulimia nervosa producing extensive palatal and incisal erosion of the upper incisor teeth. Continuing eruption has kept pace with the erosion and so the upper and lower incisor teeth are still in contact.

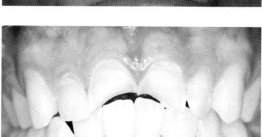

b A similar case, again caused by an eating disorder, but this time predominantly affecting the incisal edges of the upper central incisor teeth.

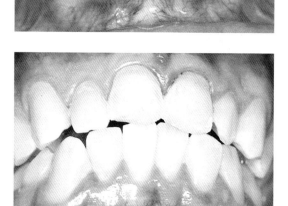

c The central incisors have been built up with composite which improves their appearance for the time being but also acts as a form of Dahl appliance which will depress both upper and lower incisor teeth. Note that the composite restorations are in contact with the lower incisors and yet the canine and posterior teeth are out of occlusion.

● The incisal teeth may be depressed and/or the posterior teeth allowed to over-erupt by conventional orthodontic treatment. The inter-incisal space created means that the worn incisal surfaces do not need to be prepared, and the gingival margins migrate upwards as the incisor teeth are intruded. This is the technique of choice in some cases, but the disadvantage is that the patient needs to wear an orthodontic appliance, which is usually visible.

● A fixed anterior bite plane, (a fixed Dahl appliance), can be cemented to the upper incisor teeth. This is designed to hold the anterior teeth apart by the amount that is needed for tooth preparation. Once cemented, the posterior teeth do not occlude, but patients cope with this very well. In three to six months the anterior teeth are intruded and/or the posterior teeth over-erupt so that they come into occlusal contact. At this stage the fixed Dahl

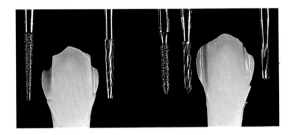

Figure 6.7

A selection of burs and the surfaces prepared by them. In all cases the bur was used entirely within the contour of the tooth and would not have damaged the adjacent tooth. *From the left*: a square-end tapered diamond bur, a square-end tungsten carbide bur, both producing narrow shoulders; a parallel-sided but pointed diamond bur, with the matching tungsten carbide finishing bur; a round-ended parallel-sided plain cut tungsten carbide bur, these last three producing chamfers.

appliance can be removed and the teeth prepared for crowns without removing any more dentine from the worn incisal edges (see Figures 4.6a to g). The original Dahl appliance was a removable cast-metal anterior biteplane retained by clasps on posterior teeth. However, this has now been largely superseded by the fixed appliance.

● The upper anterior teeth may be prepared for crowns, without removing any dentine from the worn incisal edges, and then provisional crowns made to the length and shape that is required for the permanent crowns. These will act in a similar way to the fixed Dahl appliance. However, the disadvantage is that the teeth are prepared before the tooth movement has been established.

● Restoring the worn surfaces with composite to act in the same way as a Dahl appliance (see Figures 6.6b and c).

Of these techniques, the fixed Dahl appliance is preferred whenever possible. Provisional crowns or conventional orthodontic treatment are the next best, and crown-lengthening and increasing the OVD overall should be preserved for those cases where there are specific indications for these techniques.

Tooth preparation

Choice of instruments

The major part of the preparation is carried out with the airotor. Diamond burs are preferred for preparing enamel, and either diamond or tungsten carbide burs for amalgam and dentine.

The shape of the bur or stone should be chosen to match the contour of the surface that is being prepared. This includes the shape of the margin, so that if a shoulder is being prepared, a square-ended straight or tapered bur should be used. Alternatively, if a chamfer finishing line is being prepared then an appropriately shaped bur should be chosen. Figure 6.7 shows a selection of burs set against the tooth surfaces they have prepared.

It is easier to control the preparation of the concave palatal surface of upper incisor teeth if a large-diameter diamond bur, matching the contour of the tooth, is used.

The finishing is an important stage and can take rather longer than the main bulk reduction. The purpose is to finalize the shape of the preparation, rounding-off angles where necessary, ensuring that the margin is properly located in relation to the gingival margin and is the correct contour and dimension. In addition, the small undercuts resulting from diamond score marks should be removed and the surface of the preparation left reasonably smooth. Otherwise there will be difficulty with removing a wax pattern from the die and with cementation. There is, however, no need to polish preparations: a very slight roughness helps retention (see Figure 3.7, page 49).

Slow-speed handpieces with steel finishing burs, fine stones or flexible discs can be used for finishing; however, it is more commonly done at medium to high speed with plain tungsten carbide burs, fine-grain diamonds or tungsten carbide stones.

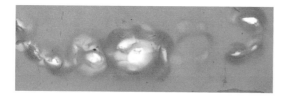

Figure 6.8

An occlusal record taken in 2 mm-thick soft wax, which does not require warming. The occlusal contacts of the unprepared first and third molar teeth can be seen together with the imprint of the second molar preparation. It is clear that there is nearly 2 mm clearance, and this is sufficient for a metal–ceramic occlusal surface.

Stages in the preparation

It is usual to prepare each surface in turn so that the amount of tooth reduction can be controlled. Establishing how much tooth has been removed can be done in a number of ways. At the margin the width of the shoulder or other finishing line can be seen directly. Where the tooth being prepared occludes with opposing teeth, and other adjacent teeth also occlude, the amount of tooth tissue removed from the occluding surface is assessed by direct observation or by the patient biting through soft wax; the thickness of the remaining wax shows how much tooth has been removed (see Figure 6.8). On other surfaces, half may be prepared first, leaving a step between the prepared and unprepared areas so indicating that amount of tooth tissue removed (similar to Figure 5.6). Alternatively, a groove may be prepared across the surface to the intended depth of the preparation and the remainder of the surface then prepared to the depth of the groove (see Figure 6.10).

The order in which the tooth surfaces are prepared will depend upon the circumstances; but some basic guidelines may be useful. Surfaces that are easy to prepare and that will improve access to more difficult surfaces should be prepared first. For example, with incisor teeth some operators prepare the incisal edge first in order to remove part of the approximal surface and improve access to the remainder of it. Similarly, the most difficult surface should be left until last.

Sometimes with a difficult path of insertion, the direction of one surface is critical. In this case it should be prepared first and the other surfaces prepared relative to it. When pins or grooves are to be used as part of the preparation, they are left until last and aligned with other prepared surfaces to form part of the overall retentive design.

Preparing teeth for complete posterior crowns

Figure 3.12 (pages 55–6) shows a typical sequence in the preparation for a complete gold crown of a posterior tooth that has been built up with a pinned amalgam core. Figure 6.9 shows a premolar with a composite core prepared for a metal–ceramic crown.

Occlusal reduction

The shape of the prepared occlusal surface should follow the general contours of the original tooth surface. In some cases, with heavily worn teeth, this will be flat, but in others the general shape of the cusps should be reproduced. This allows the crown to be of reasonably uniform thickness with minimum preparation of tooth tissue.

A convenient instrument to prepare the occlusal surface is a dome-ended parallel-sided diamond bur held on its side. With this instrument it is possible to form the cuspal inclines together with a rounded shape to the fissure pattern.

The occlusal relationships of the tooth being prepared should be studied in function. For example, in preparing a posterior tooth, if the guidance in lateral excursion is carried by the tooth being prepared, the cusp, or cusps, that carry this guidance should be prepared rather

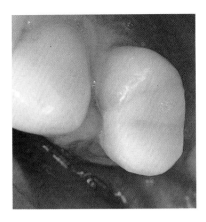

Figure 6.9

Crown preparation for a metal–ceramic crown.

a The pin-retained composite core has been present for several months. The appearance is better than an amalgam core.

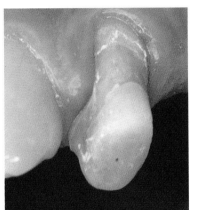

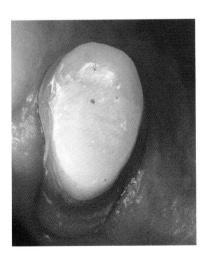

b and *c* The finished preparation.

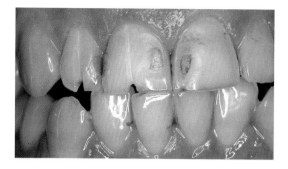

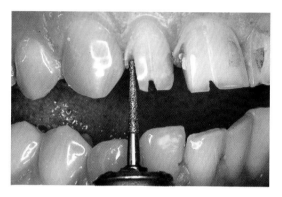

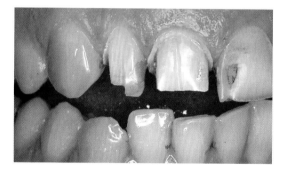

Figure 6.10

Stages in the preparation of upper incisors for PJCs. The indication for crowns was progressive erosion of the buccal surfaces and unsightly restorations that rapidly discoloured after replacement. The first three stages were carried out with a long-tapered diamond bur. Finishing was with plain-cut tungsten carbide burs in a 1:4 ratio speed increasing contra-angle handpiece. The stages in the preparation for metal–ceramic crowns would be very similar except that the palatal surfaces would be prepared with a suitably shaped bur.

a Reference grooves are cut in the buccal and incisal surfaces to establish the depth of the preparation.

b Distal surfaces being prepared. Note that a sliver of enamel has been preserved at the contact point of the lateral incisor to protect the canine from damage. This will fall away as the preparation is carried further gingivally.

c The incisal reduction of the central incisor has been completed together with half the incisal reduction of the lateral incisor.

more, so that there is a greater thickness of crown material covering them. This will produce greater strength in this stressed area and will also allow for future wear. In these circumstances the cusp in question is known as the 'functional cusp'. However, in most natural dentitions the posterior teeth disclude in lateral excursion and so none of the cusps can be described as 'functional cusps' in the same sense. Therefore they do not need to be reduced any more than the remainder of the occlusal surface.

One advantage of minimizing the reduction of the occlusal surface is to maintain the axial walls of the preparation as long as possible, thereby improving retention.

Axial reduction

Buccal and lingual surfaces   These may be prepared with parallel-sided or tapered diamonds

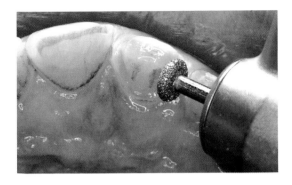

d Palatal reduction with a round-edged wheel bur in an airotor.

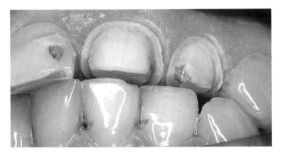

e Checking, with the teeth in occlusion, that there is sufficient clearance for porcelain.

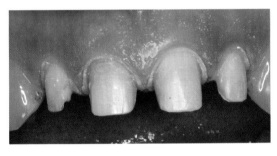

f The finished preparations. The right lateral incisor has lost a mesial composite. This defect will be made good with glass ionomer cement before the impression is taken. The finished crowns are shown in Figure 2.1a (page 26).

of appropriate length and with the end shaped to produce the required shape of margin. It may be possible to use a diamond of known taper held at a constant angle on the buccal and lingual sides, so that the taper of the preparation can be controlled. However, this often has to be modified because of the curvature of the tooth's surface, previous restorations or the presence of a core. A fairly large-diameter instrument is convenient and reduces the likelihood of vertical ridges in the preparation.

Mesial and distal surfaces These are the most difficult surfaces to prepare if there is an adjacent tooth in contact; without one, they are prepared like the buccal and lingual surfaces. Sometimes both adjacent posterior teeth are to be crowned, and then the surfaces in contact should be prepared simultaneously, the reduction of each being minimized.

Unfortunately, damage to adjacent teeth is common, with some studies showing over 90% of adjacent teeth damaged even by careful operators who knew their work would be inspected. When the preparation is finished the adjacent tooth surface should always be checked for damage, and if necessary smoothed, polished and fluoride applied.

It is almost impossible to prepare the approximal surfaces of a posterior tooth when there are teeth in contact on either side without either overtapering the preparation, removing more tooth tissue than is desirable or damaging the adjacent teeth (see Figures 3.12 and 6.7).

Very thin long tapered diamond burs are passed through the approximal surface in an attempt to leave a sliver of enamel (or core) between the bur and the adjacent tooth. Controlling the angle, position and depth of this bur without wavering or going off course is one of the most skilful procedures in operative dentistry and deserves many hours of practice on extracted teeth in models before it is attempted in the mouth.

A matrix band may be applied to the adjacent tooth to protect it, but this interferes with vision and access, and is in any case cut through very easily. A wooden wedge at the gingival margin to separate the teeth slightly may help.

Margins

The shape of the margin will be determined by the shape of the end of the bur used for the axial reduction. This may be flat, producing a shoulder, or chamfered. A knife-edge finishing line is produced by the side of the bur only being used, the tip not cutting the tooth. It is more efficient to produce the required shape of margins during the bulk preparation stage rather than as a secondary procedure.

Finishing

Suitable finishing instruments are used as described on page 115.

It is important that the angles between the axial and occlusal surfaces are rounded for reasons described in Chapter 3.

Preparing teeth for complete anterior crowns

Figure 6.10 shows stages in preparing an upper incisor tooth for a PJC. The stages of preparation

for a tooth for a metal–ceramic crown are similar, although the end result is rather different, complying with the principles described in Chapter 5. If a tapered or parallel-sided diamond bur of appropriate length and diameter is selected, the first three stages of the preparation can all be carried out with the same instrument, with only the incisal–palatal reduction and finishing left to be done with different instruments.

Incisal and proximal reduction

When only one tooth is being prepared the incisal surface can be reduced with the shank end of the tapered diamond bur and the adjacent teeth used as a guide to the amount of reduction necessary. When a series of teeth is being prepared either alternate teeth are reduced first with the unprepared teeth used as a guide, or half the incisal edge is reduced followed by the second half to the same depth.

In patients with a Class I incisor relationship the upper incisor teeth have their incisal edges inclined lingually and the lower incisals buccally. The same inclinations are preserved in the prepared teeth.

Approximal reduction may be continued with the same bur. Because so much more tooth is being removed than is necessary for a posterior gold crown and since incisor teeth are a more favourable shape and the buccal/lingual dimension at the contact point is smaller, it is much easier to prepare the approximal surfaces without damaging the adjacent teeth than in the case of posterior crowns. Passing the bur through the mesial and distal approximal surfaces (leaving a sliver of enamel) establishes the taper of these surfaces as well as the location and width of the approximal shoulders.

Buccal reduction

The contour and depth of the buccal shoulder is established with the tip of the diamond bur. A common mistake in preparing upper incisor teeth for crowns is to remove insufficient material from the buccal/incisal third of the preparation. This results either in a crown that is too thin, so that the opaque core material shows through (see Figure 3.2, page 43), or in a bulbous crown. The

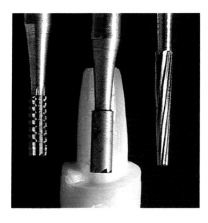

Figure 6.11

Three burs used to finish a shoulder preparation. *Left*: a steel slow-speed bur cutting both on the side and at the end. *Centre*: an end cutting bur that has produced a ledge; it would be difficult to eradicate this without lifting the bur from the shoulder. *Right*: a plain-cut tungsten carbide tapered side and end cutting bur, which is best used in a friction grip 1:4 speed increasing handpiece. The tungsten carbide bur produces the best finish most conveniently.

amount of tooth reduction in this area can be fixed by a buccal depth indicator groove being cut down the buccal surface and the remainder of the surface reduced to the same depth. With large teeth or where the alignment of the buccal surface is being altered, more than one groove may be needed. In reducing the remainder of the surface, the bur should be used at a slight angle to the depth groove to prevent it dropping into the groove and deepening it unintentionally.

Gingival–palatal reduction

The same bur is continued round the palatal surface, producing the palatal shoulder and a short gingival palatal wall nearly parallel to the buccal–gingival surface.

These three stages, using the same bur, can all be carried out very quickly provided the operator has planned the design properly and has thought through the sequence.

Incisal–palatal reduction

This surface is usually concave and is best prepared with a large-diameter instrument, for example a large wheel bur in the air turbine (see Figure 6.10d). Small instruments produce an undulating surface, which is difficult to finish smoothly. The occlusion between this surface and

the opposing teeth should be checked before the preparation starts, and constantly rechecked during preparation until sufficient space has been produced for the crown material.

Finishing

The prepared individual surfaces should be blended into each other to produce a rounded shape during the gross reduction. The axial surfaces are finished and the angles around the incisal edge rounded, using a suitable finishing instrument. An excellent finish can be produced by using a plain-cut tungsten carbide friction grip bur in a 1–4 speed increasing contra-angle handpiece. The shoulder can be finished using the same instrument or steel burs. Some dentists use end cutting burs to good effect, but these are difficult to master (see Figure 6.11).

Preparing teeth for partial crowns

Occlusal and axial reduction

The majority of the preparation is carried out as for a complete crown, except that care is taken to produce suitable finishing lines at the junction of the buccal and other surfaces. In particular, the reduction should not be carried too far round on the mesial surface or excessive metal will show.

Grooves, boxes and pinholes

Grooves and boxes are prepared with either high-speed or slow-speed burs, depending upon the difficulty of access and the operator's confidence. They are usually prepared with thin tapered plain-cut burs. If the preparation is a conventional three-quarter crown, the lingual surface of the axial grooves should be well defined, since this is the retentive surface.

Parallel-sided pinholes are prepared with a twist drill of suitable diameter for the impression technique used, usually 0.7 mm. If possible, the pinhole should be drilled once only and not in several attempts, which deepens it a little each time, but also widens and tapers it so that it becomes less retentive.

Parallel pinholes are preferable to tapered: they are more retentive, can be prepared with paralleling jigs, and even freehand are easier to prepare parallel to each other than tapered holes. When it comes to the impression there are even more important advantages (see page 135).

Preparing anterior teeth for post crowns

There are three stages:

● The shoulder or other margin is prepared
● The post hole is prepared
● Any remaining tissue between the two is reduced as necessary.

When a large part of the natural crown of the tooth remains, it may be convenient to cut this across horizontally between the midpoint and the incisal edge and remove the incisal part before these three stages are undertaken. The margin is prepared as for a PJC or metal–ceramic crown, but with more reduction so that the shoulders are wider than for an equivalent vital tooth.

Post-hole preparation

Removing the root canal filling   When the root canal filling consists of gutta percha (GP) and sealer, the coronal part may be removed with Gates–Glidden or round burs (see Figure 1.6b) or by softening it with heated metal instruments.

Provided the root filling is well condensed, a convenient method is to cut out the GP point with a slowly rotating round bur or twist drill slightly larger in diameter than the root canal. If too small an instrument is used, or too fast a speed so that the GP melts, it becomes attached to the bur and the whole of the root filling may be pulled out when the bur is removed. Using a bur or drill slightly larger than the root canal enables the root filling to be cut away from its end without the sides of the GP point becoming entangled in the bur. Extra-long-shank contra-angle burs are useful in long teeth. With normal-length burs the head of the handpiece clashes with the adjacent teeth (see Figure 6.12).

Gutta percha and most sealers are softer than dentine, and so the bur will tend to follow the root filling rather than cut into the side of the root canal, but nevertheless great care must be taken to ensure that the bur stays on course. Regular inspection of the root canal using both the mouth mirror and direct vision is essential (see Figure 6.13). Transillumination of the root canal may also help.

Some cement fillings are more difficult to remove than GP because they set to a consistency harder than dentine so that the bur tends to slip away from the root filling into the dentine. In this case the coronal end of the root filling can be removed with a long tapered bur in the airotor, but great care is needed to avoid lateral perforation of the root.

It is almost impossible to cut down full-length silver point root fillings, and these should be removed, if possible, and replaced by GP root fillings. When the silver point cannot be removed, an alternative form of core should be used.

Shaping the post hole   The post hole needs to be shaped to match the post selected (the different types of post were described in Chapter 2). When the post is to be parallel-sided, a twist drill may be used from the outset, and the root filling is removed and the post hole shaped in a single operation. In some cases, once the root filling is removed, it may be decided that a larger-diameter post is needed, and so the next size of twist drill is then used to shape the post hole (see Figure 6.14).

For a tapered post hole for a cast-metal post, an instrument such as that shown in Figure 6.12e is used. This not only produces the taper but may

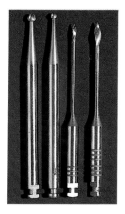

a

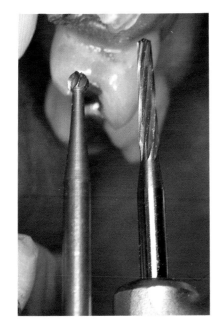

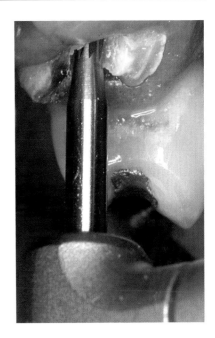

b   c

Figure 6.12

Post-hole preparation.

a Long-shank round burs (*left*) and Gates–Glidden burs for removing gutta percha from root canals.

b and c Extra-long-shank contra-angle burs allow access without the head of the hand piece clashing with adjacent teeth. They also improve visibility.

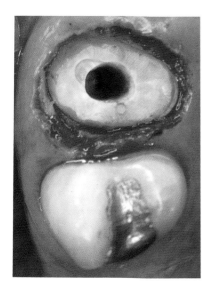

Figure 6.13

Looking up the post hole with direct vision. Note the oval shape of this post hole will resist rotation of the post within the hole. Note too that the crown margin has been exposed using electrosurgery. This was necessary here because of caries beneath the previous crown.

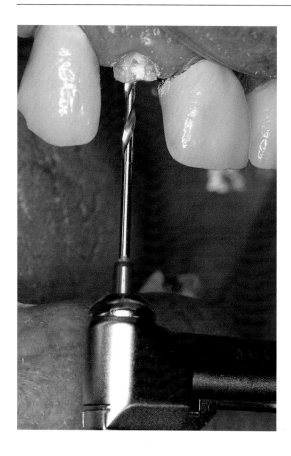

Figure 6.14

a A handpiece-driven twist drill to prepare a parallel-sided post hole.

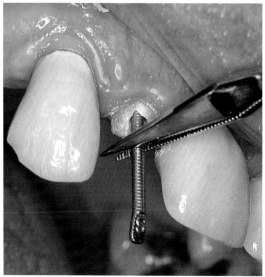

b The prepared post hole and a preformed stainless-steel post being tried in.

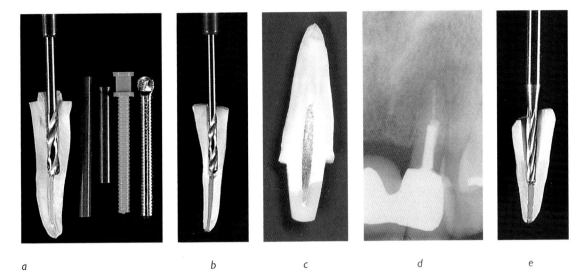

a   b   c   d   e

Figure 6.15

a A sectioned, extracted tooth showing the preparation for a parallel sided post hole. The system being used is the same as that shown in Figure 2.4b. This is a 1.75 mm diameter drill. It is rather too big for this size of tooth and is veering towards the side. Ideally the post hole should be longer but, if continued in this direction, there would be a risk of lateral perforation of the root.

b This tooth is thinner and the drill is 1.25 mm diameter. However it is progressing down the centre of the tooth with less risk of lateral perforation.

c A sectioned, extracted tooth with a stainless steel post and composite core in place. The composite core is about half the preparation. (The stainless steel post is parallel and longer but part of it and the root filling have been lost in the sectioning process.)

d A radiograph of a post in a root filled upper lateral incisor tooth. The tooth is an abutment for a bridge and the bridge had been present for many years. The length and diameter of the post are suitable for this size and shape of root.

e A tapered post hole cutter with good side cutting ability. It has been tilted back and forth to produce a tapered post which is larger at the neck than the diameter of the bur. This is often necessary when caries has progressed down the root canal or when a previous post was present. An impression and cast post will be necessary. As this preparation inevitably weakens the tooth, the root face has been prepared with an external bevel so that a complete diaphragm can be cast together with the post and core.

also be moved side to side to produce an oval-shaped canal, following the shape of the tooth. This increases the strength of the post while leaving a uniform thickness of root (see Figure 6.13). A selection of instruments, and sections of the teeth prepared using them, are illustrated in Figure 6.15.

Finishing the preparation

Once the margin, the remaining axial walls and the post hole have been prepared, there may remain a substantial collar of dentine, some spurs or none at all. Substantial amounts of dentine should be left, since they lengthen the post hole and define the margins. Fragile fragments, however, should be removed.

Completed post crown preparations with posts and cores in place are shown in Figure 3.15 (page 60).

Temporary crowns

For a description of the difference between 'temporary' and 'provisional' crowns and bridges, see page 128. Temporary crowns are described at this stage because in a normal clinical sequence, once a crown preparation has been started, it must be completed at least in terms of gross reduction at the same visit and a temporary crown fitted. Often it will be possible to proceed to impressions and other stages at the same visit, but these can be deferred if necessary. The temporary crown, however, cannot be deferred.

Preformed temporary crowns

Polycarbonate temporary crowns

The appropriate size of a temporary crown has already been selected during the planning stage, and Figure 6.16 shows the stages in preparing and modifying a polycarbonate crown for an upper incisor tooth. Here the crown is relined with a higher acrylic produced specially for temporary crowns by acrylic resin – poly(methyl methacrylate) – may also be used.

Once the polycarbonate crown has been relined, it can be adjusted for incisal length, occlusion and marginal fit. It does not matter if the polycarbonate is ground right through, as long as a layer of the lining material remains.

Stainless-steel temporary crowns

These are difficult to adapt and often do not produce good contact points or occlusal contact. They are, however, hard and durable and can be left in place for some time. The margins are trimmed with stones and contoured with pliers, and the temporary crown is then cemented, usually with a rigid cement such as zinc phosphate or a reinforced zinc oxide eugenol cement.

Aluminium crown forms

Being softer, these are more readily adapted to fit contact points and occlusal contacts, but the margins are irritant to the soft tissues unless extreme care is taken in contouring them, and some patients complain of a metallic taste. Although they are quick to make, they are generally less satisfactory than acrylic temporary posterior crowns.

Chairside techniques

Pouring techniques

The higher acrylics go through a stage during setting when they can be poured or injected into a suitable mould that is placed over the prepared teeth. Only a very thin flash of excess material remains at the periphery. Conventional self-curing acrylic resin (poly(methyl methacrylate)) should not be used with these techniques because, compared with the other materials, it has a more exothermic setting reaction and is therefore more likely to produce pulp damage. It is also more chemically irritant to gingival tissues and does not go through this pouring stage, so that a thick flash is produced and more adjustment is necessary.

The mould used may be a preformed celluloid crown form, a thin PVC slip vacuum formed on the patient's study cast (or a modified study cast), or a silicone putty or alginate impression. Figure 6.17 illustrates typical techniques using an alginate impression and a PVC slip with two different higher acrylics. Figure 6.18 shows a similar technique with a putty impression of a modified study cast and a third higher acrylic in an automix gun.

Moulding techniques

Some of the higher acrylics go through a dough stage when they can be moulded rather like putty. In this consistency they can be formed into temporary crowns simply by moulding over the prepared tooth with the fingers and the patient biting into it to establish the occlusion. Gross excesses will be present, but these can be removed by rough carving in the mouth and then with an acrylic bur in a straight handpiece once

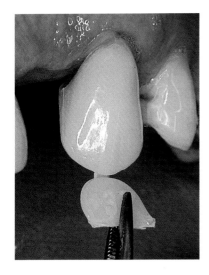

Figure 6.16

Polycarbonate temporary crowns.

a Temporary crown being tried-in.

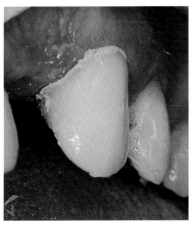

b Trimmed and relined with a temporary crown and bridge higher acrylic.

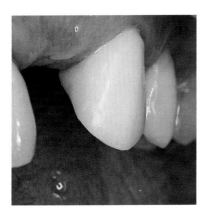

c The temporary crown two weeks later.

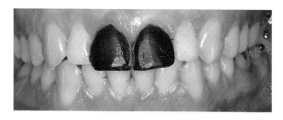

Figure 6.17

Chairside temporary crowns: pouring techniques.

a The patient shown in Figure 6.10; the buccal surfaces of the central incisors are reshaped with wax in the mouth.

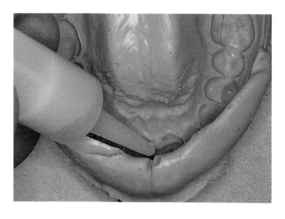

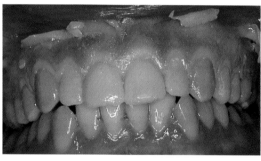

b A temporary crown and bridge higher acrylic reinforced with nylon fibres being injected into an alginate impression of the modified teeth.

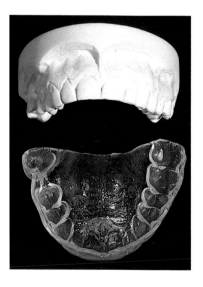

c The temporary crowns before being removed from the mouth. Note the thin flash.

d Flexible PVC slip vacuum-formed to the study cast for a different patient.

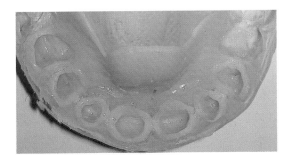

e The partly set material (in this case a different higher acrylic) is removed from the mouth still in the mould.

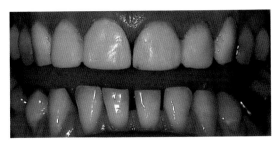

f The completed temporary crowns for the second patient.

the crown has been removed and has become hard (see Figure 6.19). This is a useful technique, particularly for posterior teeth where the shape of the tooth to be prepared (often a core) is to be changed and so is not suitable for the pouring technique.

A temporary crown made by this moulding technique will have better contact points, occlusal contact and marginal adaptation than an aluminium crown form. There is no need to modify the study model or make a vacuum-formed PVC slip and so it is an effective and efficient technique.

Temporary-post crown techniques

Some manufacturers supply temporary posts with their kits. An example of an aluminium temporary post is shown in Figure 6.15. Otherwise, temporary posts may be made from wire modified with a conventional or higher acrylic before the temporary crown is added to the wire by one of the techniques described in the previous section (see Figure 6.20).

Other techniques

Build-up techniques Temporary partial crowns, particularly pin-retained partial crowns, are very weak and tend to break up and become lost. It is also difficult to form pins by any of the techniques described so far. Temporary partial crowns can be made by placing plastic pins into the pinholes and building up a temporary crown in self-curing conventional or higher acrylic, using a paintbrush.

Copper ring and amalgam A robust posterior temporary crown that can be left in situ for some time may be made by adapting a copper ring to the margins of the preparation, cutting it short of the occlusion and filling it with amalgam carved to form occlusal contacts. If an amalgam core is present, the preparation should be lubricated with petroleum jelly to avoid any risk of new amalgam becoming attached to the preparation. These temporary crowns are easily removed by slitting the copper ring.

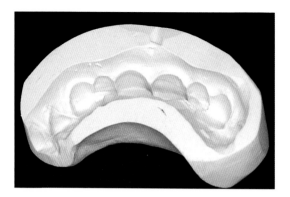

Figure 6.18

a–d A similar technique to Figure 6.17 but this time using a mould produced in a laboratory silicone putty material and a newer type of higher acrylic temporary crown and bridge material mixed in an automix gun and injected directly into the impression.

a The silicone mould made on a study cast modified with wax.

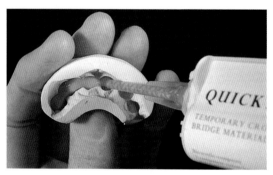

b The automix gun with a very fine nozzle.

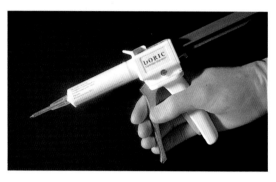

c Inserting the material.

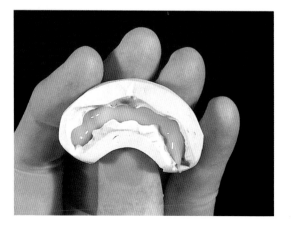

d Ready to be placed in the mouth.

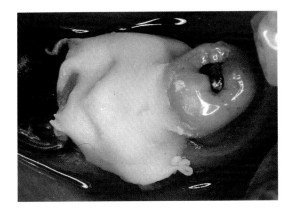

Figure 6.19

Chairside temporary crowns: moulding technique.

a A temporary crown and bridge higher acrylic mixed to a dough consistency is moulded over the prepared tooth and the patient is asked to occlude into it.

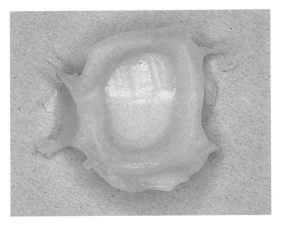

b When nearly set it is eased off the preparation and out of the undercuts between adjacent teeth. In this case the fit surface was satisfactory; in others it may need to be relined with a further mix of material after the exterior surface has been trimmed.

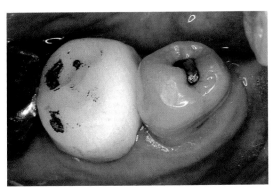

c The temporary crown trimmed to a good fit at the margins. Articulating paper is being used to adjust the occlusion.

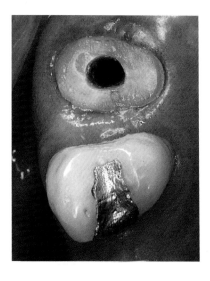

Figure 6.20

Temporary-post crowns.

a The same preparation as shown in Figure 6.13 after initial gingival healing.

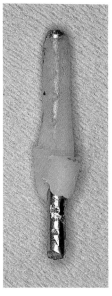

b The thickest possible length of serrated German silver wire is tried in the root canal, coated with a higher acrylic and inserted into the post hole. When nearly set it is withdrawn and reseated a number of times to prevent the possibility of the post jamming and not coming out. After excess material has been trimmed, the coronal part of the temporary crown is added using one of the techniques described earlier. In this case the polycarbonate temporary crown is illustrated in Figure 6.16.

Differences between temporary and provisional crowns

It is useful to make a distinction between 'temporary' and 'provisional' crowns (and bridges). Temporary restorations are made to last for a short while to protect the prepared dentine, to maintain the appearance, and to prevent tilting or overeruption of the prepared tooth by maintaining contact points and occlusion. Because they are temporary, they are usually made by one of the relatively simple chairside techniques described above and are cemented with a temporary crown and bridge cement.

Provisional restorations also have all these functions, but are made to last for a longer period while other treatment is being provided before the permanent restorations can be made or when a period of assessment is necessary. For example, if the patient has periodontal disease associated with poor margins on existing restorations, provisional restorations may be made with well-adapted margins and left for some time until the treatment of the periodontal disease is completed. Similarly, when the occlusion is being modified, for example by increasing the OVD, provisional restorations will be left in place for some months to assess the patient's tolerance of this change before the new occlusion is finally established by permanent restorations. During this time, the occlusion can be modified by occlusal adjustment or by additions to the restorations.

Laboratory-made provisional restorations

Some of the newer temporary crown and bridge acrylics are capable of lasting in the mouth long enough to function as provisional restorations. They can therefore be made at the chairside by the same techniques as have been described for temporary restorations.

Alternatively, the teeth are prepared, an accurate impression taken and temporary restorations made at the chairside. The impression is then used to make heat-cured acrylic restorations in the laboratory, or sometimes a simple casting is made to which acrylic or composite is added (see Figure 11.9). These will last for six months or a year without serious deterioration, although they should be checked periodically, particularly for marginal leakage and occlusal wear, which will allow the prepared tooth to over-erupt.

Cementation of temporary and provisional crowns

The retention of the temporary or provisional restoration and the likely dislodging forces should be assessed and a cement of appropriate strength selected. The following list of temporary cements and their appropriate use is arranged in ascending order of strength:

● A non-setting mixture of petroleum jelly and zinc oxide powder – used for short periods between appointments, for example, for cementing temporary crowns when teeth are prepared and impressions taken in the morning and laboratory-processed acrylic provisional crowns fitted with a stronger cement in the afternoon
● Temporary crown and bridge cement with a high proportion of modifier to reduce the strength – used when several temporary crowns are joined together, giving considerable overall retention; this may be done even though the permanent crowns will be separate (see Figure 6.17)
● Unmodified temporary crown and bridge cement – used for individual complete crowns that will have to stay in place for periods of up to two to three weeks
● Reinforced zinc oxide eugenol cement – used when a stronger cement is required, for example, with partial crowns or when complete crowns have to last for periods longer than about three weeks
● Polycarboxylate and zinc phosphate cements – used with poorly fitting temporary crowns, for example aluminium temporary crowns, or where the temporary crown has to last for an extended period, for example laboratory-made provisional crowns fitted during periods of orthodontic or periodontal treatment.

After temporary crowns have been cemented, it is important that surplus cement is removed, otherwise irritation of the gingival margin and plaque retention will produce gingival inflammation.

The working impression

The working impression is the very accurate impression from which a cast with removable dies is made. The crown is made on the removable die of the prepared tooth. The impression should include not only an accurate impression of the prepared tooth but also the adjacent teeth so that the contact points and occlusal surfaces of the crown may be contoured. It should also include the remaining teeth in the arch so that the working cast can be articulated against the opposing cast. This usually means that it should be a full arch impression.

Impression materials (Figure 6.21)

There are two groups of materials used for crown and bridge impressions: elastomeric materials (silicone, polyether or polysulphide (see Figures 6.21a,b and c)) and reversible hydrocolloid (see Figure 6.21d). The elastomeric materials set by a chemical reaction when two materials, usually two pastes, are mixed together. The reversible hydrocolloid is based on agar agar. It is melted in a water bath and sets on cooling. The teeth must be dry for elastomeric impressions, but may be wet with reversible hydrocolloid.

Silicone impression materials

These may be divided into two groups. The early type of silicone material set by a condensation reaction, leaving a residual alcohol by-product, which evaporated from the impression, causing shrinkage. These earlier condensation silicones should not now be used.

The second group of silicone materials was developed much later, and they set by an addition reaction, leaving no volatile end-product. They are very stable and can be kept for extended periods before casting. It is safe to send them through the post.

Most manufacturers supply addition-curing silicones in a range of five viscosities: putty, heavy-body, regular, light-body and wash. This means that a whole range of techniques is possible using combinations of these materials with or without special trays. Light body material is usually inserted into the mouth from an automix gun (see Figure 6.21f and g) and the medium or heavy body either mixed in a second gun or on a pad. Putty is kneeded by hand.

The material does not wet tooth preparations well. In compensation, it is very clean to use. Toxic and allergic reactions have not been reported.

The automix gun used with an extra fine nozzle has several advantages in placing the light-body material directly around the preparations (see Figure 6.21g). The material is thoroughly mixed without air bubbles, and the mix is very fresh when it is applied to the tooth preparations. With light- and heavy-body materials mixed on pads, the dental nurse usually mixes one material and the dentist the other. Timing of the two mixes, loading the syringe and then drying and isolating the preparations requires very good timing, and

the mixed, light-body material may start to set before it is properly in place. With the automix system the dentist maintains the prepared teeth in a dry and isolated state and starts to inject the light-body material at the point where the nurse is loading the tray.

Polyether impression material

Polyether is convenient since the same material may be used in the syringe and the tray, only one mix being required, although light and heavy viscosities are also available. It is also best used in thick sections, and so should be used in stock trays; or if a special tray is used, it should be made with extra thick space between one study cast and the tray.

An automatic mixing machine is available for polyether (see Figures 6.21h and i).

Polysulphide impression material

This is rarely used now. It is supplied in two viscosities: light- and heavy-body. The light-body material is used in the syringe and the heavy-body material in the impression tray. The more viscous heavy-body helps to drive the light-body material into the details of the prepared tooth and into the gingival crevice. It should be used in an unperforated rigid special tray to achieve the maximum pressure on the unset light-body material.

Polysulphide material has the advantage of a longer working time than the other elastomeric materials, but it also has a longer setting time. It is a sticky material that wets the tooth preparation well and so adapts to it, but this stickiness is a nuisance in inexperienced hands. The patient, assistant, operator and surgery can all end up in a messy condition after attempts at taking polysulphide impressions. Some patients complain of the taste and smell of the material; it is usually an unappealing brown colour.

Reversible hydrocolloid

This was available long before the elastomeric materials were developed, and it largely fell into disuse with their introduction. However, there has now been a revival of interest in the material. It has the advantage of being usable in a wet environment. The material is relatively inexpensive, although the conditioning bath (a heated water bath with three chambers) is costly and is a necessary part of the equipment. It is used in special water-cooled trays.

The hydrocolloid contains water that evaporates when the impression is stored, and so it has to be cast almost immediately after it is taken. There is also a reaction with the artificial stone used to make the working cast, and so the surface of the hydrocolloid impression must be conditioned with potassium sulphate before the cast is made.

Impression techniques

Single-stage technique (e.g. polyether)

When a single-viscosity material is used, the material is mixed, and part of it placed in an impression syringe and the remainder in the impression tray, usually a stock tray. The material is syringed over the dry tooth preparation and the tray immediately seated in place. With a stock tray that has no occlusal stops, it is important to localize the tray carefully and avoid seating it too far so that it does not contact the prepared tooth.

Two-stage technique Light- and heavy-body materials (e.g. light- and heavy-body silicone or hydrocolloid)

Two sets of material are mixed: a low-viscosity material that is syringed around the preparations, and a heavier-viscosity material used in the impression tray and seated in the mouth before the light-body material has set. The light-body material is thus forced into intimate contact with the preparation and gingival crevice.

A special tray with occlusal stops is usually used with the elastomeric materials, and occlusal stops are set into the water-cooled trays used for hydrocolloid.

Putty and wash (e.g. silicone)

This is a modification of the two-stage technique, but in this case a low- or medium-viscosity material is used in the syringe and a putty material in the tray. Because of the viscosity of the putty material, a stock tray is usually used. This technique is therefore popular because the cost of a special tray is saved. The very thin wash material does not work well with this technique since it tends to drop off the prepared teeth before the putty material can be seated.

Polymer materials

One disadvantage of putty materials is that some of the gloves worn by dentists react with the material and prevent it setting. It is therefore often necessary for the dentist or nurse who will be mixing the putty material to remove their gloves and wash their hands before mixing it. The most convenient method is to use one of the polymer materials available in an automix gun.

An alternative technique is to take a putty impression before the tooth is prepared. This is then trimmed to remove undercut areas and escape channels are cut in the sides of the impressions of all the teeth. The impression is set on one side while the tooth is prepared, and it is then relined with a very light-bodied wash material, which can also be syringed round the tooth preparation. The putty impression is then reseated in the mouth and in effect forms a very accurate close-fitting special tray. The considerable difference in the viscosities of the two materials reduces the risk of the primary impression becoming distorted through pressures generated in the reseating.

This technique should not be used when the viscosity of the two materials is close. In particular, an impression taken in any rubber material should not be relined with the same material once set without extensive modification to remove all the undercuts (see Figure 6.22).

A variation on this technique is to take a putty impression with a spacer of flexible material. For example, polythene sheet may be placed over the unset putty material before it is seated in the mouth. This reduces the amount of modification of the putty impression.

Gingival retraction

The ideal is to start with gingival health and supragingival crown margins. Gingival retraction is not then needed, impression taking is easier and more reliable, but most importantly, gingival

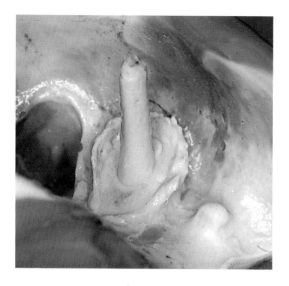

Figure 6.21

Impressions for crowns and bridges in various materials.

a The impression of the patient shown in Figure 6.20 in addition-curing silicone: light- and heavy-body technique. For the impression of the post, the light-body material is spun down the post hole with a spiral root canal paste filler. This is rotated during removal. A thin reinforcing wire is inserted to stiffen the impression and prevent it bending when the die is cast.

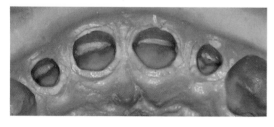

b A different brand of addition-curing silicone showing the impressions for the patient in Figure 6.10.

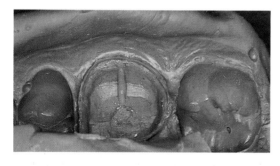

c An impression in polyether in a stock tray.

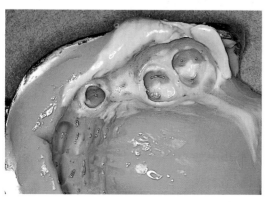

d Reversible hydrocolloid in a water cooled tray.

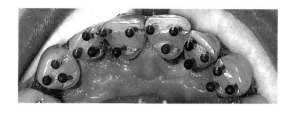

e Parallel plastic impression pins in place. These will be incorporated in a rubber impression. (This is the patient shown in Figure 12.9)

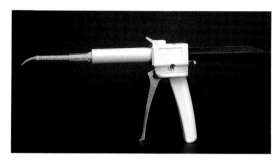

f An automix gun with a standard nozzle adapted with a fine curved tip for direct use in the mouth.

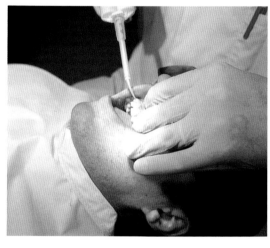

g The automix gun being used in the mouth.

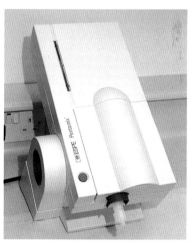

h A mixing machine for polyether impression material.

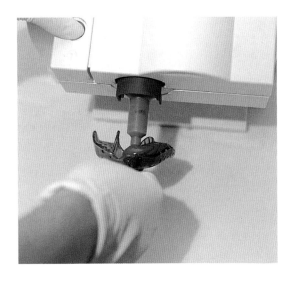

i Material being delivered directly into a stock tray.

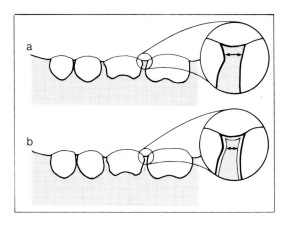

Figure 6.22

Elastomeric impressions should not be relined with a further mix of material once they are set unless all the undercut areas are cut away.

a A preliminary impression taken without a spacer.

b If this impression is relined with a second mix of material, distortion will occur: the second layer of material in the undercut areas of the unprepared teeth will distort the original material while it is in the mouth. When the impression is removed this will return to its original shape, distorting the impression of the prepared tooth. For a two-stage technique, a spacer of polythene or similar material should be used. Alternatively the primary impression should be cut back with a scalpel or burs, and in particular all the interdental areas and impression of any undercut surfaces removed.

health is easy for the patient to maintain. However, it is often necessary to retract the gingival tissues in order to obtain an impression of the tooth surface beneath the gingival margin. This will always be necessary if the preparation margin is subgingival. It will also be desirable if it is close to or at the gingival margin. This is because the crown contour at the periphery should be in line with the tooth surface to avoid a plaque retentive crevice at the margin. This can only be achieved if an impression of the tooth surface is obtained for some distance beyond the preparation margin.

There are four ways of retracting the gingival margins (in ascending order of destructiveness):

● Blowing the impression material into the gingival crevice with vigorous blasts of air
● Temporarily retracting the gingival margin with cord
● Using cords impregnated with chemicals
● Electrosurgery.

Compressed air (see Figure 6.23a,b) With a healthy gingival margin undamaged by the preparation it is usually sufficient to blow the impression material into the crevice with air. This technique works best with polysulphide impression materials and with some silicones. The viscosity and wetting ability of the material are critical.

Cord and impregnated cord (see Figure 6.23c) If cord is to be used, it is usually impregnated either with adrenaline, which acts as a vasoconstrictor assisting in gingival retraction and in arresting any minor gingival haemorrhage, or with an astringent material such as aluminium trichloride, which functions in a similar way. However, some operators prefer plain unimpregnated cord.

Cords are available in various thicknesses, both twisted and braided. Braided cords are preferred since they do not unravel while they are being inserted.

A cord of appropriate diameter is pressed lightly into the gingival crevice with a suitable instrument, for example a flat plastic type or one of the special instruments designed for the purpose (see Figure 6.23d and e). It may not be necessary to retract the gum all the way round the tooth if part of the preparation margin is sufficiently supragingival. The cord is left in place for two or three minutes and then removed before the impression is taken. If it is left for too short a time, gingival retraction is inadequate; if it is left for too long, the chemicals diffuse and become inactive. Too much force should not be used, or permanent damage to the gingival tissues may result.

It is possible to use a very thin cord pressed into the base of the gingival crevice and a thicker cord placed on top of it. Only the thick cord is removed before the impression is taken. This technique is not recommended, since it can be unnecessarily destructive. The cord, being inelastic, often becomes attached to the rubber impression, and may cause a distorted die to be made. If there is enough room for two layers of cord in the pocket, perhaps the patient should have periodontal treatment before permanent crowns are made!

Electrosurgery (see Figures 6.13 and 6.20a) Electrosurgery can be used to arrest gingival haemorrhage before impression taking and to establish a distinct gingival crevice, exposing a subgingival preparation margin. This technique should be reserved for unusual situations, for example where a tooth has been fractured with the fracture line extending subgingivally and an impression is required in order to make a post core and diaphragm. Further gingival recontouring may be carried out surgically once the crown is fitted if necessary.

Impression of pinholes

Tapered plastic pins are available that match the size of standard tapered burs. These are inserted into the pinhole and become incorporated into the elastomeric impression. The problem is they sometimes don't – they either wedge in the tapered pinhole and are left behind, or they float out during the syringing procedure and are lost in the bulk of the impression. These tapered plastic pins were in fact produced to be incorporated in direct wax patterns made in the mouth. They were not intended originally for the indirect technique, and so it is not surprising that these problems arise. They should no longer be used.

Parallel-sided pinholes avoid these problems. The impression pins are longer and it is easier to syringe impression material around them without dislodging them. Plastic parallel pins have heads that lock them into the impression material (see Figure 6.21e). Either a plastic pin 0.1 mm smaller than the hole is used in the wax patterns or, if these are not available, pinholes in the die may be slightly enlarged by gently turning the twist drill in the hole with the fingers. Then pins the same size as the impression pins can be used. These burn out with the wax so that the pin is cast together with the rest of the casting (see Figure 6.24).

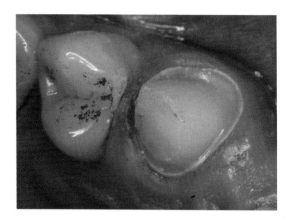

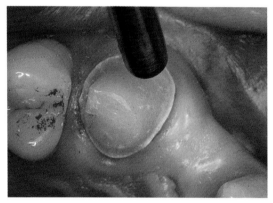

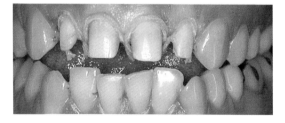

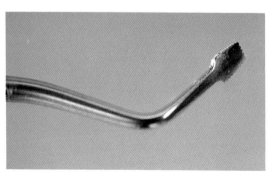

Figure 6.23

Gingival retraction.

a A crown preparation with the mesial margin level with the gingival margin.

b The mesial–gingival margin being retracted solely by blowing air into the gingival crevice. With light-bodied elastomeric impression materials this is often all the retraction that is needed.

c Gingival retraction with adrenaline-impregnated braided cord. These are the preparations shown in Figure 6.9f. The palatal margins are supragingival, and gingival retraction is only necessary on the buccal and proximal surfaces.

d An instrument designed to insert gingival retraction cord.

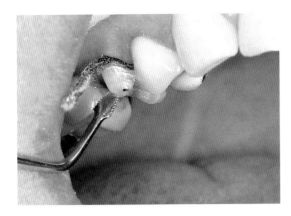

e The instrument in use.

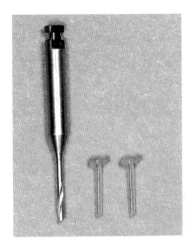

Figure 6.24

a A 0.7 mm diameter twist drill with two headed, burnout plastic pins. These are also 0.7 mm diameter but will go into the drilled pin holes because, prepared freehand, the pin holes are always slightly larger than the drill.

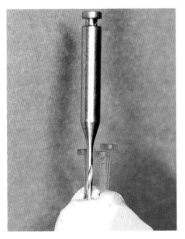

b The working cast has been poured and the impression pins removed from the pin holes. They cannot, however, be reinserted as they are too tight a fit. The pin hole can be slightly enlarged by turning the drill in the pin hole with the fingers so that the same size plastic pins can be used as part of the pattern.

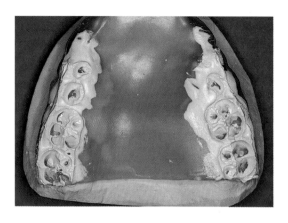

Figure 6.25

Occlusal records.

a A full arch wax occlusal record modified by the addition of a rapidly setting temporary crown and bridge cement to the upper and lower surfaces. Note that the wax extends across the palate, supporting the two sides.

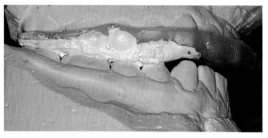

b Excess cement is trimmed away with a scalpel so that when the casts are seated, very precise location of them within the record can be seen. Note that this patient has an anterior open bite, making location of the casts without an occlusal record difficult.

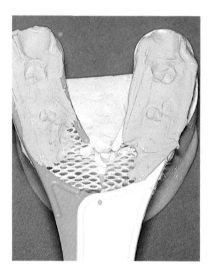

c Hard-setting zinc oxide occlusal registration paste used on a specially designed adjustable plastic frame with gauze mesh.

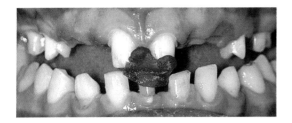

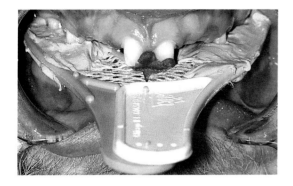

d and e When many or all of the teeth are to be prepared, an acrylic resin index may be used to record the OVD. In this case the teeth were prepared and long-term provisional restorations placed at a new increased OVD. When the patient had become accustomed to this, the anterior provisional restorations were removed and an acrylic index made to the height established by the posterior provisional restorations. Then these were removed and the occlusal relationships recorded for the whole arch with zinc oxide eugenol, with the acrylic index still present (e).

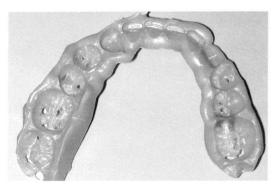

f An elastomeric polymer occlusal record. This is placed in the mouth by an automix gun as a wide strip of material laid over the lower teeth. The jaw is closed into whichever position is being registered (eg ICP or RCP or a lateral excursion record). The material sets quickly to a firm but still elastic consistency. It should be trimmed with a scalpel for the same reason described in b above.

Occlusal records

An occlusal record is not always necessary (see Chapter 4). In some cases an intercuspal position (ICP) record is all that is required. In others a combination of retruded contact position (RCP) and left, right and protrusive excursion records, together with a facebow, may be needed.

The intra-occlusal records may be taken in a polymer material, in wax, or a zinc oxide eugenol paste on a suitable frame.

In most cases the modern polymer materials, delivered by means of an automix gun, are the materials of choice. Some of these guns have a shaped nozzle so that a flat, broad band of material can be laid directly from the gun over the occlusal surfaces of the lower teeth.

If the automix material is not available, any of the elastomeric impression materials can be used to produce occlusal records, and there are fast-setting rubber materials specially produced for the purpose.

The disadvantages of some of the older occlusal registration polymers is that, being rubber, the casts tend to spring out of it and have to be held firmly in place while being articulated.

Because of its elasticity, this older material is not suitable when all the posterior teeth on one side have been prepared or are missing.

Wax occlusal records

Pink wax is softened in a flame or in hot water and shaped to the approximate size of the study cast. It is laid on the lower teeth and the jaw closed into the required position. The wax is allowed to cool or is chilled with water and then removed.

Wax records are liable to distort and may need to be readapted. This may be done by thorough cooling outside the mouth and relining with a temporary crown and bridge cement (see Figure 6.25).

The problem with the wax record is that firm pressure is needed to seat the working and opposing casts into it, and this can distort it, particularly if all the teeth have been prepared or are missing on one side of the arch. Conversely, knowing of this risk, the technician may not press the casts into the record firmly enough, and so they are left slightly unseated. These problems can be avoided if the buccal part of the record is cut away so that the fit of the casts into the record can be clearly seen (see Figure 6.25).

Zinc oxide eugenol paste record

A special hard setting zinc oxide eugenol occlusal registration paste avoids some of the problems of wax records. It is spread on to a gauze mesh in a plastic frame (see Figure 6.25). This does not distort, can be trimmed with a scalpel out of the mouth and resists firm pressure in seating the casts. It is, however, a rather time-consuming, messy and expensive technique.

Trying-in the crown

Safety precautions

Small slippery objects like crowns tend to slip out of the gloved fingers, especially when wet. They are even more prone to slip out of tweezers, which should never be used.

The dangers of dropping a crown down the patient's throat are obvious. If it is inhaled, this is a serious medical emergency and the patient should be rapidly inverted and encouraged to cough. If this is not successful, the patient should be immediately taken to hospital for the crown to be removed.

If the crown is swallowed, this is less dangerous – and also less dangerous than swallowing a sharp instrument such as an endodontic file. However, radiographs should usually be taken and if possible the crown recovered by the patient when it is passed to reassure the patient it has passed safely. The patient should be advised to use a sieve and running water to find the crown in the faeces. Figure 6.26 shows an abdominal radiograph with a crown in the colon.

Various precautions are possible:

● With practice and experience it is possible to control even small inlays and crowns by keeping the gloves dry and the tooth well isolated and dry. One finger should be kept behind the crown at all time. A competent dental nurse with a wide-bore high-volume aspirator should be at the ready.
● Gauze or sponge packs may be placed behind the area where the crown is being tried in. These are theoretically a good idea, but with some patients the irritation at the back of the mouth makes them consciously suppress the cough reflex so that if a foreign object drops behind the pack, the risk of it being inhaled rather than swallowed may be increased.
● The patient may have treatment in an upright position and be told to lean forward, if the crown drops, and cough it out.
● In some cases it is advisable to try-in crowns under rubber dam, but it is difficult to assess the margins if clamps are used, and impossible to judge the gingival relationship or occlusion.

The checking procedure

As pointed out in Chapter 5, a gold crown is tried in, adjusted if necessary and then cemented.

A conventional PJC is tried-in with its platinum foil in place, adjusted, stained and reglazed if

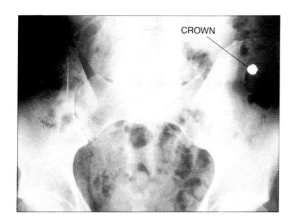

CROWN

Figure 6.26

A crown that has been swallowed at the try-in stage. It is now at the top of the descending colon, and was passed 24 hours after this radiograph was taken. It was recovered, sterilized and cemented.

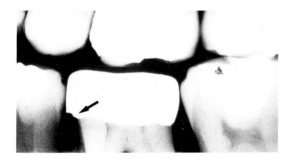

Figure 6.27

a A crown with a large positive ledge or overhang. This should not be cemented in this condition. The distal margin is a better fit, but the surface is bulbous and overcontoured, encroaching on the embrasure space. Compare the contour of the distal surface of the crown with the mesial surface of the tooth behind.

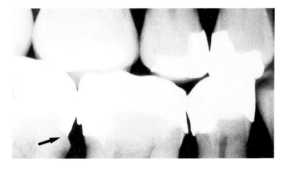

b A negative ledge or short crown margin. There is no gap. All the other restoration margins on this radiograph are also overhanging or defective in some way.

necessary, and then the foil is removed before the crown is cemented.

The metal part of a metal–ceramic crown may be tried-in before the porcelain is added and then returned to the laboratory and retried with the porcelain before being finally cemented.

At the try-in stage the following checks should be made, together with any necessary adjustments.

Checking and adjusting the fit

The marginal fit is checked by eye and with a sharp probe. Gaps, overhanging margins (positive ledges) and deficiencies (negative ledges) may be present (see Figure 6.27).

A uniform gap all the way round indicates that the crown is not fully seated. Having checked for retained temporary cement or trapped gingival

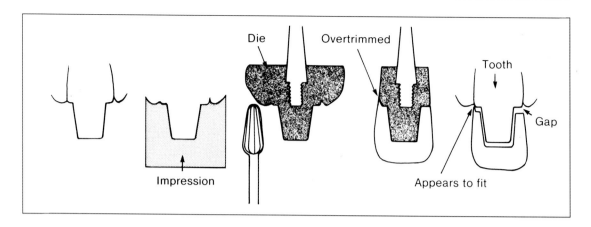

Die   Overtrimmed   Tooth

Impression   Appears to fit   Gap

tissue, a firmer seating force should be applied, and if the gap persists, the contact points should be checked. If, after any necessary adjustment to these, the crown still does not seat, it should be removed and the fit surface inspected. If it is metal, burnish marks on the axial walls may show where the crown is binding. These are ground lightly with a bur or stone and the crown retried.

If there is some improvement but not complete seating, the fit surface should be lightly sand-blasted and reseated. If no burnish marks appear, it is likely that the margins or occlusal surface are preventing complete seating. A common cause is a slightly overtrimmed die (see Figure 6.28). If the occlusal surface is suspected, disclosing wax (a very soft wax) is melted into the crown, which is seated before the wax sets. When the crown is removed, high spots will show as perforations of the opaque wax.

Fine powder suspensions in aerosol sprays or painted colloidal graphite are also used to show where tight crowns are binding, but they are very untidy materials.

If there is a gap around only one part of the crown, it may be seating unevenly because of a tight contact point; otherwise the impression or die may have been distorted.

A positive ledge should be adjusted until the probe passes smoothly from tooth to crown without a catch. A negative ledge is a bigger problem and often means that the crown has to be remade.

A PJC made for a very parallel-sided preparation may not seat fully without forces being

Figure 6.28

A common cause of crowns not seating. The impression clearly shows the margin of the preparation but does not extend very far beyond it. It is often more difficult to distinguish the margin on the stone die than on the impression, particularly when dust from the trimming obscures vision. This leads to an overtrimmed die. To be on the 'safe side', the technician extends the crown beyond the margin, producing a bevel. This fits the die well, but when tried in the mouth the tiny bevel perches on top of the prepared margin, preventing the crown from fully seating. It may appear to fit in the overtrimmed area, but a gap will be present elsewhere.

applied that would risk the crown being fractured. If the shade and other aspects of the crown are satisfactory, the platinum foil should be removed, and the crown will usually then seat completely.

Checking retention

A crown should not feel tight. A crown for a long preparation with optimum taper, which will have excellent retention when cemented, may simply drop off the preparation when tried in. A feeling

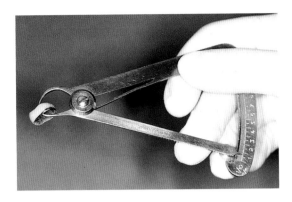

Figure 6.29

A pair of callipers which magnify 1:10 being used to measure the thickness of the occlusal surface of a metal ceramic crown. It is about 1 mm thick at this point.

of tightness is the result of unnecessary roughness of the preparation or a casting that has been distorted. Tightness of fit is not a reliable test of retention, and tight crowns may be more difficult to cement, resulting in an open margin.

The crown should be tested for a tendency to tilt or pivot when rocked from side to side. Tilting of the preparation clearly reveals an unretentive design. Small pivoting movements show that the crown is not fully seated and is rocking about the contact points or on high spots on the fit surface – in which case the margins should be checked again. Alternatively, there is too much space between the crown and the tooth. This may be due to the excessive use of die relief (a varnish spacer painted on to the die, avoiding the margins), a poorly adapted platinum foil, an over-expanded casting or one that has had its fit surface ground.

Checking and adjusting contact points and axial contours

Dental floss should be used to check that the contact points are neither too tight nor too slack. Tight contacts can be lightly ground a little at a time and polished; any deficiency in porcelain should have more porcelain added.

Buccal and lingual contours should not be too bulbous, the marginal area should be in line with the tooth surface to reduce plaque retention and the surface should look natural. Again, adjust-ments may be made by removing or adding materials and repolishing or glazing.

Checking and adjusting the shade

Shades that are slightly too light (the chroma too low) can be darkened by adding stain of appropriate colour and refiring. Stain can also be used to add missing characteristics such as crack lines or mottled areas. However, if the basic hue is wrong or the chroma too dark, or the fault lies in the colour of the opaque core material or the 'dentine' porcelain, it is often not possible to change the shade sufficiently. The crown has to be remade if it is a PJC or the porcelain removed and replaced if it is a metal–ceramic crown.

Checking and adjusting the occlusion

See Chapter 4 for details of occlusal adjustments. If reduction is necessary, the thickness of the occlusal surface should be checked with magnifying callipers (see Figure 6.29).

Cementation

When all the checks and adjustments are complete, the crown is permanently cemented.

Choice of cements

The range of cements used for permanent cementation include:

- Glass ionomer cement
- Zinc phosphate cement
- Resin-based adhesive cements
- Polycarboxylate cement.

Glass ionomer cements

Glass ionomer luting cements have now been available for long enough for one to be able to say that they are a good choice for many crowns. Glass ionomer cement adheres to dentine and enamel, it has a low solubility, it leaches fluoride and is relatively non-irritant to the pulp.

Zinc phosphate cement

Zinc phosphate has been in use as a luting cement for much longer than all the others. Although its acidity must be irritant to the pulp, literally millions of crowns have been cemented with it, with a very low proportion of clinically detectable ill-effects. Patients sometimes complain of transient discomfort when the cement is setting if a local anaesthetic is not used, but most patients need a local anaesthetic for crown cementation anyway and so this is not a major problem. However, the irritant nature of the cement remains an anxiety. The pulps of some teeth fitted with crowns do become inflamed and eventually necrotic. This also happens occasionally with other cements, and it is difficult to identify the cause of pulp death. Was it the cement, the effects of preparing the tooth, or the original condition for which a crown was necessary?

Zinc phosphate has two major advantages which probably account for its continued popularity. It has a long, controllable working time and it produces the thinnest cement film, which can be as little as 10 μm. Of course, this is still ten times the diameter of the micro-organisms that lodge at the periphery of the cement film to form plaque.

Resin-based and adhesive cements

A variety of resin-based luting materials are now available. They are still not commonly used with conventional crowns for a number of reasons. First the truly adhesive cements containing either 4-META or a phosphonate derivative are inhibited from setting by the presence of oxygen. The margins of the restoration therefore have to be coated with an aqueous jelly material until the cement sets, and then cleaning up the surplus cement is difficult. A second reason is that, although they are initially more adhesive than the established luting cements, they have not been used for long enough for one to be sure of their long-term success.

Therefore the resin-based and adhesive cements are used for luting porcelain veneers and minimum-preparation bridges (see Chapter 8), but are not yet recommended for cementing conventional crowns, although this advice may change in the future.

Polycarboxylate cement

This has a relatively low compressive strength and high cement-film thickness. It also absorbs water to a greater extent.

Despite a low pH when set, it is less irritant than zinc phosphate cement and adheres to enamel and to a lesser extent to dentine. However, its disadvantages probably outweigh its advantages, and it is not used by the majority of dentists.

Cementation technique

Preparing the crown

The crown should be completely cleaned of all traces of polish, disclosing wax, saliva and so on. This is best done in an ultrasonic cleaning bath, or if this is not available by scrubbing with a toothbrush and detergent. The crown should be thoroughly dried with tissues and blasts of air.

Preparing the tooth

The tooth should be thoroughly washed with water spray and gently dried with air; it should not be overdried, since this may damage the pulp by desiccation. The washing and drying should be left until the last minute to avoid contamination of the surface by saliva or gingival exudate.

Mixing and applying the cement

The cement should be mixed according to the manufacturer's instructions. Glass ionomer cement is mixed by incorporating powder into water on a glass slab or paper pad, or encapsulated versions are mixed mechanically. In the case of zinc phosphate cement, slow mixing of small increments of powder on a cool glass slab, over a wide area, will increase the working and setting time. This will also allow the pH to rise a little before the cement is applied to the tooth.

The cement is applied to the hollow part. With a complete crown this is the fit surface of the crown, while with a pin it is the pinhole in the tooth. When the opposite member is inserted into the hollow, the cement coats it and is extruded from the margins. If the other surface is coated with cement, for example the tooth preparation for a complete crown, it may be scraped off the surface when the crown is seated, and part of the surface left bare of cement.

The walls of a post hole may be coated using a rotary paste filler or reamer.

Nothing is gained by coating both surfaces. Time is lost, so that the cement becomes more viscous by the time the crown is seated, resulting in a thicker cement layer. Only if both parts have hollow features, such as in a complete crown preparation with additional pin retention, should both surfaces be coated.

The entire surface should be coated quickly with plenty of surplus cement. Any benefit that might be gained by applying a thin, even coat of cement is lost through the extra time taken to achieve this.

Inserting the crown

The crown should be seated quickly and pressed home with firm, continuous force to extrude all the excess cement from the margins. The pressure may be applied by the operator or by the patient biting on a suitable prop, such as a cotton wool roll. Pressure should be maintained and the area kept dry with cotton rolls or absorbent pads and aspiration until the cement has set. Excess cement is also left until the set is complete and it is then removed.

Burnishing crown margins

Finely bevelled gold crown margins may be burnished and so distorted to provide a close fit at the margin. The value of this procedure is doubtful for a number of reasons: the distortion may produce a plaque retentive groove at the margin; the sites where burnishing may be most valuable since they are the least accessible for oral hygiene procedures are also the least accessible for burnishing (for example interproximal areas); the harder modern casting alloys, including many metal–ceramic alloys, cannot be burnished successfully; and finally, modern impression and casting techniques are very accurate, so that the benefits of burnishing are less than they were at one time.

If margins are burnished nevertheless, this should be done while the cement is setting. If done beforehand, the tightly adapted margins would prevent the escape of cement unless a vent (or hole) were prepared in the occlusal surface of the crown. If burnishing were to be done after the cement had set, the cement at the margin would be crushed and leakage would follow.

Oral hygiene instruction and maintenance by the patient

A final and important stage is to teach the patient how to clean and maintain the crown, and in particular how to clean the marginal area. Dental floss and an appropriate toothbrush technique should be advised.

Some patients already have excellent oral hygiene, and too much emphasis on the importance of cleaning around the crowned tooth may result in over-enthusiastic cleaning, causing damage to the gingival tissues or to the tooth.

Recall, assessment, maintenance and repair

Assessment

A systematic assessment of all crowns should be made at each recall examination. This should include evaluation of the following:

Oral hygiene

Plaque levels and gingival inflammation around the crown should be compared with similar teeth elsewhere in the mouth. If the crowned tooth is worse, the reason should be investigated and dealt with. In any case, when it is present periodontal disease should be treated.

Margins

The crown margins should be examined for positive and negative ledges and gaps, and preparation margins should be examined for secondary caries and signs of abrasive wear.

Structure of the crown

This should be examined for fractures and wear, including occlusal perforations.

Appearance

The appearance of the crown or the adjacent teeth may have altered since it was fitted. Any change should be assessed as acceptable or unacceptable. In the latter case the crown will usually have to be replaced: apart from grinding, little can be done to alter the crown's appearance once it is cemented.

Adjustments and repairs to crowns in situ

These are dealt with in Chapter 13, together with bridges.

Practical points

● Good records in the form of study casts and photographs before preparation are useful for planning and later reference.

● Examine the whole mouth and use different lighting conditions when selecting the shade for the crown.

● Prepare each tooth surface in turn so that the amount of reduction can be controlled; the order depends on individual circumstances.

● Gross reduction, at least, must be completed in one visit and a temporary crown fitted.

● The working impression should include an accurate impression of both the contact points and occlusal surfaces of the adjacent teeth as well as the prepared tooth itself and the remaining teeth in the arch.

● Good temporary crowns are necessary to protect the prepared tooth and to prevent tooth movement.

● Special care is needed when trying in the crown to avoid the risk of losing it down the patient's throat.

● After cementation, careful instruction to the patient on oral hygiene and maintenance is of paramount importance.

Part 2 Bridges

7 Indications for bridges compared with partial dentures and implant-retained prostheses

Although the number of crowns made in the UK National Health Service more than doubled in the decade between 1980 and 1990 (see Chapter 1), the number of bridges increased nearly twenty-fold in the same period. Figures for bridges made under private contract are not available, but it seems almost certain that the increase has been of similar magnitude. Large increases are also reported in many other countries.

It can be assumed that this dramatic change is the result of a number of factors: a general growth in dental awareness and expectation, changes in undergraduate and postgraduate dental education, and the introduction of new, simpler techniques and materials. Many patients reject the idea of wearing partial dentures, and the demand for bridges, despite the high cost, is likely to rise.

General terminology

The terminology used in bridgework is sometimes rather loosely applied, and in different parts of the world the same terms are used to describe different things. The word 'bridge' itself is used in the UK to describe a fixed appliance only, whereas in parts of the world it also includes certain tooth-borne removable appliances.

The following names will be used for the various appliances. The terms in parentheses are those commonly used in the USA, although American terminology is rather variable.

- A **bridge** (fixed partial denture) is an appliance replacing one or more teeth that cannot be removed by the patient (see Figure 7.1a). The general term 'fixed bridge' is avoided since it implies one of the specific designs of bridge (see Chapter 8). Substantial tooth preparation is necessary for a conventional bridge. The bridge usually occupies no more space than the original dentition.
- A **minimal-preparation bridge** (resin-bonded bridge, adhesive bridge, Maryland bridge) is attached to the surface of minimally prepared (or unprepared) natural teeth and therefore occupies more space than the original dentition (see Figure 7.1b).
- A **removable bridge** is very much the same as a bridge in that it is retained by crowns, is entirely tooth-supported, does not replace soft tissue, and, unless it is examined closely, appears to be the same as a bridge. However, it can be removed by the patient (see Figure 7.2).
- A **precision-attachment partial denture** is retained by proprietary attachments and is removable by the patient. Soft-tissue elements are replaced and the appliance usually has structures that pass across the oral tissues, for

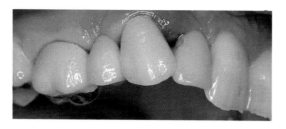

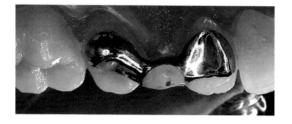

Figure 7.1

Bridges.

a A conventional bridge replacing the upper right lateral incisor with a single artificial premolar tooth filling the space between the canine and first molar teeth. The bridge has just been cemented. The gingival condition around the molar abutment is good, but around the canine it is inflamed buccally as a result of irritation from a broken temporary bridge in this area.

b A minimal-preparation bridge attached to the surface of the lateral incisor and second premolar, with a single artificial tooth filling the space between this. This fixed-fixed design is now less popular (see page 175).

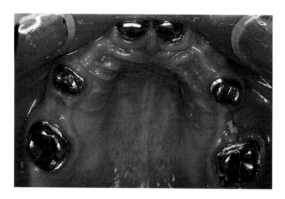

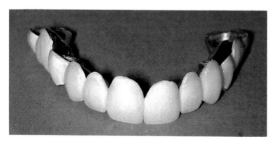

Figure 7.2

A removable bridge.

a Cast copings permanently cemented to the remaining teeth. The external surfaces of these are milled parallel to each other in the laboratory.

b The removable bridge, which the patient can take out himself.

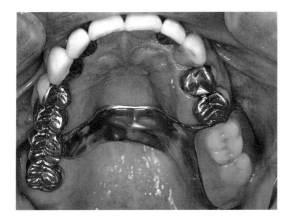

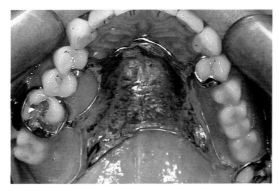

Figure 7.3

Partial dentures.

a A precision-attachment retained partial denture. In this case the two premolar teeth on the right of the picture are splinted together and an intra-coronal precision attachment is incorporated into the distal surface of the second premolar. The first molar on the left is an artificial tooth – part of a bridge – and it too contains a precision attachment. The partial denture retained by these two attachments can be removed by the patient.

b A conventional cobalt-chromium partial upper denture that is tooth-supported with rests, clasps and a major palatal connector. None of the metal work is visible from the front of the mouth.

example across the palate or around the lingual alveolus. Natural teeth have to be prepared and crowns or other restorations made for them, incorporating part of the precision attachment (see Figure 7.3a).

- A **partial denture** may be rested entirely on teeth, or be supported by the soft tissues, or by a combination of these two. Rest seats are commonly used, but otherwise it is usually not necessary to prepare the natural teeth extensively. Partial dentures are retained by clasps, by adhesion to the soft tissues, or by dental or soft tissue undercuts (see Figure 7.3b).

- An **implant-retained prosthesis** is one retained by osseointegrated implants (see Figure 7.4a). A single implant may support a single tooth prosthesis (see Figure 7.4b,c and

d) or a series of implants may support a prosthesis replacing a number of teeth. This is usually known as an implant-supported bridge. The patient cannot remove it, but in some cases the dentist can, by undoing the screws holding the prosthesis to the implants (see Figure 7.4e,f and g). Implant supported bridges may be small, replacing only one or two teeth, or may be larger, including replacing all the teeth in one arch. Implants may also be used to support a bar (or other attachments) on to which a removable complete overdenture can be clipped. Overdentures are beyond the scope of this book.

The term 'fixture' is sometimes used to describe the osseointegrated part of the implant,

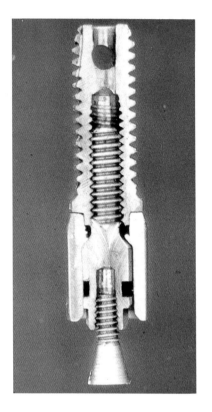

Figure 7.4

a A cross section through a typical implant. Systems vary and so this one will not be described in detail but it is typical in having four elements: from the top down the coarsely threaded screw is the fixture which is screwed into a tapped hole in the bone and then covered to osseointegrate; the transmucosal abutment is smooth sided and retained into the osseointegrated fixture by the middle sized screw; the small screw at the bottom holds the prosthetic elements to the fixture. There are now a wide range of prosthetic elements which will not be described here.

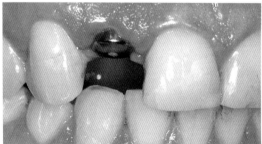

b, c and *d* A single tooth implant replacing the upper right lateral incisor.

b Shows the stage after the second surgical procedure to expose the fixture and to place the healing abutment. The healing abutment is in place and the incision line mesial and distal to it can still be seen.

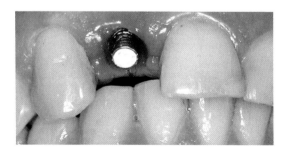

c The healing abutment has been replaced by the transmucosal abutment (TMA).

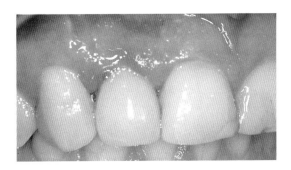

d A crown has been fitted to the TMA.

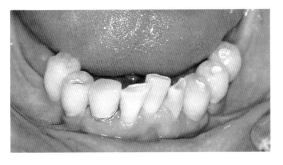

e Four fixtures in the lower jaw.

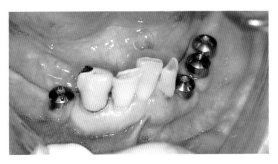

f A three unit 'bridge' has been attached to the three implants on the left and on the right, a three unit cantilever bridge retained by the natural canine tooth and the implant has been extended with a cantilever premolar pontic.

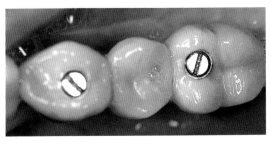

g A three unit bridge retained by two fixtures showing the screws which can be undone if necessary by the dentist. These are covered with composite until it is necessary to gain access to the screws.

but is also sometimes used to describe the whole implant assembly. It is helpful to use the following terms:

- **Fixture** to describe the part that osseointegrates and that is buried beneath the gingival tissues (in most systems) for a period of months before exposing it and inserting the
- **Transmucosal abutment (TMA)**, which is the part of the implant that attaches to the fixture and passes through the gingival tissues to the mouth. To this, is attached the
- **Prosthesis**, which replaces the missing tooth or teeth.

General advantages and disadvantages of replacing missing teeth

It is not always necessary to replace missing teeth, and in some cases there are positive disadvantages in doing so. At one time there was a rather naive, simplistic view that the mouth was a 'functioning machine' and that if part of it was missing, it was rather like a tooth or teeth missing from a cogwheel in a piece of machinery such as a car gearbox. This is not the case because the human body is much more adaptable and flexible than machinery engineered by man. In fact there is reasonably good evidence that, with a modern diet, it is perfectly possible to function with no molar teeth at all provided the first and second premolar teeth and incisors are all present in the upper and lower jaws and are in good occlusal contact. Despite this evidence, many patients would prefer to have at least some of their missing teeth replaced. It is the dentist's role, as a professional adviser, to advise the patient whether or not it is really in their best interest to have a tooth or teeth replaced. In some cases it is wise for a dentist to refuse to replace missing teeth, particularly by means that are likely to give rise to problems elsewhere in the mouth, or if the prosthesis has a poor prognosis, even if the patient attempts to insist that a replacement should be made. This is primarily for the patient's benefit but also for the dentist's. There have been a number of dento-legal cases in which dentists have been successfully sued for making prostheses, particularly bridges and implant-retained

prostheses, when it was against the dentist's better judgement and the prosthesis has subsequently failed.

The first big decision that therefore must be made jointly by the dentist and patient is 'should the missing tooth/teeth be replaced or not?'

It is necessary for both the dentist and the patient – and in some cases a third party financially involved with the transaction – to be convinced that the replacement will produce *significantly* more benefit than harm. The following questions must be asked:

1 How will the patient's general or dental well-being be improved by the replacement?
   – What disadvantages will the replacement bring with it?
   – What is the ratio of these advantages and disadvantages?

2 If the balance is strongly in favour of replacement, should the replacement be by means of:
   – A bridge
   – A removable bridge
   – A precision-attachment partial denture
   – A partial denture
   – An implant-retained prosthesis
   (Of these, a bridge or a partial denture are by far the most common.)

Advantages of replacing missing teeth

Appearance

For many patients with teeth missing in the anterior part of the mouth, appearance is an overriding consideration. For them a replacement is certainly necessary. Just as with crowns, it is also necessary to judge the appearance of gaps further back in the mouth, taking account of the anatomy and movement of the patient's mouth.

Occlusal stability

This was discussed in Chapter 4; and it was also made clear that in many cases, although occlusal stability is lost initially when teeth are extracted, tilting and over-eruption usually eventually lead to an occlusal relationship that, although it may not be satisfactory and may contain occlusal interferences,

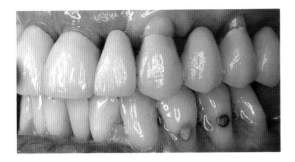

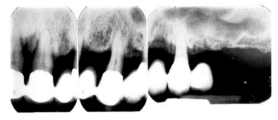

Figure 7.5

a A 12-unit bridge supported by 6 teeth with considerably reduced periodontal support. Several teeth were uncomfortably mobile before the provisional bridge was fitted. The patient was able to maintain good oral hygiene following periodontal therapy, and the provisional bridge was replaced after a year by this permanent bridge, which has now been in place for 12 years. The patient understood the reasons for the visible supragingival margins and accepted them.

b Radiographs of the three abutment teeth on the left-hand side for the patient shown in *a*.

is nevertheless stable. If the missing teeth can be replaced before the tooth movements occur and when tooth movements are likely, this may well be sufficient justification for the replacement. In many cases, however, the patient is first seen some years after the extraction and has a new stable relationship. A replacement for the missing teeth would not improve the stability and so is not justified (see Figure 7.15). Special occlusal considerations are discussed under orthodontic retention and alterations to the OVD.

Ability to eat

Many patients manage to eat quite successfully with large numbers of teeth missing. Patients with no lower molar teeth who are fitted with well-designed and well-constructed partial lower dentures frequently leave them out because they claim that it is easier to eat without them. Some patients, though, have a genuine and persistent feeling of awkwardness if they are deprived of even one posterior tooth. As with appearance, the patient's concept of the problem is as important in deciding on a replacement as the problem itself. Generally though, the more teeth that are missing, the more important is a replacement.

Other advantages

The three advantages listed above are by far the most common indications for replacing missing teeth. The following, though less common, can be extremely important for individual patients:

Speech Patients concerned about the quality of their speech are usually also concerned about their appearance. The upper incisor teeth are the most important in modifying speech, and so when they are missing they will usually be replaced to improve both speech and appearance.

Periodontal splinting Following the successful treatment of advanced periodontal disease, it may be necessary to splint uncomfortably mobile teeth. In order to produce a cross-arch splinting effect it is necessary to bridge any gaps to provide a continuous splint – whether or not there are any other indications for replacing the missing teeth (see Figure 7.5).

A feeling of 'completeness' Some patients believe, or have been told, that there is a major disadvantage to having teeth missing, even when they have no problems of appearance, occlusal stability or with eating. These patients appear to

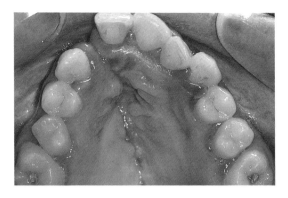

Figure 7.6

A surgically repaired cleft lip and palate with missing lateral incisor. The palatal gingival inflammation is exacerbated by the temporary denture – an additional indication for a bridge. Other indications, as well as improving the appearance by replacing the lateral incisor, are to change the shape of the central incisor and stabilize the relationship of the abutment teeth either side of the cleft.

receive considerable comfort from a bridge – less from a removable appliance. This feeling should not be discounted if it is held with conviction, even though the dentist may not be equally convinced of the benefits of a bridge. However, such attitudes should not be encouraged.

Orthodontic retention Most orthodontic treatment is stable, but it is occasionally necessary to provide a bridge partly to maintain an orthodontic result. A common example is in cases where the lateral incisors are congenitally missing and the upper canines have been retracted to recreate space for them. The main reason for replacing the missing lateral incisors is, of course, appearance, but a second reason is to prevent the canine teeth relapsing forwards again, and so the bridges must be designed to serve this purpose. The resulting appearance is usually better than attempts at converting the appearance of the canines to lateral incisors.

Another example is in patients with cleft palates who have been treated orthodontically as well as surgically (see Figure 7.6).

Orthodontic retention is a special example of an indication for tooth replacement for reasons of occlusal stability. In almost all patients who have taken the trouble to have orthodontic treatment, appearance will also be important.

Restoring occlusal vertical dimension
Occlusal collapse with excessive wear or drifting of the incisor teeth sometimes follows the loss of a number of posterior teeth. This is a difficult

problem to treat, but in some cases the posterior teeth are replaced by bridges or removable dentures that not only replace the missing teeth but restore the lost occlusal vertical dimension, creating space for the upper incisors to be retracted or crowned as necessary.

Wind-instrument players Players of brass or reed instruments contract the oral musculature to form what is known as the embouchure. This allows for the proper supply of air to the instrument. Even minor variations in the shape of the teeth can affect the embouchure, and missing teeth can have a disastrous effect on the music produced by some players.

With some instruments the mouthpiece is supported indirectly by the teeth, via pressure on the lip. Clearly with these patients not only is the replacement of any missing teeth essential but a bridge will usually be necessary. This must be designed very carefully to reproduce as much of the original contours of the missing teeth as possible.

Disadvantages of replacing missing teeth

Damage to tooth and pulp

In preparing teeth for conventional bridges or precision-attachment partial dentures, it is often necessary to remove substantial amounts of healthy tooth tissue. This damage, although it may be justified if the indications are powerful enough, should not be undertaken lightly. The problem is less serious if the teeth to be used to support the bridge are already heavily restored or crowned.

Whenever a tooth is prepared, there is a danger to the pulp, even if proper precautions such as cooling the bur are followed. There is sometimes an additional threat to the pulp when teeth are prepared for bridges. With some designs, preparations for two or more teeth have to be made parallel to each other, and if the teeth are slightly out of alignment, the attempt to make the preparations parallel may involve more reduction in one part of the tooth than normal and so endanger the pulp.

With the falling incidence of caries in many countries, and a more conservative approach to restorative dentistry, situations arise more and more commonly in which the logical abutment teeth for a bridge are sound and unrestored or have minimal restorations. To prepare these teeth would be very destructive, and this is one reason why the minimal-preparation bridge and implant-retained prostheses are becoming so popular.

Secondary caries

As with all restorations, bridges carry the risk of microleakage and caries. This risk is more significant (particularly dento-legally) if the restoration is an elective one rather than the result of caries.

Failures

Chapter 13 contains a black museum of failures among crowns, bridges and implant-retained prostheses. Provided the bridge is well planned and executed and the patient is taught proper maintenance and is conscientious, the chances of failure are small. However, there is always an element of risk, and this must be explained to the patient.

Patients often ask how long the bridge will last. This is an impossible question to answer, since most bridges do not wear out, neither do the supporting teeth. Failure is the result of an isolated incident, a progressive disease process, or bad planning or execution in the first place. Isolated incidents such as a blow cannot be predicted and may occur on the day the bridge is fitted, in 40 years' time or never. The prevention of caries and periodontal disease is largely under the control of the patient, as explained above, assisted and monitored by the dentist and hygienist. Changes affecting caries and periodontal disease likewise cannot be predicted. These include dietary changes, drugs producing a dry mouth and geriatric changes that make cleaning difficult.

A number of long-term surveys of bridge success and failure have produced results varying from very low to high rates of failure. It is possible to calculate from the published figures an average life expectancy of a bridge, but this is not the proper statistic to use, and it should not be quoted to patients unless the statistical significance is thoroughly understood by both dentist and patient. Some bridges are failures from the day they are inserted and some last for over 40 years. To quote an 'average' of 20 years is meaningless.

In the more recent surveys more sophisticated statistical methods have been used to describe survival rates of bridges. In addition, a number of factors affecting the survival rate have also been analysed, including the design of the bridge, the number of teeth being replaced, the periodontal support for the abutment teeth, the vitality of the abutment teeth, and factors to do with the patient such as age and gender. Some of the surveys show a survival rate that remains high for the first ten years or so with more than 90% of the bridges still in place at that time. After this, the survival rate declines, with 60–70% of bridges still in place at 15 years. There are not sufficient studies to establish the number of years at which the survival rate is 50%, in other words when there is an even chance that the bridge will still be in place. However, looking at the published survival curves and extrapolating them, the figure is likely to be between 30 and 40 years survival for small, well-made conventional bridges.

One of the difficulties in interpreting these surveys is the fact that many of the bridges were made a long time ago using techniques, materials and concepts that are now regarded as out of date.

There is therefore no reliable, consistent figure which can be given to a patient when they ask: 'How many years will the bridge last?'. It is often necessary to give the patient a fairly detailed explanation of why such a figure cannot be given or to say something more vague such as (depending on the patient's age, condition of the abutment teeth, etc.): 'A bridge made for you may have to be replaced with another bridge or an alternative prosthesis once (or twice) during a normal lifetime, at times that cannot be predicted.' However, because the prognosis for a bridge cannot be guaranteed, potential failure should be regarded as a disadvantage and balanced against the advantages. It is not realistic to ignore the possibility of failure, and its financial implications for patient and dentist must be recognized.

The considerations and survey evidence of success and failure in relation to removable appliances and implant-retained prostheses are rather different and will not be pursued here.

Effects on the periodontium

There is ample evidence that subgingival crown margins, whether or not as part of a bridge, increase the likelihood of gingival inflammation. Although there is less evidence that this progresses to destructive periodontal disease, it is an unwelcome factor. Even poorly maintained supragingival crown margins can produce periodontal effects, as can restrictions of embrasure spaces and reducing access by the presence of a bridge. The average partial denture is capable of causing even more significant periodontal damage.

Some patients, given extensive courses of treatment, even if without special oral hygiene instruction, still improve their plaque control. Presumably their increased dental awareness improves their motivation. Although this change seems to have long-lasting effects, it is obviously not a justification on its own for making bridges.

Cost and discomfort

Many patients regard these as the most important disadvantages in any tooth replacement. Bridges, denture and implant-retained prostheses cannot be made other than by the individual attention of the dentist and the technician. Personal service of this type will always be expensive. The cost of partial dentures does not rise in proportion to the number of missing teeth, whereas the cost of a bridge tends to do so.

Implant treatment is usually charged per fixture, irrespective of the number of artificial teeth supported by each fixture. The charges are currently significantly higher than those for bridges, which are in turn higher than those for partial dentures. The reason for this ratio is more to do with the perception by both patient and dentist of the skill and training required of the dentist and technician for each of the procedures, together with a concept that the more 'sophisticated' procedures must cost more. This approach is based on historical and traditional views and is not particularly logical. There is nothing intrinsically more difficult or demanding about any of the techniques as compared with the others. If anything, bridges are more demanding because, once they are permanently cemented, it is difficult to make any significant modifications. However, removable dentures and implant-retained prostheses that can be unscrewed and removed by the dentist give more potential for modifications after they are fitted.

Comparing typical fees and calculating approximate fees per hour for the three treatment methods of partial dentures, bridges and implant-retained prostheses, and taking the cost for replacing one tooth with a partial denture as the baseline figure, replacing it with a bridge would cost two to three times as much and with an implant-retained prosthesis three to four times as much, even allowing for the additional items that must be purchased for the implants.

Dental treatment is much less painful than some patients imagine, but there is nearly always some discomfort, such as holding the mouth open for long periods and difficulty in controlling fluids in the mouth. If the treatment is carried out under sedation, there are the disadvantages of the patient needing to be accompanied, being unable to drive after the appointment, and so on.

The choice between fixed and removable prostheses

General considerations

Patient attitude

Patients show different degrees of enthusiasm for fixed and removable prostheses. Unless the patient is particularly anxious to have a bridge or implant-retained prosthesis and fully understands the implications, it is often better, particularly when a number of teeth are missing, to make a partial denture first to see how the patient responds. It may be that the denture is satisfactory, both aesthetically and functionally. If so, the destructive and irreversible tooth preparations that may be necessary for a bridge or surgical procedures for implants can be avoided, or at least deferred.

Alternatively, if the patient is unhappy with the partial denture, he or she will enter into the arrangements for making a bridge or implant-retained prostheses with greater enthusiasm and commitment. Patients should never be persuaded to have bridges or implants against their wishes, and they must give fully informed consent, including, in most cases, time to reflect.

Age and sex

Similar arguments apply to bridges as to crowns (see Chapter 3). However, whereas there may be no satisfactory alternative to a crown for an old or young patient, a partial denture may make a very satisfactory alternative to a bridge or implant-retained prostheses. This is particularly true for very young patients, who may not fully appreciate the lifelong implications of bridges or implants. It is often better to make a minimal-preparation bridge or partial denture until the patient is mature enough to assess the relative merits of the alternatives. But a teenager with a missing incisor who cannot be fitted with a minimal-preparation bridge may be desperately unhappy about wearing a partial denture. In this case, the provision of a conventional bridge or single tooth implant as early as possible may make a remarkable psychological difference (see Figures 7.4b,c and d and 7.7).

At the other end of the age scale, no patient, however old, should be written off as being past bridgework. Figure 9.4d shows a bridge made for a spritely 76-year-old who would have been appalled at the idea of wearing a partial denture. Many patients 10 years older than this would have the same attitude. Figure 9.4d was published in the first edition of this textbook, and the patient is still well and is still happily wearing the permanent bridge made when the two lower incisor

sockets had fully healed. The bridge has so far lasted for more than 12 years and, like the patient, is still going strong.

Confidence

Many patients feel more confident with a bridge than with any form of removable appliance. However retentive a partial denture, some patients never lose the anxiety that it will become dislodged during speaking or eating. Others are not prepared to remove partial dentures at night.

Many patients do tolerate partial dentures very well, however, and it is often difficult to tell beforehand what the response will be to either form of treatment. The majority of patients who have had both partial dentures and bridges prefer the latter.

Occupation

Sports players and wind-instrument players have been referred to earlier (see Chapter 3). Although sports players should be provided with crowns when necessary, it may be better to defer making an anterior bridge or implant-retained prostheses until the patient gives up the more violent sports, and meanwhile to provide a partial denture.

Although wind-instrument players usually need a bridge replacement for their missing anterior teeth, there are some who find that air escapes beneath and between the teeth of a bridge. They are better able to maintain a seal with a partial denture carrying a buccal flange.

Public speakers and singers who make more extreme movements of the mouth often need the confidence that comes from wearing a bridge.

General health

Both bridges and partial dentures are elective forms of treatment, and need not be provided for people who are ill. When tooth replacement is necessary for someone who will have difficulty tolerating it because of poor health, or when there are medical complications such as with patients who require antibiotic cover for every appointment, it is better to consider the simpler, less time-consuming form of treatment first.

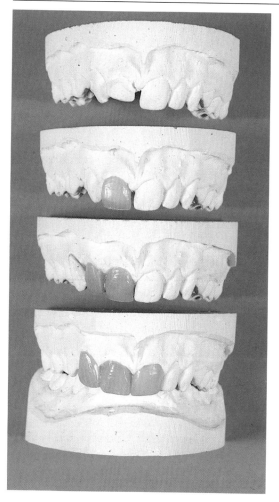

Figure 7.7

a Original study cast and diagnostic wax-ups for a patient who lost the upper right central incisor in an accident in his early teens. Rather than maintain the space, the lateral incisor was moved into the position of the central incisor and the canine tooth into the position of the lateral incisor. On the patient's left the first premolar was extracted since the teeth were crowded, and so the midline was maintained. This study cast was made when the patient was 16 and was becoming very concerned about his appearance. The shape of the lateral incisor had been modified with composite, but this and the canine tooth were still unattractive. The appearance of simply crowning the lateral incisor to make it resemble a central incisor is shown in the first diagnostic wax-up. This is also not satisfactory, and so the second diagnostic wax-up shows the effects of extracting the upper right first premolar, retracting the canine tooth and the lateral incisor orthodontically and making a bridge to replace the central incisor tooth. However, the patient was not prepared to have further orthodontic treatment to achieve this ideal result, and so the bottom diagnostic wax-up shows the appearance that would be achieved by extracting the lateral incisor and making a conventional three-unit fixed-fixed bridge. This is a very destructive approach, but was justified in this case in view of the patient's considerable anxiety over his appearance.

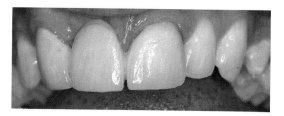

b The bridge in place. The patient is happy with this appearance and considers the treatment to be successful.

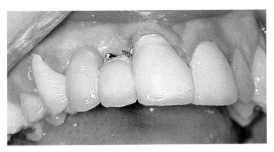

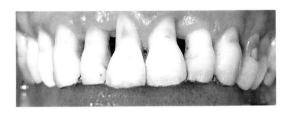

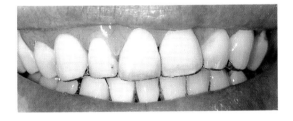

Figure 7.8

a and *b* A bridge with separate acrylic buccal prosthesis.

a The lateral incisor and canine were lost in a road accident together with a substantial amount of alveolar bone. The teeth have been replaced by means of a bridge, and a horizontal precision attachment has been set into the neck of the lateral incisor.

b The unilateral gingival prosthesis in place, retained by the precision attachment. In this case the main purpose is to pad out the lip contour rather than change the appearance of the gingival margins. The lip, when not retracted, conceals the necks of the teeth.

c and *d* A fixed partial crown splint (see Chapter 12 and Figure 12.9)

c The unsightly appearance following gingival recession and surgery.

d A removable acrylic gingival prosthesis in place.

Having missing anterior teeth replaced, though, can boost the morale of patients recovering from long illnesses or facial trauma.

Appearance

When a tooth is lost, alveolar bone and gingival contour are also lost, and it is never possible to disguise this fact entirely (see Figures 7.1a and 9.9a). Thus no artificial replacements ever look exactly like the natural teeth, although some may be sufficiently realistic to deceive all except the dentist with his bright light and mouth mirror. In some cases dentures with flanges achieve this object better than bridges; in others bridges have the better appearance. When a substantial amount of alveolar bone is

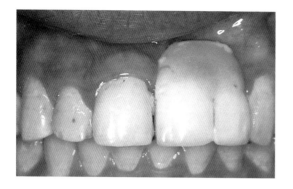

Figure 7.9

a A minimum preparation bridge with a very unsightly and unsatisfactory flange in pink porcelain which does not match the patient's gingival pigmentation. It is also unhygienic.

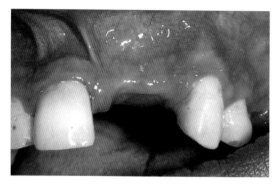

b After removing the bridge the thin receded ridge can be seen.

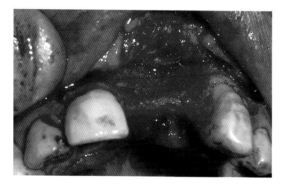

c The alveolar ridge is exposed.

lost in one area, the combination of a bridge with a separate removable buccal flange sometimes gives the best appearance (see Figure 7.8).

When the loss of alveolar bone is significant and the lipline is such that it shows and is difficult to disguise easily, the ridge may be augmented surgically and the tooth or teeth replaced by a bridge or implant. The preferred material is autogenous bone usually taken from somewhere within the patient's mouth, often the chin or the maxillary tuberosity, but freeze-dried bone or other artificial materials are available (see Figures 7.9 and 7.10).

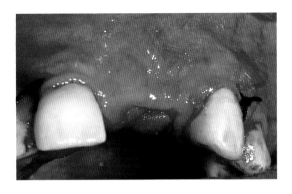

d After augmentation and suturing.

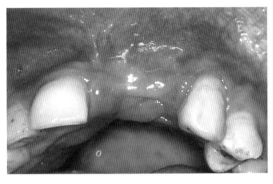

e The ridge healed.

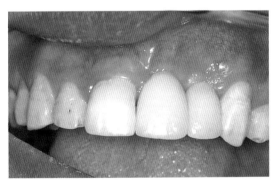

f A new minimum-preparation bridge with an improved appearance of the pontics and the augmented ridge. It is also more cleansable.

General dental considerations

Questions of oral hygiene and periodontal health were dealt with in relation to crowns in Chapter 3 and similar considerations apply to bridges. However, when there are strong indications for replacing missing teeth in a case where there has been periodontal disease and alveolar bone loss, provided the periodontal disease is under control it is preferable to provide a bridge whenever possible rather than a partial denture. This is because a number of abutment teeth splinted together as part of a bridge have a better prognosis than individual teeth with reduced alveolar

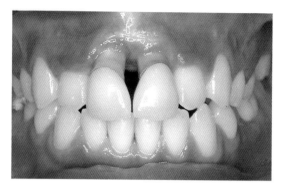

Figure 7.10

Localized alveolar bone loss treated by ridge augmentation and implants.

a The upper central incisor teeth have been crowned but in taking the impression, electrocautery had been used and had damaged the alveolar bone. A sequestrum of bone had subsequently been exfoliated. This photograph was taken three years later at which time the gingival recession had become aesthetically unacceptable and the central incisor teeth were beginning to drift forwards.

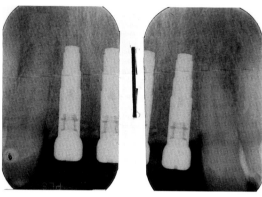

b Radiographs of the fixtures in place helping to support an alveolar bone graft taken from the chin.

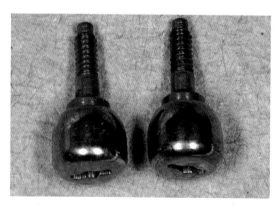

c The healing abutments.

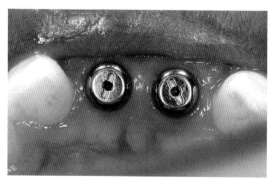

d The healing abutments in place after second stage surgery.

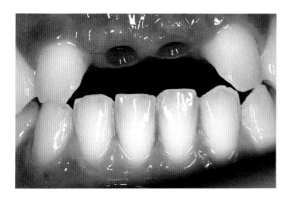

e After healing and removal of the healing abutments.

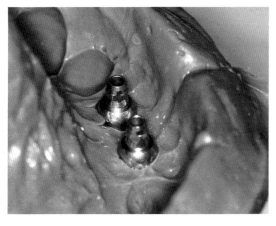

f The impression.

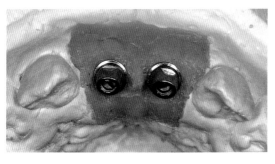

g The working model with a silicone ridge and the TMA analogues.

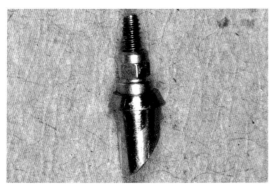

h The TMA and prosthetic core.

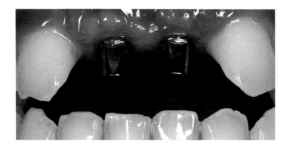

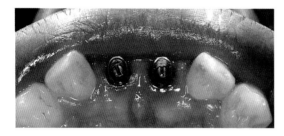

i Two prosthetic cores screwed into place.

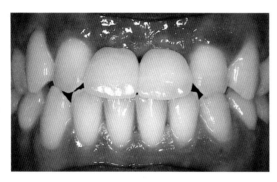

j A palatal view showing the screws.

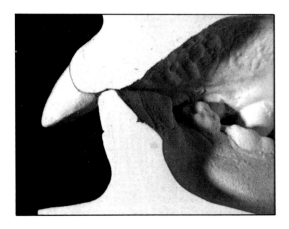

k Immediately after inserting the two crowns. Further healing of the gingival tissues is anticipated now that the patient no longer wears a temporary partial denture.

Figure 7.11

Sectioned study casts of a patient with a complete overbite, with the lower incisors occluding against the palate. A denture would not be possible without altering the occlusion, shortening the lower teeth or providing orthodontic treatment.

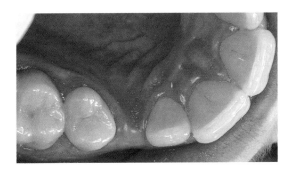

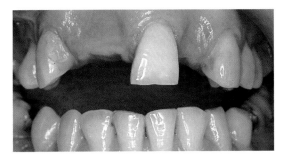

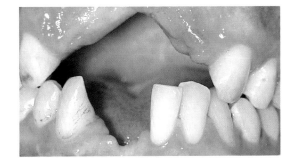

Figure 7.12

Cases illustrating indications for bridges.

a A small but visible space in an otherwise-healthy and unrestored arch. The indication here is to improve the patient's appearance and prevent any further mesial movement of the posterior teeth, which have already reduced this two-unit space to less than a single tooth width. Orthodontic treatment to complete the closure was not possible. A minimal-preparation bridge was chosen (see Figure 7.1b). The construction is shown in Figure 11.12 (page 234).

b The patient, a professional singer, had tried a succession of partial dentures of various designs. She did not like the appearance of any of them and did not feel secure about their retention when singing. The bridge, which is shown in Figure 9.4e (page 197), has been present for more than 20 years and has solved her problems.

c Substantial alveolar bone loss together with the loss of several teeth following a motorcycle accident in an 18-year-old girl. The soft-tissue support is not ideally suited to dentures. The patient was very depressed about her other facial injuries and felt unable to cope with dentures. The preparations for the lower bridge are shown in Figure 3.14f (page 59) and the finished bridge, together with the preparations for the upper bridge, in Figure 8.1a (page 174).

support, which may be mobile, used as denture abutments.

When only one or two teeth are missing in the arch, a bridge is usually considered the better restoration. When large numbers of teeth are missing, particularly when there are free-end saddles, partial dentures or implant-retained prostheses are a more logical choice. In some cases the preferred treatment is to replace one or two missing anterior teeth with a bridge and the posterior teeth with a partial denture. This has the advantage that the patient is not embar-

rassed to leave the denture out at night and is more confident when wearing it during the day.

Occlusal problems may indicate a bridge rather than a partial denture. For example, a missing upper incisor in an Angles Class II Division I malocclusion with the lower incisors occluding against the palate would be difficult to replace by means of a partial denture without increasing the occlusal vertical dimension or providing orthodontic treatment. A bridge would be more straightforward (see Figure 7.11).

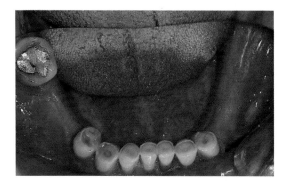

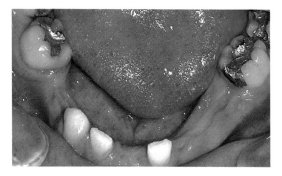

Figure 7.13

Indications for partial dentures.

a A heavily worn dentition with short clinical crowns and no posterior teeth on one side. A partial denture is the obvious choice here.

b Several teeth missing as a result of hypodontia in a 19-year-old patient. In view of the recent extraction of the deciduous teeth together with the apparently high caries incidence judged from the number and size of amalgam restorations, and the small size of the anterior abutment teeth, a partial denture was provided. An additional problem in providing a bridge would have been the lingual inclination of the first lower molar teeth, making parallel preparation difficult. Eventually though, the patient found the denture intolerable, and a bridge was made. One stage in its construction is shown in Figure 11.11 (page 232). Implants would have been a possibility, probably with ridge augmentation, but at the time funding was not available for this patient.

In both *a* and *b* the indications for replacing the missing teeth are both aesthetic and functional.

Local dental considerations

The condition of the teeth adjacent to and opposing the missing teeth may help to determine whether a fixed or removable prosthesis is indicated. When the prognosis of teeth adjacent to the space is doubtful it may be better to provide a partial denture – at least in the short term until the prognosis is clearer. The doubtful tooth could then either be used as a support for a bridge or extracted and a larger bridge or denture constructed. If the angulation or size of the teeth adjacent to the space make them unsuitable to support a bridge, it may be better to provide a partial denture rather than design an unnecessarily elaborate and complex bridge.

Examples of specific indications for bridges, dentures and implant bridges

Figure 7.12 shows three cases in which bridges were preferable, and Figure 7.13 one where a partial denture was the chosen treatment and one where it might have been. Figure 7.14 shows patients for whom implant-retained bridges are

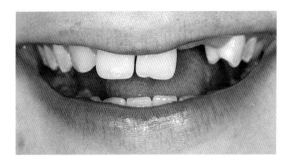

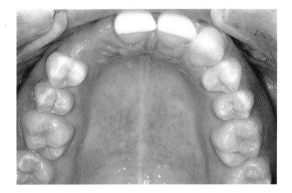

Figure 7.14

Indications for implants.

a and *b* The upper left lateral incisor and canine teeth have been lost through trauma. The mouth is very clean and well cared for with no caries or restorations. The ridge is substantial (confirmed by appropriate imaging).

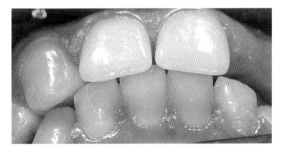

c The occlusion of the patient shown in a and b. It is unfavourable for a minimum preparation bridge. Therefore all the indications in this case are for an implant retained prosthesis.

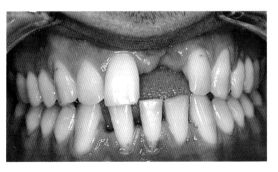

d In this case only one central incisor tooth is missing but the gap is much greater than the other central incisor. The patient had previously had a midline diastema with which he was content. The mouth is well cared for with few restorations and a single tooth implant is indicated.

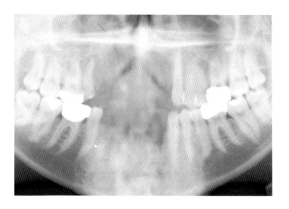

e, f, g and h A patient who was severely injured in an accident in which, amongst other injuries, she lost six upper and six lower teeth together with a significant amount of alveolar bone.

e The condition after initial healing.

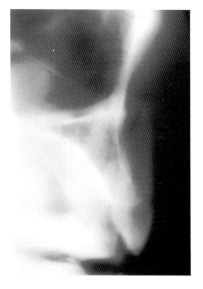

f and g A Scanora (a three dimensional imaging system which involves less radiation than computerized tomography – CT) profile of the upper left lateral incisor region.

f The radiograph.

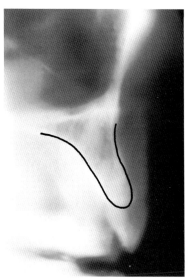

g A tracing of the outline of the ridge. The original magnification is 1:1.7. Imaging either by Scanora, CT or a similar imaging system is usually necessary to determine the quality and amount of bone available for placing implants. In this case ridge augmentation would have been preferable but the patient had had so many operations following her accident that she refused to have further operations for ridge augmentation.

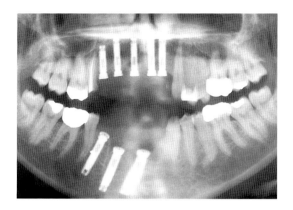

h The implants in place, some at a compromised position. However they have all satisfactorily osseo-integrated and the patient has been wearing the prostheses for five years and has recovered from her other injuries.

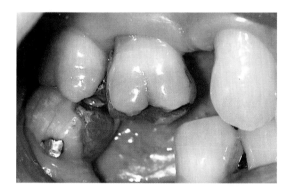

Figure 7.15

This patient had had these spaces for many years, and, despite some mesial drift of the lower molar tooth and considerable mesial movement of the upper molar teeth – so that space for both premolar teeth was now less than half a unit – she was not concerned about the appearance, had no difficulty eating, and even these extensive tooth movements had not produced occlusal interferences. There therefore seemed insufficient justification to replace any of the missing teeth.

indicated. Figure 7.15 shows a case where it would be better to leave the patient with no prosthesis.

Scope of this book

This chapter has dealt with the decisions to be made about whether the tooth or teeth should be replaced, and, if so, whether the replacement should be by a partial denture, bridge or implant-retained prosthesis. All these alternatives need to be considered equally at the planning stage and so are included here in some detail. However, the remainder of this book is to do with bridges only, and the section on further reading guides the reader towards texts on partial dentures and implant prostheses.

Practical points

- When teeth are missing, the first decision is whether replacing them will do more good than harm.

- If the decision is for replacement, the second consideration is whether the prosthesis should be a partial denture, a bridge or an implant-retained prosthesis.

- If the decision is for a bridge, it is necessary to consider what design should be used.

- The patient's attitude, general health, occupation and age should all be taken into consideration.

- The state of the teeth and the whole mouth will affect the final decision as to whether a bridge will be successful.

8 Types of bridge

The appliances used to replace missing teeth were defined in Chapter 7. Some of the terms used in bridgework are also used in relation to partial dentures.

- An **abutment** is a **tooth** to which a bridge (or partial denture) is attached.
- A **retainer** is a **crown** or other restoration that is cemented to the abutment. The terms 'retainer' and 'abutment' should not be confused or used interchangeably.
- A **pontic** is an **artificial tooth** as part of a bridge.
- A **span** is the space between natural teeth that is to be filled by the bridge.
- A **pier** is an abutment tooth standing between and supporting two pontics, each pontic being attached to a further abutment tooth.
- A **unit**, when applied to bridgework, means either a retainer or a pontic. A bridge with two retainers and one pontic would therefore be a three-unit bridge.
- A **connector** (or joint) connects a pontic to a retainer, or two retainers to each other. Connectors may either be fixed or allow some movement between the components that they join.

Conventional and minimal-preparation bridges

Conventional bridges involve removing tooth tissue, or a previous restoration, and replacing it with a retainer. This may be destructive of tooth tissue and will certainly be time-consuming and expensive. The alternative, minimal-preparation bridge involves attaching pontics via a metal plate to the unprepared (or minimally prepared) lingual surfaces of adjacent teeth. The attachment is made by a composite resin material, retained by the acid-etch technique to the enamel. Obviously these bridges can be used only when the abutment teeth have sufficient intact enamel.

Basic designs, combinations and variations

There are four basic designs of bridge, the difference being the type of support provided at each ends of the pontic. The same name is given to the design, however many pontics there are in the span and abutment teeth splinted at one end of the span (see Figure 8.1).

The four basic designs are the same whether the bridge is a conventional or a minimal-preparation type. It is possible to combine two or more of the four basic designs and to combine conventional and minimal-preparation retainers in the same bridge (the hybrid bridge – see page 179).

Of the four basic designs, the first three may be either conventional or minimal-preparation types. It would be unusual to have a minimal-preparation version of the spring cantilever bridge.

The four basic designs (see Figure 8.1)

Fixed–fixed bridge

A fixed–fixed bridge has a rigid connector at both ends of the pontic. The abutment teeth are therefore rigidly splinted together, and for a conventional bridge must be prepared parallel to each other so that the bridge, which is a minimum of three units, can be cemented in one piece. The retainers should have approximately the same retention as each other to reduce the risk that forces applied to the bridge will dislodge one retainer from its abutment, leaving the bridge suspended from the other abutment.

To minimize this risk, it is also important for the entire occluding surface of all the abutment teeth for a conventional bridge to be covered by the retainers. The opposing teeth cannot then contact the surface of an abutment tooth, depress it in its socket and break the cement lute. If this

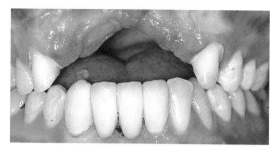

Figure 8.1

Four basic bridge designs of conventional bridges.

a **Fixed–fixed design** Both upper and lower bridges will be fixed–fixed, the lower retained by full crowns on the canine tooth and central incisor (see Figures 7.12c, page 167 and 3.14f, page 59 for the pre-operative condition and the preparations). The upper bridge will be retained by the canine teeth only (see page 209 for the rationale for this design). The bridge was made before implants were generally available.

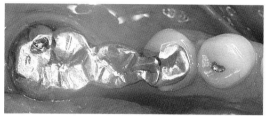

b **Fixed–movable design** with DO inlay in the lower second premolar and full crown on the molar tooth. This bridge has been present for 20 years – in fact so long that the occlusal surface of the crown has worn through (see Chapter 13). The movable joint can be seen between the pontic and the minor retainer. It would not normally be as obvious as this.

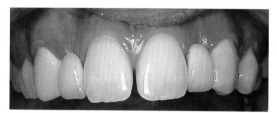

c **Cantilever design** Both lateral incisors are pontics supported by crowns on the canine teeth. Both bridges are conventional all-porcelain, and the right one had been present for 14 years at the time this photograph was taken. The left one fractured after 7 years and was replaced with another all-porcelain bridge.

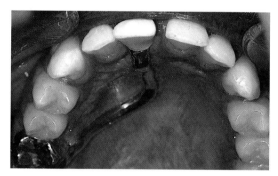

d **Spring cantilever design** with the first molar tooth as abutment. There is a midline diastema, and a diastema between the lateral incisor and canine on the side of the missing central incisor. Any other bridge design would have involved closing one or both of these spaces. Today a single-tooth implant would be the preferred solution to the problem.

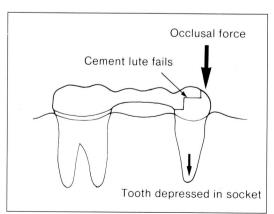

Occlusal force

Cement lute fails

Tooth depressed in socket

Figure 8.2

An unsatisfactory design for a fixed–fixed bridge.

A conventional fixed–fixed bridge should have all the occluding surfaces of the abutment teeth protected by the retainers. Otherwise an occlusal force directed at the unprotected area will depress the abutment tooth in its socket while the retainer is held by the bridge and the other abutment tooth. This will break down the cement lute, causing leakage. The retainer is held in place by the bridge, and so secondary caries develops rapidly (see Figure 13.5, page 261).

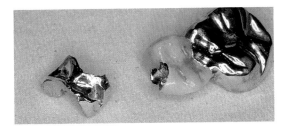

Figure 8.3

Fixed–movable bridges.

a A conventional bridge with an MOD gold inlay as the minor retainer and a full gold crown as the major retainer.

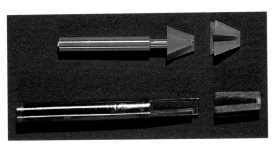

b Acrylic burn out patterns for moveable connectors. The blue is very tapered, the red more parallel-sided.

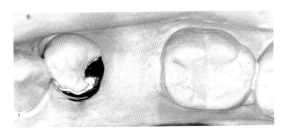

c and *d* A minimum-preparation fixed–movable bridge.

c Shows the minor retainer in place with a depression, rather than a slot, in the distal rest. The preparation for the minor retainer is within enamel.

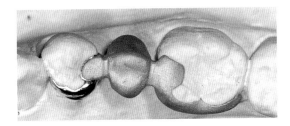

d Shows the finger from the pontic resting on the minor retainer. This will resist axial forces on the pontic which would tend to tilt the molar abutment tooth fowards. It does not resist lateral forces but these can be made insignificant by contouring the occlusion of the pontic

should happen, the retainer will not appear loose since it will still be held in place by the rest of the bridge. However, oral fluids will enter the space between the retainer and the abutment preparation, and caries will rapidly develop (see Figure 8.2).

This rule does not apply to minimal-preparation bridges in which the bond between the retainer and the abutment tooth is much stronger. However, it is sometimes not strong enough, and debonding sometimes occurs as a result of a mechanism similar to that shown in Figure 8.2. This probably partly accounts for the higher incidence of retention failure with minimal-preparation bridges than with conventional bridges, particularly with the fixed–fixed design. Initially, the most popular design of minimal-preparation bridge was fixed–fixed. This was because in the early days of the minimal-preparation design, it was thought that as much retention as possible should be obtained by using at least two abutment teeth. Since then, a number of success-and-failure surveys have shown that the cantilever design of minimum-preparation bridge with one abutment tooth is more successful, particularly with anterior bridges.

At one time it was thought that the support for the abutment teeth at each end of a fixed–fixed conventional bridge should be similar. In other words, the root surface area of the abutments should be approximately the same. Today this is not considered necessary (see Chapter 10).

Fixed–movable bridge

A fixed–movable bridge has a rigid connector, usually at the distal end of the pontic, and a movable connector that allows some vertical movement of the mesial abutment tooth. The movable connector should resist both separation of the pontic from the retainer and lateral movement of the pontic (see Figure 8.3a and b).

Occasionally the fixed and movable connectors are reversed, but this has a number of disadvantages. The retainer with the movable connector (the minor retainer) is smaller and less visible and so is better in the more anterior abutment tooth. Posterior teeth commonly tilt mesially, and this tends to unseat distal movable connectors, but is resisted by mesial ones.

The movable connector can be separated before the bridge is cemented, and so the two parts of the bridge can be cemented separately. The abutment teeth do not therefore have to be prepared parallel to each other and the retention for the minor retainer does not need to be as extensive as for the major retainer. Neither does it need full occlusal protection. Occlusal forces applied to the tooth surface not covered by the retainer will depress the tooth in its socket, and there will be movement at the movable joint rather than rupturing of the cement lute (see Figure 8.2).

A fixed–movable minimal-preparation bridge cannot have the movable joint within the contour of the original abutment tooth unless this is prepared sufficiently for the movable connector, or there is sufficient occlusal clearance, which is

sometimes the case following tilting of the minor abutment tooth. The fixed–movable design for minimal-preparation bridges has become popular in recent times, and early results suggest that it is more successful than fixed–fixed. This is presumably because it can accommodate individual movement of the abutment teeth and the risk of debonding is therefore reduced (see Figure 8.3c and d).

Cantilever bridge

A cantilever bridge provides support for the pontic at one end only. The pontic may be attached to a single retainer or to two or more retainers splinted together, but has no connection at the other end of the pontic. The abutment tooth or teeth for a cantilever bridge may be either mesial or distal to the span, but for small bridges they are usually distal.

Two conventional cantilever bridges are shown in Figure 8.1c. These were made before the minimal-preparation design of bridge was in use and would now be considered unnecessarily destructive. However, they are sometimes still used (see Figure 8.4a). Figures 8.4b,c and d also show minimal-preparation cantilever bridges which are less destructive and have a good record of success.

Spring cantilever bridge

Spring cantilever bridges are restricted to the replacement of upper incisor teeth. Only one pontic can be supported by a spring cantilever bridge. This is attached to the end of a long metal arm running high into the palate and then sweeping down to a rigid connector on the palatal side of a single retainer or a pair of splinted retainers. The arm is made long and fairly thin so that it is springy, but not so thin that it will deform permanently with normal occlusal forces (i.e. exceed the elastic limit). Forces applied to the pontic are absorbed by the springiness of the arm and by displacement of the soft tissues of the palate so that excessive leverage forces do not disturb the abutment teeth. The abutments are usually the two premolar teeth splinted together, or a single premolar or molar tooth.

Spring cantilever bridges are seldom made these days and have been replaced either by

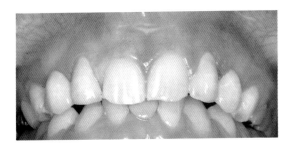

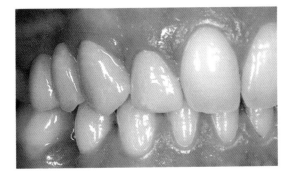

Figure 8.4

a All porcelain cantilever bridges similar to Figure 8.1c but made more recently of a stronger ceramic material (Inceram). In this case the lateral incisor teeth were congenitally missing and the deciduous canine teeth remained with good long roots. They were therefore used as abutments for these cantilever bridges until such time as the deciduous canine teeth are lost. The patient is in her early twenties and this may not be for a decade or two when implants will probably be the treatment of choice but will have to last for less time, assuming the patient has a normal lifespan.

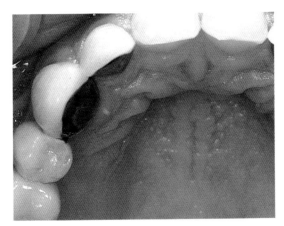

b and *c* A minimum-preparation cantilever bridge replacing the lateral incisor retained by the canine tooth.

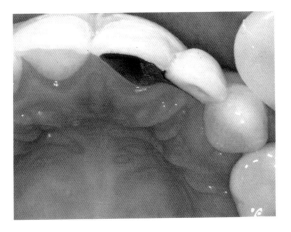

d A similar cantilever bridge but this time retained by the central incisor tooth.

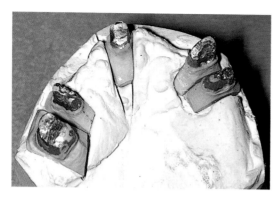

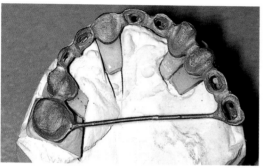

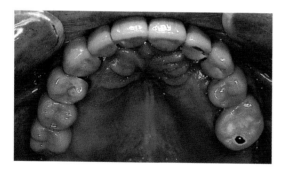

Figure 8.5

A large splint/bridge with cantilevered pontics.

a The working dies.

b The metal framework, showing two cantilevered pontics on the right of the picture.

c The completed restoration in the mouth (photographed in a mirror so that the cantilevered pontics are shown on the left).

minimal-preparation bridges or by single-tooth implants. The two commonest reasons for making spring cantilever bridges used to be to preserve intact anterior teeth when posterior teeth needed crowning in any case and also to preserve diastemas between the anterior teeth. The minimal-preparation bridge now allows the first of these objectives to be met and the single-tooth implant solves the second problem. Both these

designs are preferable to the spring cantilever bridge, which is difficult to clean and maintain.

Combination designs

The four basic designs can be combined in a variety of ways. In particular, the fixed–fixed and

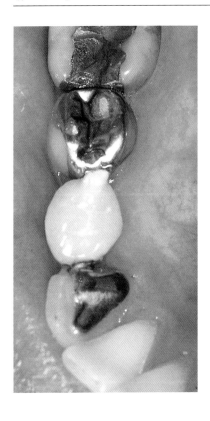

Figure 8.6

A hybrid bridge with a conventional retainer (an inlay in the premolar tooth carrying a movable connector for a fixed–movable bridge). The other retainer on the canine is of the minimal-preparation type. Hybrid bridges should only be made fixed–movable and with the movable joint in the conventional retainer.

cantilever designs are often combined (see Figure 7.1a). In larger bridges additional cantilever pontics may be suspended from the end of a large fixed–fixed section (see Figure 8.5). Similarly, it is possible to combine fixed–fixed and fixed–movable designs.

It is possible to combine a bridge with a removable buccal flange that replaces lost alveolar tissue (see Figure 7.8).

Hybrid design

This term refers to a bridge with a combination of conventional and minimal-preparation retainers. There are three different hybrid designs:

- Fixed–fixed with one conventional and one minimal-preparation retainer.
- Fixed–movable with a minimal-preparation retainer carrying the movable connector.

- Fixed–movable with the conventional retainer carrying the movable connector.

The first design *should not be used* and the second only rarely. In either case, if the minimal-preparation retainer becomes debonded then it will not be possible to re-cement it without removing the conventional retainer, which may well involve destroying the bridge.

The third design is acceptable and may well be the one of choice given circumstances in which one of the abutment teeth (usually the mesial one) already has a restoration that could be replaced by means of an inlay or other conventional retainer and the other abutment tooth is unrestored or the restoration does not involve the surfaces to be covered by a minimal-preparation retainer (see Figure 8.6). These circumstances occur surprisingly often, and so this design of bridge is increasingly being used.

Variations

Removable bridges

All the designs described so far are permanently cemented in the patient's mouth. With large bridges there are disadvantages in permanent cementation in that the maintenance and further endodontic or periodontal treatment of abutment teeth is difficult, and if something goes wrong with one part of the bridge or with one of the abutment teeth, usually the whole bridge has to be sacrificed. For this reason, larger bridges, including full arch bridges, are sometimes made so that they can be removed by the patient. The advantage of this is that cleaning around the abutment teeth and under the pontics is much easier. The bridge has to withstand handling by the patient, and so it is usually made with acrylic facings (see Figure 7.2, page 150). The acrylic facings are less liable to chip if the bridge is dropped. They can also be replaced without the risk of distorting the framework as would be the case with porcelain.

Advantages and disadvantages of the four basic designs

A comparison of conventional fixed–fixed, fixed–movable and cantilever bridges is shown on page 182. Spring cantilever bridges are not included, because they are now seldom made and should not be attempted by inexperienced dentists.

A comparison of minimal-preparation fixed–fixed, fixed–movable and cantilever designs is shown on page 183.

Choice of materials

Metal only

Many posterior bridges, both conventional and minimal-preparation can be made entirely of cast metal, whether they are fixed–fixed, fixed–movable or cantilever. If the retainers or pontics do not show when the patient smiles and speaks then an all-metal bridge is the best choice with conventional bridges – the material necessi- tates the least destruction of tooth tissue and, depending on the choice of metal, may be the least costly. The margins are also easier to adapt to the preparations.

Metal–ceramic

When the strength of metal is required together with a tooth-coloured retainer or pontic, metal–ceramic is the best material. This has now replaced all other crown and pontic facing materi- als, including acrylic, except in special circum- stances, such as patient-removable bridges. Proprietary ceramic pontic facings have also been superseded by metal–ceramic pontics.

A range of composite crown and bridge facing materials is now available, but it is too early to say whether these have no advantage over metal–ceramic materials for permanent bridges.

Ceramic only

The all-ceramic bridge is limited by its relatively poor strength to two-unit cantilever bridges or three-unit fixed–fixed bridges. All-porcelain bridges made from conventional feldspathic porcelain can have a very satisfactory appearance (see Figure 8.1c, page 174). However, with improvements in metal–ceramic materials, these all-porcelain bridges have now fallen into disuse. The newer cast-ceramic and reinforced porcelain materials (see Figure 8.4 page 177) have produced a new generation of all-ceramic bridges.

One advantage of the all-ceramic bridge is the 'fuse-box' principle (see Chapter 2). All-ceramic bridges, if properly designed and constructed, have sufficient strength to survive normal functional forces, but will break if subjected to excessive forces. This potential for fracture may save the roots of the abutment teeth from fracturing if the bridge receives a blow. It is not uncommon for patients who lose a tooth as a result of an accident to have a further accident, either because of their occupation or sport or because, with a Class II Division I incisor relation- ship, their upper incisors are vulnerable to trauma. A broken bridge is better for the patient than broken roots.

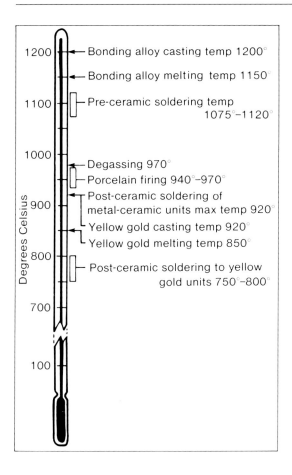

Figure 8.7

Typical temperature ranges for the metal–ceramic process. These vary according to the metal, porcelain and solder used, and with the type of furnace, in particular its rate of temperature rise.

Combinations of materials

Many combinations are possible, but three deserve special mention. The first two are common.

- A metal–ceramic retainer and pontic with a movable connector to a gold inlay or other minor retainer.
- An all-metal retainer (a full or partial crown) towards the posterior end of the bridge with anterior metal–ceramic units.

Soldering standard casting alloys to metal–ceramic alloys after the porcelain had been added was difficult at first, and failures were common. With improved materials and techniques, however, this is no longer the same problem. The solder joint is made in a low-fusing solder after the porcelain has been added, and the bridge cannot be returned to the furnace for further adjustments to the porcelain after it has been made. Figure 8.7 shows the range of temperatures of the various components in the metal–ceramic system.

- A framework of standard casting alloy and separately constructed porcelain crowns cemented to them; this type of construction is now uncommon, but they are still seen in a number of patients and need to be maintained, sometimes by the replacement of fractured crowns (see Figure 13.11h, i, page 269).

COMPARISON OF CONVENTIONAL BRIDGE DESIGN

ADVANTAGES

Fixed–fixed

- Robust design with maximum retention and strength
- Abutment teeth are splinted together; this may be an advantage, particularly when teeth are uncomfortably mobile following bone loss through periodontal disease
- The design is the most practical for larger bridges, particularly when there has been periodontal disease
- The construction is relatively straightforward in the laboratory because there are no movable joints to make
- Can be used for long spans

Fixed–movable

- Preparations do not need to be parallel to each other, so divergent abutment teeth can be used
- Because preparations do not need to be parallel, each preparation can be designed to be retentive independently of the other preparation(s)
- More conservative of tooth tissue because preparations for minor retainers are less destructive than preparations for major retainers
- Allows minor movements of teeth
- Parts can be cemented separately, so cementation is easy

Cantilever

- The most conservative design when only one abutment tooth is needed
- If one abutment tooth is used, there is no need to make preparations parallel to each other; if two or more abutment teeth are used, they are adjacent to each other, so it is easier to make the preparations parallel
- Construction in the laboratory is relatively straightforward
- Most suitable in replacing anterior teeth where, if the occlusion is favourable, there is little risk of the abutment tooth tilting.

DISADVANTAGES

Fixed–fixed

- Requires preparations to be parallel, and this may mean more tooth reduction than normal, endangering the pulp and reducing retention; the strength of the prepared tooth may also be reduced
- Preparations are difficult to carry out, particularly if several widely separated teeth are involved; the preparation is slow and the parallelism has to be constantly checked, or alternatively (and wrongly) the preparations are over-tapered to ensure that there are no undercuts and so retention is lost
- All the retainers are major retainers and require extensive, destructive preparations of the abutment teeth
- Has to be cemented in one piece, so cementation is difficult

Fixed–movable

- Length of span limited, particularly with mobile abutment teeth
- More complicated to construct in the laboratory than fixed–fixed
- Difficult to make temporary bridges

Cantilever

- With small bridges the length of span is limited to one pontic because of the leverage forces on the abutment teeth; if more teeth are to be replaced with a cantilever bridge, a large number of abutments widely spaced round the arch must be used
- The construction of the bridge must be rigid to avoid distortion
- Occlusal forces on the pontic of small posterior bridges encourage tilting of the abutment tooth, particularly if the abutment tooth is distal to the pontic and is already predisposed to tilting mesially.

COMPARISON OF MINIMAL-PREPARATION BRIDGE DESIGNS

ADVANTAGES

Fixed–fixed

- A large retentive surface area
- A single casting and so relatively simple in the laboratory

Fixed–movable

- Independent tooth movement is possible, particularly for the minor abutment tooth (with the movable joint). The major retainer can be designed for optimum retention, sometimes incorporating intra-coronal as well as extra-coronal elements replacing restorations
- The retention of the minor retainer need not be substantial, particularly if the movable joint consists only of a rest seated in a seat on the minor retainer. In this case there are few displacing forces on the minor retainer
- The retention of the two retainers can be very different, usually with the major retainer distally and the smaller, minor retainer attached to a premolar tooth. The retainer can be made very small, and its appearance is similar to a small amalgam restoration
- Prevents a posterior abutment tooth tilting as is sometimes the case with a cantilever bridge. The movable joint merely acts to prevent this rather than to provide any retention for the bridge

Cantilever

- The most conservative of all designs, usually only involving a single minimal-preparation retainer
- Ideal for replacing upper lateral incisors, using the canine tooth as the abutment, provided the occlusion is favourable
- Suitable posteriorly when the span is short
- Easy for the patient to clean with floss passed through the contact point between the pontic and the unrestored adjacent tooth
- No need to align preparations
- Easy laboratory construction

DISADVANTAGES

Fixed–fixed

- Because part of the occlusal surfaces of both abutment teeth are usually opposed by teeth in the opposing jaw, there is a tendency for them to be dislodged from the retainer, thus debonding the bridge
- With tilted abutments it is sometimes difficult to achieve an adequate retentive surface without substantial tooth preparation
- The retention of both retainers should be approximately equal. This is difficult to achieve when one retainer is a molar tooth and the other a premolar

Fixed–movable

- Not suitable for anterior bridges
- More difficult to make in the laboratory, requiring two separate castings
- Not suitable for longer-span bridges, where a conventional fixed–movable bridge would be satisfactory. This is because the movable joint is seldom large enough to resist lateral forces on the pontic, but will only resist axial forces by means of the rest on the minor retainer

Cantilever

- Relatively small retentive area, and vulnerable to debonding through torquing forces

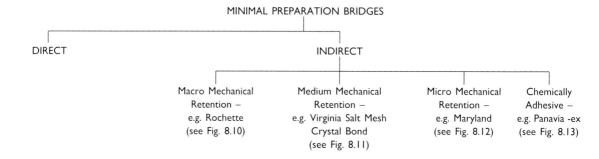

MINIMAL PREPARATION BRIDGES

DIRECT   INDIRECT

| Macro Mechanical Retention – e.g. Rochette (see Fig. 8.10) | Medium Mechanical Retention – e.g. Virginia Salt Mesh Crystal Bond (see Fig. 8.11) | Micro Mechanical Retention – e.g. Maryland (see Fig. 8.12) | Chemically Adhesive – e.g. Panavia -ex (see Fig. 8.13) |

Figure 8.8

A simple classification of minimal-preparation bridges.

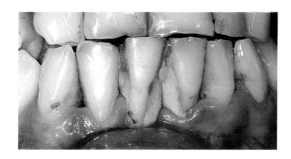

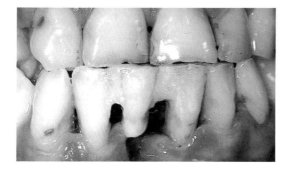

Figure 8.9

Minimal-preparation direct bridge.

a This patient presented with periodontal disease and gross calculus. As an initial phase in his treatment following removal of the calculus, the mobile lower incisor was splinted to the adjacent teeth with acid-etch retained composite. However:

b It was decided later that the prognosis of this tooth was hopeless, and the root was resected and removed.

Types of minimal-preparation bridge

Figure 8.8 shows a simple classification of minimal-preparation bridges; variations of this technique are shown in Figures 8.9–8.13.

● Direct bridges may be made using the crown of the patient's own tooth. This can often be done as a simple and rapid way of replacing a

tooth lost through injury (which cannot be reimplanted) or which has to be extracted urgently. Sometimes metal mesh or wire is added to the lingual surface to increase strength, but this is not always necessary. If the natural crown of the tooth is not available or is not suitable, an acrylic denture tooth can be used in the same way (see Figure 8.9).

● Macro-mechanically retentive bridges (Rochette,

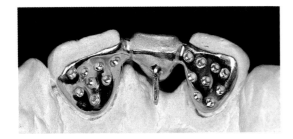

Figure 8.10

A Rochette (macro-mechanically retentive) bridge replacing one central incisor. The porcelain is yet to be added, and the palatal spur on the pontic will act as a handle until the bridge is finished, when it will be removed. This design is still used when the bridge (or splint) is likely to be removed in the future. The composite is drilled out of the holes, and the bridge can be removed with less trauma to the abutment teeth than with other methods.

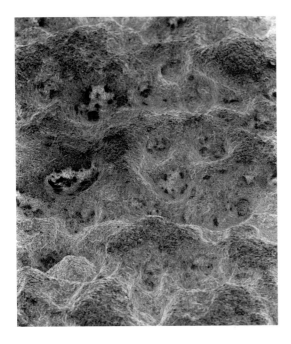

Figure 8.11

Four types of medium-mechanically retentive surfaces. All are bulky and with poor retention. They are now seldom used.

a A scanning electron micrograph (SEM) of the retentive metal surface produced by the Virginia salt technique. Salt is applied to an adhesive on the die and then a pattern is built up in either wax or acrylic. This is removed from the die and the salt dissolved in water. The pattern is then cast, leaving depressions where the salt crystals were. Field width equals 900 μm.

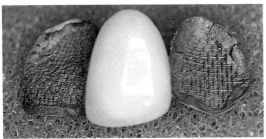

b A cast-mesh bridge. It is difficult to achieve good adaptation of the mesh over the entire retainer surface, and neither of these retainers has retentive features right up to the periphery. The added thickness of the retainer can also be seen.

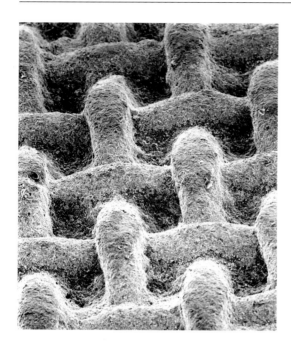

c SEM of a cast-mesh surface. Note that the undercuts form only a small proportion of the surface and that there are thick, non-undercut elements. Field width equals 900 μm.

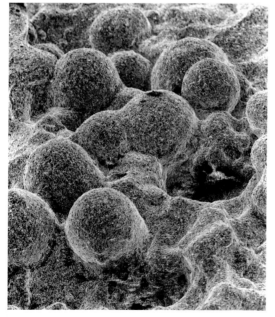

d SEM of a cast-metal surface resulting from a proprietary mixture of acrylic beads and salt, producing both spheres (from the acrylic beads) and depressions (from the salt). Again this has large unretentive elements. Field width equals 900 μm.

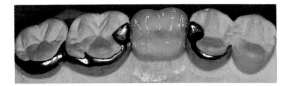

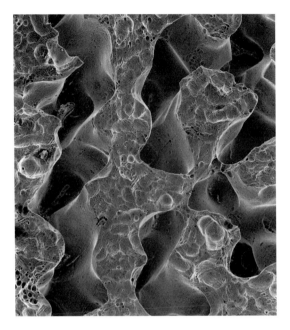

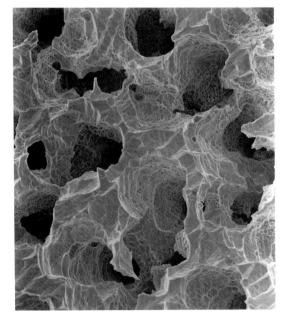

Figure 8.12

a A minimum-preparation bridge: the design is unsatisfactory in that the extension distally onto the third molar tooth to increase retention would give rise to an impossible cleaning problem between the second and third molars. This is a technique bridge, not made for a patient. It is shown to illustrate a common design error.

b SEM of a cast nickel–chromium metal surface etched in the laboratory. The very retentive but delicate etch pattern is much smaller in scale than the retention systems shown in Figure 8.10a, c and d. Field width equals 90 μm, i.e., the magnification is 10 times greater than Figures 8.10a, c and d.

c SEM of a surface chemically etched at the chairside. Field width equals 90 μm.

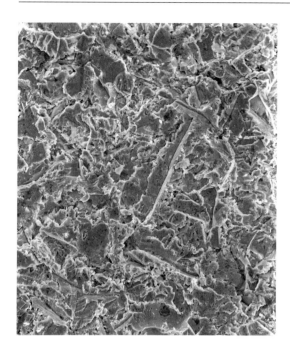

Figure 8.13

SEM of a cast nickel–chromium metal surface blasted with 50-μm aluminium oxide particles. The surface has no physical undercuts but is irregular. This is the recommended metal finish for the chemically adhesive cementing resins. Field width equals 90 μm.

see Figure 8.10) have large undercut perforations through the cast-metal plate, through which the composite flows. These holes are cut in the wax or acrylic pattern with a bur and are then countersunk.

● Medium-mechanical retentive systems all involve retentive features cast as part of the metal framework (see Figure 8.11). They all add significantly to the cement-film thickness in some areas, at least, of the retainer and they all produce large, non-undercut lumps of metal on the fit surface that do not contribute to retention but necessitate a relatively thick retainer. They are therefore no longer used, but patients with this type of bridge may present with the bridge debonded. It is usually not worth trying to re-attach it.

The size of the retentive features is intermediate between those of macro- and micro-mechanical retentive systems.

● Micro-mechanical retention is produced by casting the metal retainer and then etching the fit surface by one of two methods:

electrolytic etching in acid in the laboratory or chemical etching with a hydrofluoric acid gel either in the laboratory or at the chairside. Although these two systems produce different etch patterns, they are all very retentive (see Figure 8.12). The size of the retentive features is approximately one-tenth that of the medium-mechanical retentive systems, and the retentive features are undercut from the surface. The smaller size of these etch pits and the absence of any unnecessary non-retentive features (as in the medium-mechanical retentive systems) allow thinner metal retainers and a thinner cement-film thickness.

● Chemically retentive resins are now available. Several have been marketed, and some (e.g. Panavia 21) have performed well in laboratory and short-term clinical trials. They adhere chemically to recently sandblasted metal surfaces and are retained on the tooth by conventional acid-etching of the enamel (see Figure 8.13).

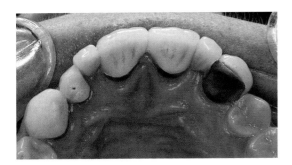

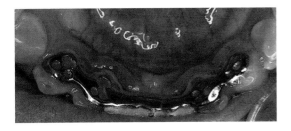

Figure 8.14

a and *b* The upper conventional bridges and the lower Rochette bridge were all made five years before these photographs were taken. Note that the patient has managed to maintain good oral hygiene and periodontal health round the conventional bridges, but has had much more difficulty around the lower Rochette bridge.

Comparison of indirect minimal-preparation retention systems

A number of laboratory studies and clinical trials have shown that micro-mechanical and chemical adhesive systems are the most retentive. The chemical adhesive systems have been available for a number of years and are proving the most successful of the systems. However, longer-term clinical trials are still necessary. The more recently introduced materials are claimed to have better retentive properties than earlier materials, but time will tell. An advantage of using the chemical adhesive materials is that the laboratory only needs a sandblaster rather than etching equipment, and the health and safety hazards of etching in an acid solution or using hydrofluoric acid gel are avoided. The adhesive cement is easy to mix and use and has a good working time, so that the bridge can be fully seated without too much hurry. Rubber dam should always be used and the margins of the restoration coated with a gel material to prevent air contacting the setting cement, since its setting is inhibited by oxygen.

A disadvantage of the micro-mechanical retention system is that the metal framework should not be tried in the mouth after the surface has been etched. This is because the very delicate etch pattern may well be damaged or clogged by deposits from saliva (see Figure 8.12). This means that the ideal is to try-in the unetched framework and then either return it to the laboratory for etching or etch it at the chairside. This takes time and therefore adds to the cost.

The macro-mechanical retentive design (Rochette) overcomes this problem but is less retentive in most cases, and, because it is cemented with a conventional composite (rather than one specifically designed for cementing minimal-preparation retainers, see page 233) and the composite comes through the perforations to the mouth, it is prone to degradation over a period of years. However, the main advantage of the Rochette bridge is that it can be removed from the mouth fairly easily. The composite is drilled out from the holes, and the bridge can usually be removed without too much force. For this reason, the Rochette bridge is still used when the abutment teeth have a poor prognosis and when further modifications are likely to be necessary – for example when one lower incisor is being replaced for periodontal reasons and the other teeth are still receiving periodontal treatment. The Rochette design is also used for immediate insertion bridges so that the bridge can be removed when the tissues have healed and the pontic adapted to the ridge or the bridge remade.

Historically, the medium-mechanical retentive systems were developed after the Rochette and Maryland designs in an attempt to overcome the disadvantages of these described above. However, they have disadvantages of their own in being less retentive than the micro-mechanical system and yet having thicker metal retainers and a thicker cement film. One advantage, however, is that they can be made in any metal, including precious metals, whereas the etched systems can only be made in base metal alloys that are etchable. However, despite this, they are no longer used.

Disadvantages of minimal-preparation bridges in general

As the metal plate is added to the surface of the tooth or only replaces part of it, the thickness of the tooth is increased, and may (for example in a normal Class I incisor relationship) interfere with the occlusion unless space is created orthodontically or by grinding the opposing teeth (see Chapter 11).

The margin of the retainer inevitably produces a ledge where plaque can collect. This is a problem, especially in the replacement of lower incisors. Here plaque and calculus deposits are common on the lingual surface towards the gingival margin, and the presence of such a ledge can only make it more difficult for the patient to clean in this area (see Figure 8.14) Another example of a design that would prevent good oral hygiene is shown in Figure 8.12a.

Practical points

● The four basic bridge designs differ in the support provided at each end of the pontic.

● The basic designs can be combined to give, for example, a fixed–fixed/cantilever design.

● Minimal-preparation bridges are useful, particularly in younger patients, and – where practical – are often the design of choice.

● With conventional bridges, the fixed–movable design is preferred to fixed–fixed where possible.

● With minimal-preparation bridges, the preferred design is cantilever, followed by fixed–movable rather than fixed–fixed.

● Bridges that are made to be removable by the patient make further endodontic or periodontal treatment possible and also make cleaning easier.

9 Components of bridges: retainers, pontics and connectors

Each part of the bridge should be designed individually, but within the context of the overall design. This chapter should therefore be read in conjunction with the next, since in practice the two processes – designing the bridge and its components – are done together, although it is clearer to describe them separately.

Retainers

Major or minor

As described in Chapter 8, all fixed–fixed, cantilever and spring cantilever bridges have only major retainers. Fixed–movable bridges have a major retainer at one end of the pontic and a minor retainer (carrying the movable joint) at the other.

Major retainer preparations must be retentive and, with conventional bridges, must cover the whole occluding surface of the tooth. It is important to recognize the difference between the occlu*ding* and the occlu*sal* surface.

A **major retainer** for a conventional posterior bridge should not be less than an MOD inlay with full occlusal protection. For incisor teeth it is usually a complete crown, although partial crowns are still sometimes used.

Minor retainers do not need full occlusal protection: a minor retainer may be a complete or partial crown, or a two- or three-surface inlay without full occlusal protection (see Figures 8.1b and 8.3 pages 174 and 175). Minimal-preparation minor retainers are also used for minimal-prepa-ration bridges where the occlusion is favourable (see Figure 8.3c and d).

Complete crown, partial crown, intra-coronal or minimal-preparation retainers?

The choice between complete or partial crown retainers in the past was governed by the techniques and materials available. Before the air rotor and metal–ceramic techniques were available, three-quarter crowns were popular as bridge retainers, partly because less enamel had to be removed and partly because it was not necessary to provide a tooth-coloured facing. With the air rotor, complete crown preparations became easier, and there was a swing towards complete crown retainers. Once metal–ceramic and elastomeric impression materials became generally available, the swing was accelerated.

The choice between complete and partial crown retainers for posterior conventional bridges should depend upon a proper consideration of all the circumstances of the case, and should not be made from habit. It will be found that even after a full assessment, 80–90% of conventional bridge retainers will be full crowns, but for the remaining 10–20% there are sound reasons for choosing a partial crown. (See Chapter 2 for a comparison of complete and partial crowns.)

Intra-coronal retainers are used only as minor retainers except for very retentive MOD protected cusp inlays.

With the reported reduction in caries and with a more conservative approach to cavity preparation, an increasing number of potential abutment teeth have sufficient enamel available for minimal-preparation retainers to be considered. When

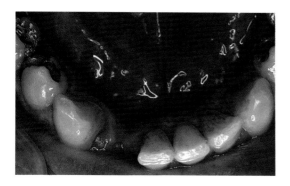

Figure 9.1

Non-parallel abutment teeth. It would not be possible to make a fixed–fixed bridge with complete crowns on the central incisor and canine. Even if one of the teeth were devitalized to align an artificial core with the other abutment, this would not work. If the canine were devitalized, the core would have to be so prominent to be parallel with the central incisor that it would interfere grossly with the occlusion. If the central incisor were devitalized, the retainer would tilt lingually and would be both uncomfortable and unaesthetic. The design chosen was a simple cantilever. The preparation of the canine tooth and finished bridge is shown in Figure 10.3.

this is so, they are usually the retainers of choice, provided that the other conditions for their use are met (see later). This is because they are the most conservative retainers, and it is wise to preserve as much natural tooth tissue as possible, even at the cost of a slightly increased risk of retention failure.

Partial crowns are now seldom used for anterior bridge retainers. When the tooth is intact a minimal-preparation retainer is more conservative of tooth tissue than a complete crown, and so is the preferred choice whenever possible.

Materials

Minimal-preparation retainers are usually made in base metal alloys so that they can be etched and also because these alloys are strong in thin sections. Of the conventional retainers, an all-metal retainer is the most conservative of tooth tissue, and the simplest and usually the least expensive to produce. When appearance permits, this should be used in the posterior part of the mouth. In the anterior part of the mouth metal–ceramic is the most suitable material.

Criteria for choosing a suitable retainer

In some cases the type of retainer will be obvious. For example, if a root-filled tooth that already has a post crown is to be used as a bridge abutment,

there is little choice but to use another post-retained crown, whether as a major or minor retainer. In other cases, the full range of choice is available, and the decision on the type of retainer cannot be divorced from the decisions on the overall design and which abutment teeth to use. These three sets of considerations are dealt with separately (in Chapters 8, 10 and here), but in reality the decision-making process is not so clear-cut, and thoughts on possible abutment teeth, retainers and the overall design intermingle in the operator's mind and influence each other until a final decision on all three emerges.

The criteria for selecting a particular retainer will include:

- Alignment of abutment teeth and retention
- Appearance
- Condition of abutment teeth
- Conservation of tooth tissue
- Occlusion
- Cost

Alignment of abutment teeth and retention

When the abutment teeth are more or less parallel to each other and a fixed–fixed conventional bridge is being considered, either complete or partial crown retainers can be made. If the abutment teeth are not parallel (see e.g. Figure 9.1), complete crown retainers with a common

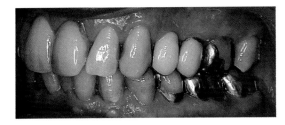

Figure 9.2

The appearance of retainers.

a The canine tooth has a partial crown retainer that is barely visible from the front. The bridge has been present for many years.

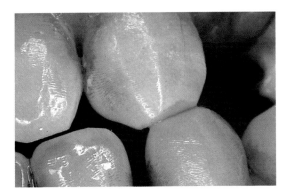

b The upper canine tooth has an extensive incisal wear facet and pronounced buccal striae. The buccal surface would be difficult to reproduce in porcelain if a complete crown retainer were used, and a large amount of gold would show if the wear facet were protected by a partial crown retainer. The design of the bridge in this case was therefore fixed–movable with a distal palatal gold inlay in the canine tooth.

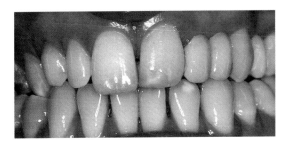

c The upper central incisors both have minimal-preparation retainers. The blue 'metal shine-through' can be seen. The incisal edge of the upper left central incisor has been restored with composite, which is beginning to lose its polish. 'Metal shine-through' can be reduced by finishing the retainer short of the incisal edge, but this also reduces its retention. The problem can be minimized using opaque luting cements.

path of insertion are not feasible. They could not be made independently retentive without one or other of the teeth being devitalized. This is sometimes necessary, but it is a very destructive approach.

The solution will usually be to employ a minimal preparation bridge or a design other than fixed–fixed so that the teeth do not have to be prepared parallel to each other.

It is impossible to give in absolute terms the amount of retention necessary for any one retainer. It is reasonable to assume that the retention for a bridge retainer should be at least as great as for a similar restoration made as a single unit. When it is necessary to reduce a

retentive feature, for example to over-taper a preparation to provide a single path of insertion with another preparation, it is advisable to add some further retentive feature such as grooves or a pin.

Appearance

In some cases a complete crown will have a better appearance, in some a partial crown, and in others a minimal-preparation retainer. Sometimes none of these types will be completely satisfactory. Figure 9.2 shows examples of partial crown, inlay and minimal-preparation retainers where the appearance of the buccal surface is better than would be expected with a full crown. Figure 9.2c also shows an example of 'metal shine-through', which sometimes occurs with minimal-preparation retainers.

When several teeth are to be crowned or replaced as pontics, there is an aesthetic advantage to the bridge retainers and pontics being made in the same material (usually metal–ceramic), at least giving consistency of appearance.

The condition of the abutment tooth

Frequently a minimal-preparation or partial crown retainer cannot be used because of the presence of caries or large restorations involving the buccal surface, or because of the loss of the buccal surface from trauma or other cause. In these cases a complete crown retainer is chosen.

Conservation of tooth tissue

There is a natural reluctance to remove sound buccal enamel and dentine from a healthy intact tooth. This weakens the tooth, destroys its natural appearance and endangers the pulp. Therefore minimal-preparation retainers should be used whenever possible. However, if there are sound indications for a complete crown, the operator should not allow his or her clinical judgement to be influenced by an overprotective attitude to dental enamel.

Occlusion

In some cases the abutment teeth are sound but there is insufficient space for a minimal-preparation retainer. The choice therefore is between creating space by reducing the opposing teeth, preparing part way through the enamel of the abutment teeth, moving the abutment teeth orthodontically or a combination of these approaches. Often the best way to achieve a small amount of axial tooth movement is to use a fixed Dahl appliance (see Figure 4.6, pages 72–3). If none of these methods are acceptable then a conventional retainer will be necessary.

Cost

Partial crowns and complete metal crowns may be less expensive than metal–ceramic crowns (see Chapter 2), and minimal-preparation retainers are the least expensive. When there are no other overriding factors affecting the choice, this is obviously of considerable importance.

Pontics

Principles of design

Pontics are designed to serve the three main functions of a bridge:

- To improve appearance
- To stabilize the occlusion
- To improve masticatory function.

In different areas of the mouth the relative importance of these will alter. The principles guiding the design of the pontic are:

- Cleansability
- Appearance
- Strength.

The compromise often necessary between cleansability and appearance will also vary in different parts of the mouth.

Cleansability

All surfaces of the pontic, especially the surface adjacent to the saddle, should be made as cleansable as possible. This means that they must be smooth and highly polished or glazed, and should not contain any junctions between different materials. In a metal–ceramic pontic the junction between the two materials should be well away from the ridge surface of the pontic.

It is important too that the embrasure spaces and connectors should be smooth and cleansable. They should also be as easy to clean as possible. Access to them and the patient's dexterity should be taken into account in designing pontics.

When a conflict exists between cleansability and appearance, priority should be given to cleansability.

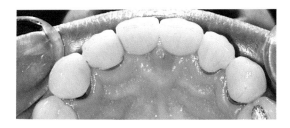

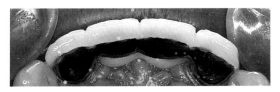

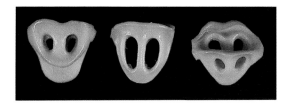

Figure 9.3

The strength of metal–ceramic pontics.

a The central incisor pontics in this case have no metal visible on the palatal surface.

b When the palatal reduction of the abutment teeth is only sufficient for a layer of metal, this is often carried along the pontics as well, leaving an occluding surface entirely in metal. The porcelain, however, is carried right under the pontics so that only porcelain contacts the ridge.

c Preformed wax patterns for metal–ceramic pontics. The porcelain is condensed through the holes.

Appearance

Where the full length of the pontic is visible, it must look as toothlike as possible. However, in the premolar and first molar region it is often possible to strike a happy compromise between a reasonable appearance for those parts of the pontic that are visible and good access for cleaning towards the ridge.

Strength

All pontics should be designed to withstand occlusal forces; but porcelain pontics in the anterior part of the mouth may not of course be expected to withstand accidental traumatic forces.

The longer the span, the greater the occlusal gingival thickness of the pontic should be. Metal–ceramic pontics are stiffer and withstand occlusal forces better if they are made fairly thick and if the porcelain is carried right round them from the occlusal to the ridge surface, leaving only a line of metal visible on the lingual surface or none at all (see Figure 9.3a, b). Preformed wax patterns for pontics designed to give maximum strength with a minimum of metal are available (the reinforced porcelain system – RPS) (Figures 9.3c and 8.5b, page 178).

The surfaces of a pontic

A pontic has five surfaces:

● The ridge
● The occlusal
● The approximal
● The buccal
● The lingual.

Some of these will be similar to the natural tooth being replaced; others will be very different.

The ridge surface

This surface of the pontic is the most difficult to clean, and yet it also has a considerable influence on appearance. There are four basic designs of ridge surface (see Figures 9.4 and 9.5).

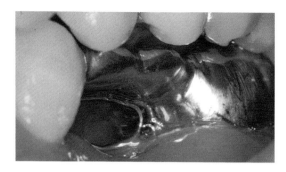

Figure 9.4

The four designs of pontic ridge surface.

a A wash-through pontic with a concave mesio-distal contour.

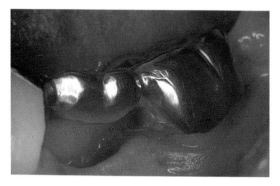

b Wash-through pontic, convex mesio-distally.

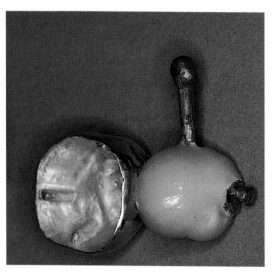

c and *d* Dome-shaped pontics. *c* A molar dome-shaped pontic with the male part of a movable connector and a lingual handle to localize the pontic while soldering to the gold crown. This handle will be removed after the bridge is tried in.

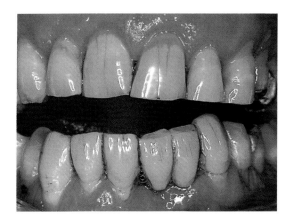

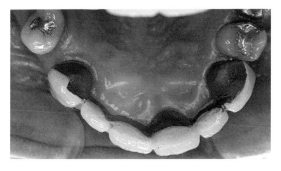

d An acrylic provisional bridge fitted as an immediate replacement for the lower left central and lateral incisors, showing an application of the dome-shaped pontic.

e and *f* Ridge-lap pontics. *e* This bridge has been satisfactory, but the patient complains of food impaction under the single lateral incisor pontic. She can sweep the other side clean with her tongue since the span is longer.

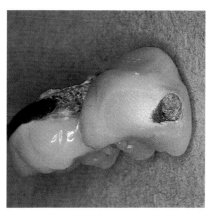

f A modified ridge-lap pontic with contact over the buccal half of the ridge but cut away lingually. The bridge has failed because of a fractured solder joint (see Chapter 13).

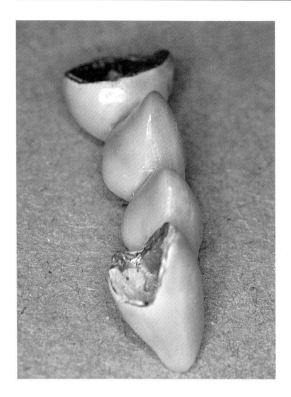

g Typical ridge-lap pontics on another failed bridge. This time the failure was due to loss of retention. Despite the design and the smooth porcelain surface, the ridge beneath these pontics was moderately inflamed.

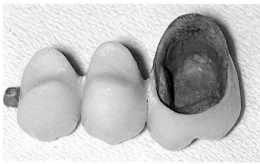

h Saddle-shaped pontics with well-contoured, cleansable connectors.

Wash-through Other terms used for this type of pontic are hygienic and sanitary, but the term wash-through is more descriptive and less suggestive of vitreous china bathroom fittings. The wash-through pontic makes no contact with the soft tissues and so is the easiest to clean. It is used where a pontic is required for functional purposes rather than appearance and is most useful in the lower molar region. Of the two designs shown in Figure 9.4a and b, the concave mesiodistal design is preferred. It is sufficiently strong, uses less metal and leaves a large space for access for the toothbrush or other cleaning aid. The other design derives historically from an early type of proprietary 'sanitary' pontic, which is now obsolete.

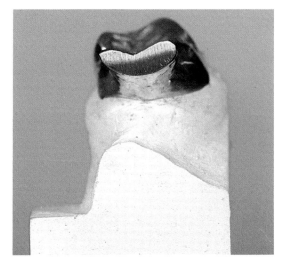

a

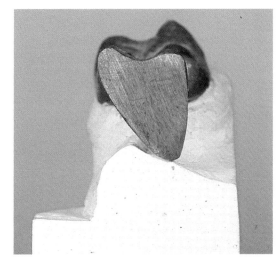

b

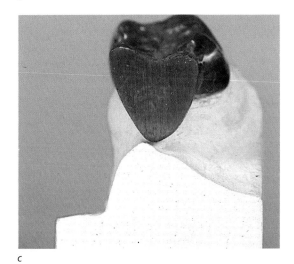

c

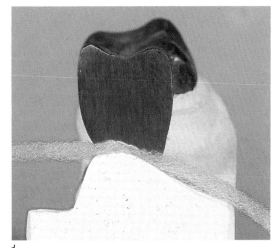

d

Figure 9.5

Four sectioned casts of the same patient, showing the profile of the midpoint of a lower molar edentulous area where a bridge is to be made. The profiles of four pontics are shown:

a A wash-through pontic with no contact with the ridge.
b A dome pontic making point contact on the tip of the ridge.
c A partly modified ridge-lap pontic with a buccal surface resembling a natural tooth but with minimal ridge contact. The difficulty of cleaning the lingual aspect near the ridge is obvious.
d A full-saddle pontic that, if well polished on the gingival surface, would be cleansable with superfloss.

Dome-shaped (see Figure 9.4c, d)   This is the next easiest to clean and is used where the occlusal two-thirds or so of the buccal surface of the pontic show, but not the gingival third. It is commonly used in the lower incisor and premolar regions and sometimes in the upper molar region.

This has also been described as torpedo-shaped or bullet-shaped, but the less aggressive term, dome-shaped, is preferred.

Ridge-lap and modified ridge-lap (see Figure 9.4e, f, g)   The principles of this design are that the buccal surface should look as much like a tooth as possible right up to the ridge, but the lingual surface should be cut away to provide access for cleaning.

Ideally the pontic should have a completely convex lingual surface, making only a line contact along the buccal side of the ridge. But this is often impractical because of the shape of the ridge, and so the modified ridge-lap pontic, which has minimal contact with the ridge from the point of contact on the buccal side up the crest, is often used (see Figure 9.4).

These designs, particularly if the pontic is fairly narrow mesio-distally, as in the case of an incisor or premolar pontic, are sometimes unpopular with patients because they find that food impacts into the space on the lingual side and cannot be readily removed with the tongue (see Figure 9.4e). Besides, considerable manual dexterity is needed to manoeuvre dental floss, tape or other cleaning aid, holding it first against the pontic and then in a secondary cleaning movement against the ridge (see Figure 9.5).

These pontics were designed at a time when there was a lot of concern about the effect of pontics on the soft tissues but before the significance and nature of plaque were as well understood as they are today. They are still commonly used, perhaps through habit and convention. Other designs should also be considered.

Saddle   The saddle pontic is so named because of its shape. It has by the far the largest area of surface contact with soft tissue, and so, although it was popular in the early days of bridgework, it became much less so as dentists became more concerned about the effects of pontics on ridges. Now that it is recognized that plaque can cause inflammation however small the surface area of contact and must be removed in all cases, the emphasis in pontic design has shifted. Accessibility for cleaning and patient comfort and convenience are the important criteria, rather than the size of area of contact. Many patients prefer the saddle-shaped pontic since the lingual surface feels more like a tooth than any other design. With modern cleaning aids, such as superfloss, the ridge surface of properly designed and constructed saddle pontics is relatively easy to clean. This also requires less manual dexterity by the patient than ridge-lap pontics (see Figure 9.5d).

A saddle pontic should closely follow the contour of the ridge but should be smooth on the under surface. It should not displace the soft tissues or cause blanching when it is inserted, but should make snug contact.

The effects of pontics on the ridge
Sometimes when bridges are removed the area of the ridge that was in contact with the pontic has a red appearance. Biopsy studies have shown that there are always some chronic inflammatory cells in this region, but the main explanation for the redness is probably the reduction in keratinization. The surface does not have the normal stimulation from food and the tongue that stimulates keratinization elsewhere. Unless clearly inflamed or ulcerated, the redness is of little clinical consequence (see Figure 9.6).

The occlusal surface

The occlusal surface of the pontic should resemble the occlusal surface of the tooth it replaces. Otherwise it will not serve the same occlusal functions and may not provide sufficient contacts to stabilize the occlusal relationships of its opponents.

In some cases, when occlusal stability is less important (for example when the pontic is opposed by another bridge), the pontic may be made narrower bucco-lingually to improve access for cleaning. Other arguments for narrowing pontics are less convincing (see Chapter 10).

The approximal surfaces

The shape of the mesial and distal surfaces of the pontic will depend upon the design. With fixed–fixed bridges the approximal surface will consist partly of a fixed connector. It is important that the embrasure space between the connector and the gingival tissue be as open as

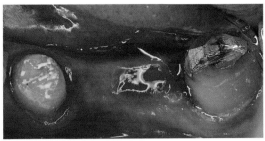

Figure 9.6

a Mucous-membrane reactions under pontics. This area of reduced keratinization under a pontic produced no symptoms. There was no ulceration or bleeding on flossing under the pontic. Although inflammation requiring treatment at the gingival margin of the abutment teeth is present, it is doubtful whether the changes in the remainder of the ridge have had any real significance.

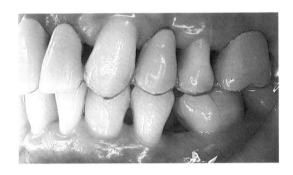

b A much more serious case, with ulceration and a very inflamed mass of granulation tissue. This must clearly be treated in the first place by removal of the bridge. In fact no further treatment was necessary. The inflammation resolved over a three-week period.

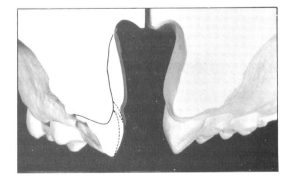

Figure 9.7

Well-contoured open embrasure spaces.

Figure 9.8

Sections through both the lateral incisor areas of the same patient. *Left*: the lateral incisor is present. *Right*: it is missing and the alveolus has resorbed. The profile of the resorbed side has been superimposed on the other to show the extent of the resorption and three ways in which a pontic might be modified to overcome this problem.

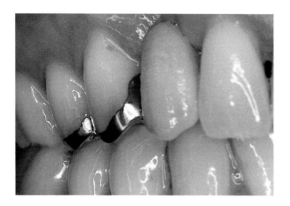

Figure 9.9

Buccal pontic–ridge relationships.

a A pontic replacing an upper canine, where the neck of the pontic has been curved inwards to meet the resorbed alveolar ridge at the correct vertical position. The incisal two-thirds of the buccal surface have been contoured in line with the adjacent teeth so that all the compensation for the missing alveolar bone is in the gingival buccal third. (Note the excessive amount of gold shown by these two partial crowns, in contrast with those in Figure 9.7.)

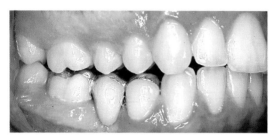

b The same compromise has not been made with this lower premolar pontic, which instead looks too long. This would also create difficulty in cleaning under the pontic.

possible to ensure that there is good access for cleaning, particularly if the pontic is a ridge-lap or saddle pontic (see Figure 9.7). The gingival side of a movable joint is more difficult to leave entirely smooth, and so it is again important that there should be good access for cleaning.

The approximal surface of a cantilever bridge on its free side will simply make normal contact with the adjacent tooth, or in some cases there may be a diastema with no contact. Occasionally, where the span is very short, a cantilever pontic may be made to overlap the adjacent tooth to improve its appearance. In this case the pontic surface in contact with the natural tooth should be as smooth as possible, although it may be slightly concave. If the patient is taught to clean with dental floss, the natural tooth surface should not be any more susceptible to caries than with a normal contact point.

The buccal and lingual surfaces

The buccal surface of a wash-through or dome-shaped pontic does not resemble the shape of a natural buccal surface, particularly gingivally. With ridge-lap and saddle pontics the buccal surface is intended to look as much like a tooth as possible for its entire length. The problem is that when a tooth is missing, so also is some of the alveolar bone that supported it. This means that the alveolar contour where the pontic touches the ridge never looks entirely natural, and the pontic must also be shaped unnaturally to meet the resorbed ridge. Figure 9.8 shows, by means of sections through a study cast, how the ridge contour in a resorbed saddle area necessitates a compromise pontic appearance. Figure 9.9a shows an obvious example of this where an upper canine is missing. Figure 9.9b also shows an example of a case in which this compromise has not been made. The aesthetic result is not good and there is greater difficulty than necessary in cleaning.

No ridge–pontic relationship can ever appear entirely natural, even when the ridge has not resorbed significantly. But at the normal distance from which teeth are seen, the illusion that the tooth emerges from the gum can be sufficiently

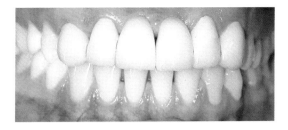

Figure 9.10

An acceptable appearance for a bridge – or is there more than one bridge?

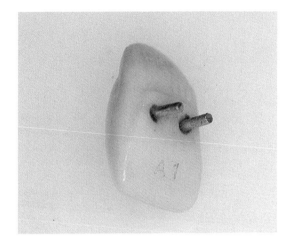

Figure 9.11

A long-pin porcelain pontic facing. The two pins protrude from the palatal surface. The neck (*above*) and the incisal edge are ground to shape before the backing is waxed up to the pontic facing. When the backing is cast, the facing is cemented and the pins cut slightly long and riveted over into two small countersinks on the lingual surface.

convincing: which are the pontics and which are the retainers in Figure 9.10?

The lingual surface of a pontic will be designed as a result of deciding the ridge surface. With ridge-lap pontics, the lingual surface should be smooth and convex.

Materials

The choice for pontics is the same as for retainers. At one time there was also the choice of a number of proprietary pontic facings.

Proprietary pontic facings

Well after the introduction of metal–ceramic materials, until dentists and technicians became more confident with them, many pontics were made with proprietary ceramic pontic facings. Nowadays, however, these facings are not used, and so will not be described in detail. It is only necessary for the practising dentist to recognize the common types and have some idea about maintenance and repair (see Chapter 13).

The commonest type of facing in recent use was the ceramic long-pin facing (see Figure 9.11). Other older types include Steele's flat-back facings in porcelain or acrylic, Trupontics and tube pontics.

The special case of the spring cantilever bridge pontic

Again the bridges are now seldom made, but many patients still have them and they may need maintenance or repair.

Spring cantilever bridge pontics may be metal–ceramic. This means either making the whole spring arm of a metal suitable for bonding to porcelain, or soldering a metal–ceramic pontic to a standard gold bar, when localization is a problem. The bar settles into the tissues for the first two to three weeks after it has been cemented, and so it is better not to complete the pontic until this has happened.

For these reasons the spring cantilever bridge pontic often consists of a separate crown cemented to a core on the end of the bar. The core should have a diaphragm so that the cement junction is not deep under the pontic and difficult to clean.

Connectors

Fixed connectors

There are three types of fixed connector:

● Cast
● Soldered
● Porcelain.

Cast connectors are made by wax patterns of the retainers and pontics connected by wax being produced so that the bridge is cast in a single piece. This has the advantage that a second soldering operation is not required. But the more units there are in the bridge, the more accurate the casting must be. Minor discrepancies in the compensation for the contraction of molten metal that may be acceptable for single-unit casting become unacceptable when magnified several times.

Cast connectors are stronger than soldered connectors, and also it is sometimes possible to disguise their appearance more effectively. For these reasons, multiple-unit bridges are often cast in several sections of three of four units divided through the middle of a pontic. The split pontics are then soldered with high-fusing solder before the porcelain is added, so that all the connectors are cast. The solder joint produced in this way is strong both because it has a larger surface area than if it were at the connector and because it is covered by porcelain, stiffening it.

Soldered connectors are used if the pontics and retainers have to be made separately. This is necessary when they are made of different materials, for example a complete gold crown retainer with a metal–ceramic pontic.

Porcelain connectors are used only in conjunction with all-porcelain bridges. The details of their construction are beyond the scope of this book, but the same principles of accessibility and cleansability still apply.

Movable connectors

Movable connectors are always designed so that the pontic cannot be depressed by occlusal forces. This means that the groove or depression in the minor retainer must always have a good base against which the male part of the attachment can seat. Sometimes, with small pontics and short spans, this is the only force that needs to be resisted, and therefore the female part of the attachment, in the minor retainer, need only be a shallow depression (see Figure 8.3c, page 175). This is the commonest design for fixed–movable minimal-preparation bridges.

However, with longer-span bridges the movable joint must also resist lateral forces applied to the pontic and (assuming the movable joint is mesial) distal forces on the pontic, which would separate the components of the movable connector. In these circumstances the connector is designed as a tapered keyhole-shaped slot so that the pin can move up and down a little and yet seat firmly against the base of the slot, but it cannot move laterally and the connector cannot separate. Examples of this type of connector are shown in Figure 8.3.

There are different ways of producing movable connectors. In the freehand method a wax pattern is produced for the minor retainer with a shallow depression or tapered groove prepared in the wax, the retainer is cast and with a groove, the shape is refined with a tapered bur. The pontic is then waxed up with a finger or ridge to fit into the depression or groove. This is cast and the two parts of the movable joint fitted together before the bridge is taken to the chairside for trying in (see Figure 8.3a).

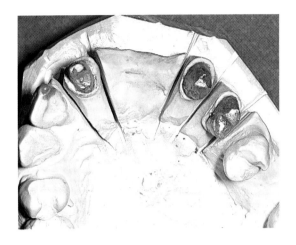

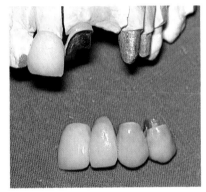

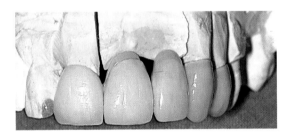

Figure 9.12

Creating a fixed–fixed design with non-parallel abutments.

a The central incisor could not be retracted sufficiently to be parallel to the other abutment teeth even if devitalized and with a post and core fitted. It would interfere with the occlusion.

b and *c* The bridge is made in two parts with separate paths of insertion, and the divided pontic connected in the mouth by cement and a screw attachment.

In some cases a depression or groove may be prepared in an existing cast restoration in the mouth and an impression taken of it together with the other prepared abutment tooth or teeth.

Acrylic, burn-out, patterns are available that may be incorporated into the pontic and minor retainer so that the whole bridge can be waxed up in one operation and the minor retainer and remainder of the bridge invested and cast separately (see Figure 8.3b, page 175).

Proprietary groove-and-ridge precision attachments in metal may also be used as movable connectors, but are generally too retentive and there is the risk that they will not permit sufficient movement. When precision attachments are used, the minor retainer should have more retention to its abutment than would be necessary if a less retentive connector were used.

Screw precision attachment connectors may be used to produce a fixed–fixed bridge by connecting two retainers that cannot be prepared parallel to each other (see Figure 9.12).

Practical points

● Components need to be designed within the context of the whole bridge.

● The criteria for selecting retainers depend on the condition of the abutment teeth, appearance, occlusion, conservation of tooth tissue and cost.

● With pontics it is often necessary to compromise between the best results for cleansability and appearance.

10 Designing and planning bridges

Criteria for selecting a bridge design

No firm rules can be given for selecting any particular design. Bridge design is complex, poorly researched and dominated by personal opinion derived from clinical experience, or lack of it. Many of the ground rules of bridge design were laid down in the first three decades of this century by teachers who were trying to rescue the subject from the purely empirical approach used until that time. Although they were a major advance on what had gone before, these ground rules were not scientifically investigated. Yet they became accepted as irrefutable and remained relatively unaltered for over 50 years, despite a growing understanding in that time of related subjects such as the supporting structures of teeth in health and disease, and of occlusion and jaw function. In this period, great developments have been made in restorative materials and techniques, so that bridges now fit better, look better and are stronger.

This increased understanding and technical development should affect traditional ideas of design to a considerable degree.

In recent years, clinical evidence has been accumulating suggesting that many of the early rules of bridge design should no longer be applied. However, this evidence is not yet sufficiently clear-cut for new, firm rules to be established, leaving today's dentists, including the author, in a state of confusion. A number of criteria may nevertheless be used in choosing a design, although the weight given to each will vary with the circumstances and the opinions held by the operator. It is to be hoped that with further clinical research (which is urgently needed) the relative importance of these criteria will become clearer.

Support

One of the best known rules for bridge design was devised by Ante and described by him in 1926. He suggested that each pontic should be supported by the equivalent of an abutment tooth with at least the same root surface area covered by bone as would have supported the missing tooth; that is, a given area of periodontal membrane could support up to twice its normal occlusal load. The root surface area of an abutment tooth covered by bone is of course reduced following destructive periodontal disease. This has been a guiding principle for many years, and other workers have calculated the average root surface area of all teeth and suggested typical bridge designs based upon these calculations.

This arbitrary, mechanical rule is similar to the engineering principles used for designing bridges across rivers. There are many reports in the literature of experiments (usually carried out in the laboratory on models or in computer simulations) relating occlusal forces to reactions in the supporting structures of teeth. The results of these experiments have tended to reinforce these mechanical ideas of how bridges should be designed.

The evidence now accumulating suggests that these principles are wrong, or at least do not tell the whole story. Provided that any periodontal disease is treated and periodontal health maintained, and provided the occlusal forces are evenly distributed, bridges can be successful with as little as one-quarter of the support advocated by Ante. Such bridges have been successful for many years.

The assumptions made by the engineering school of thought ignore the fact that the occlusal load on a bridge is determined not by extraneous influences, such as lorries driving across road bridges, but by the muscles of mastication. These

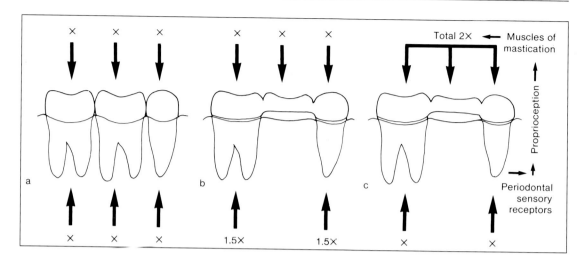

Figure 10.1

Occlusal loading of abutment teeth.

a In an intact dentition an occlusal force, X, is resisted by an equal and opposite force generated within the supporting structures of the tooth.

b When a tooth is extracted and replaced by means of a bridge, engineering principles suggest that the same force, X, delivered to each of the three occlusal surfaces would require the generation of 1.5X in the supporting structures of the two remaining teeth. This principle is no doubt true for inanimate objects but assumes that the occlusal force is constant.

c The occlusal force is of course generated by muscles of mastication, which are under physiological control and do not function independently. Therefore, if the supporting structures of the two remaining teeth are

only capable of generating a resisting force of X, and if they retain a full periodontal sensory mechanism, once force X is exceeded, the proprioceptive mechanism will suppress the contractions of the muscles of mastication so that the force delivered to the three occlusal surfaces totals 2X.

This is an oversimplified version of what happens in real life. Sometimes the sensory mechanism is not intact owing to periodontal disease and alveolar bone loss. The proprioceptive mechanism may be overridden by stimulae from higher centres, producing bruxism or other parafunctional activity. The description also ignores the effect of lateral forces which are more complex. However, the illustration serves to show that bridges should not be designed simply using engineering principles: the biological implications must be taken into account.

are under the control of the neuromuscular mechanism, itself influenced by proprioception from receptors in the periodontal membrane of the teeth supporting the bridge. Comparisons with road bridges are therefore meaningless.

There is plenty of evidence that occlusal loading is modified by the presence or absence of natural teeth and by their condition. For example, patients can generate 10 times as much force between upper and lower natural teeth as they

can between upper and lower complete dentures, where the force is resisted by mucous membrane. It is false logic to assume that increasing the occlusal area of a tooth by adding a pontic to it will inevitably increase the occlusal loading on that tooth. However, forces in an 'unnatural' direction, for example rotational or leverage forces, may not be resisted so well. There is not the same inbuilt mechanism to perceive and control these forces (see Figure 10.1).

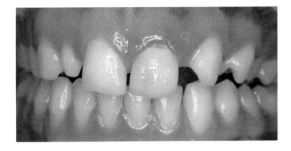

Figure 10.2

Abutment support and length of span.

a A tiny pontic is needed here, and any of the available abutment teeth, which have no alveolar bone loss, would provide more than enough support.

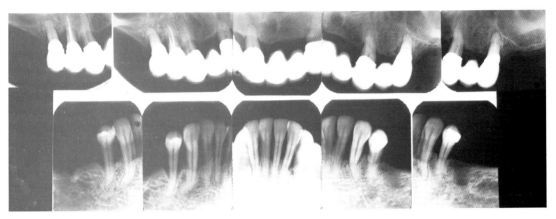

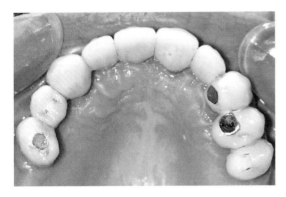

b Radiographs of the six abutment teeth supporting the 10-unit bridge in *c*. All the abutment teeth have less than half their original bone support. For the remaining lower teeth this is also much reduced, but the periodontal treatment has been successful and there has been no increase in bone loss or further mobility.

c The bridge has been satisfactory, with no further bone loss, but the terminal abutment on the left of the picture has had to be root-treated through the retainer. The bridge, which was 9 years old when this photograph was taken, is rather bulbous.

These considerations are often less important in designing small bridges than they are with large bridges. Figure 10.2a shows a case where the span is so small that any of the available abutment teeth would meet all the traditional criteria for support; while in the case of Figure 10.2b a bridge could not be provided if Ante's law were to be observed.

Figure 10.2c shows the bridge for the same patient. It has been successful for many years.

An example of a bridge design that is sometimes unnecessarily destructive because it relies in part on Ante's law for its justification is the replacement of four upper incisor teeth when the canines and first premolar teeth on both sides are used as abutments. Not only is this destructive, it also creates embrasure spaces between the splinted abutment teeth, which are difficult to clean. The premolars are less satisfactory abutments than the canines, and add little to this design. It has been said that occlusal pressure on the pontics, which are in front of a straight line between canine abutments, would produce a tilting force on the canines. However, in a canine-guided occlusion these same teeth will withstand the entire force of lateral excursions and yet often remain the firmest teeth in the arch. Figures 8.1a (page 174) and 11.3a (page 225) show two cases where the canines alone have been used very satisfactorily as abutments. This design, using the two canine teeth as the only abutments, can now be regarded as the normal design for a bridge to replace the four incisor teeth in either the upper or lower jaw. It is not necessary and may be counterproductive to include the first premolar teeth.

The best guidance that can be given for the present is that abutment teeth with healthy periodontal tissues are well able to support a (theoretical) increase in loading in an axial direction by an amount that is virtually unlimited. However, they are not so well able to withstand twisting or levering forces. This means that large bridges of fixed–fixed design can be made with very limited numbers of abutment teeth. The curvature of the bridge around the arch reduces the leverage and twisting forces so that all forces are in the long axis of the abutment teeth (see Figure 10.2c). This is the principle of 'cross-arch splinting', and it may be extended so that in ideal circumstances long cantilever extensions of several units may be carried by such bridges (see Figure 8.5, page 178). However, these long cantilevers cannot be supported by individual abutment teeth. They would produce a leverage or twisting force on the abutment tooth causing movement of the tooth in the same way as an orthodontic appliance, or they would loosen the tooth.

The application of these principles of support is illustrated in a series of examples at the end of this chapter, and more practical advice on selecting abutment teeth is also given later in the chapter.

Conservation of tooth tissue

Clearly the most conservative design is a minimal-preparation bridge. This is therefore the design of choice whenever possible, but in many cases it is not.

All conventional bridges are potentially destructive, and some are immediately so. Figures 9.1 (page 192) and 10.3 show a case in which a bridge was made before the introduction of minimal-preparation bridges. The bridge has remained stable and satisfactory. A conventional bridge necessitated extensive destruction of sound tooth tissue. Although this is unfortunate, the alternatives of leaving the space or of providing a partial denture were even more unacceptable.

It was reasonable to use a bridge design as conservative of tooth tissue as possible, at the same time being compatible with other principles. In this example a simple cantilever bridge was used with only one abutment tooth rather than fixed–fixed or fixed–movable designs that would have involved more abutment teeth.

Cleansability

Figure 9.2b (page 193) shows an example in which an upper first premolar is missing. If it is decided that a simple cantilever design using either the upper canine or the upper second premolar will not give sufficient support, the choice will be between a fixed–fixed or fixed–movable design, or a cantilever bridge using the premolar and first molar splinted together as the abutments. This latter design will be more difficult for the patient to clean than the others because of the fixed connector between the premolar and molar tooth. This consideration may determine the choice of design.

Abutment teeth towards the front of the mouth are easier for patients to clean than those further back, partly because of access and partly because the bucco-lingual width of the contact areas is greater with posterior teeth.

Appearance

The example shown in Figure 9.2b may again be used to illustrate the way in which the appearance of the bridge may be one of the factors in determining its design. If a fixed–fixed design is used, in this case it will be necessary to make either a complete crown or a partial crown

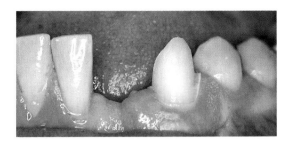

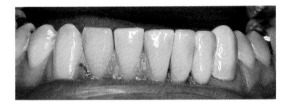

Figure 10.3

a and *b* A cantilever bridge with a single lower canine abutment tooth and two incisor pontics (only one tooth is missing). One reason for this design was to conserve tooth tissue, in particular the lower incisors. There would additionally be difficulty with preparing parallel abutments as illustrated in Figure 9.1 (page 192). This bridge was made before the days of minimal-preparation bridges or implants, which would now solve this problem. It has, however, been successful for several years, with no rotation, mobility or bone loss.

(which will have gold showing on the incisal edge) for the upper canine. Neither of these is likely to be as attractive as the natural tooth. With a complete crown it will be difficult to produce the distinctive characteristics of the buccal surface of the natural tooth. A fixed–movable design, on the other hand, can have a minor retainer that consists only of a distal–palatal inlay in the canine carrying a slot for the movable connector. This means that the appearance of the buccal surface of the canine will be left undisturbed.

Thus consideration of support, a conservative approach to tooth preparation, cleansability and appearance lead to a decision in the case illustrated in Figure 9.2b to make the bridge fixed–movable rather than fixed–fixed or cantilever.

Planning bridges

Collecting information about the patient

Chapter 5 includes a detailed review of the history and examination of a patient for whom crowns are being considered. The same approach should be taken with a patient for a bridge. There are, however, a number of additional considerations relating to bridges. These are listed below

and should be read in conjunction with the relevant paragraphs in Chapter 5.

Consideration of the whole patient

With crowns, the choice may be between crowning a tooth or extracting it, and the decision may well be to make a crown even though many factors, for example, the patient's age, attitude to treatment or oral hygiene are less than ideal. With bridges, there is often the alternative of a partial denture, a minimal-preparation bridge or a conventional bridge, and so it may not be necessary to make so many compromises. If there is any doubt, it is better to make a partial denture first.

Clinical examination

Assessing abutment teeth Any tooth that can be crowned can also be considered as an abutment tooth, but the abutment tooth may have to withstand forces from different directions than one crowned as an individual tooth (see Figure 3.6 page 48).

Teeth with active periodontal disease should not be used as abutment teeth, although many with reduced alveolar support following successful treatment of periodontal disease can be used.

They are commonly splinted to other abutment teeth to give mutual support.

Some dentists prefer to avoid root-filled teeth or teeth needing post crowns because of the chances of fracture of the roots. However, this risk exists whether or not the tooth is used as an abutment tooth. It may even be reduced if the tooth is used as one of a number of abutment teeth in a larger bridge, so that the force of a blow to the tooth is shared by the other abutments. Given the choice between a tooth with a post crown as an abutment and a perfectly sound tooth, it is more conservative of tooth tissue to use the former. Although some surveys have shown a higher incidence of failure with post crowns than other forms of retainer, these figures are similar to the failure rate for individual post-retained crowns.

There may be no suitable alternative abutment to a root-filled tooth, and the choice is then between using the tooth or not making a bridge.

Length of span   Any design of bridge may be used for short spans of one premolar or incisor width. Simple cantilever bridges may be used to replace one or even two anterior teeth with only one strong abutment tooth, provided the occlusion avoids excessive lateral forces on the pontics (see Figure 10.3). Spring cantilever bridges should not be used for more than one upper incisor pontic. Unilateral posterior cantilever bridges should be limited to one pontic and only used when the occlusion is favourable. The difference between anterior and posterior cantilever bridges is that with anterior bridges the forces on the abutment teeth are more horizontal than occlusal, and anterior teeth are better able to withstand additional lateral forces than are posterior teeth. In particular, posterior teeth tend to tilt mesially in any case, and a cantilever pontic attached to the mesial surface of the abutment tooth increases this tendency as a result of occlusal forces on the pontic. Small posterior cantilever bridges should therefore be designed cautiously, and preference given to the fixed–movable design where possible. Molar teeth are better abutments for cantilever bridges than premolars. Longer spans of cantilever pontics may be used in conjunction with large cross-arch splinted bridges.

Fixed–movable bridges are usually limited to spans of two or three premolar size units. Beyond this, movement at the movable joint may become excessive, although much longer spans have been successful.

Fixed–fixed bridges may be used for any size of span. It is common to find all four incisor teeth missing, and the design of bridge used to replace these is almost always fixed–fixed with the canine teeth as the only abutments.

Occlusion   Not only should the occlusion of the remaining teeth be assessed, as described in Chapter 4, but the potential occlusion of the pontic with the opposing teeth should also be assessed. In some cases the occlusal relationships of the potential abutment teeth will help determine which should be used and which design of bridge is suitable. Figure 10.4 shows two cases: one suitable and one unsuitable for a simple cantilever bridge replacing the upper lateral incisor, with the canine as the only abutment tooth. The difference between them is the way the lower incisors relate to the space when the mandible is moved in the protrusive lateral direction. In the second case two abutment teeth will be necessary: either the canine and the first premolar with a cantilever design, or the canine and central incisor with a fixed–fixed or fixed–movable design.

Shape of ridge   The contour of the saddle area will be taken into account in determining whether a bridge with a movable buccal veneer or a partial denture should be made (see Chapters 7 and 8), or whether surgical ridge augmentation should be considered (see Figure 7.9, pages 162–3).

When a bridge is to be made, the shape of the ridge will affect the appearance of the pontic, and if this is likely to be a critical factor, in other words if the neck of the pontic shows and the patient is very concerned about their appearance, then one of the procedures described below should be followed to ensure an acceptable final result.

Predicting the final result

The final appearance of the bridge can be predicted using the study casts, by various intra-oral trials or by means of a provisional bridge. Sometimes combinations of these methods are

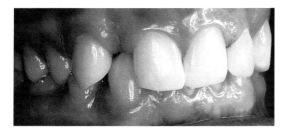

Figure 10.4

Occlusal assessment.

a A missing lateral incisor with deep overbite. The lower canine tooth touches the palate. There would be insufficient space for a minimal-preparation bridge without orthodontic treatment or extensive reduction of upper or lower teeth.

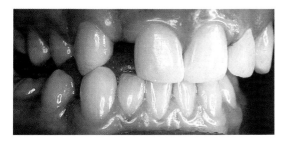

b The same patient in a right lateral excursion. The occlusion is canine-guided and the lower teeth are clear of the upper lateral incisor space, so that a simple cantilever bridge with the canine as the sole abutment would be satisfactory. The occlusion of the patient shown in Figure 8.1c (page 174) is similar.

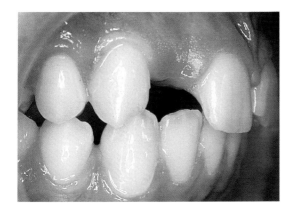

c In this case the lower incisor passes through the upper lateral incisor space in right lateral excursion, such that group anterior guidance will be inevitable, with pressure on the palatal surface of the pontic unless it is shortened or proclined to an aesthetically unacceptable degree. A cantilever bridge with one abutment tooth would carry the risk of acting as an orthodontic appliance and rotating the abutment tooth.

necessary. In straightforward cases the dentist and technician will have a good idea of what the final bridge will look like, but the patient will be less clear. The prediction is therefore for the patient's benefit. In other cases where there are unusual features, the dentist and technician may not realize the full aesthetic implications of attempting to make a bridge, or their understanding may be different. In these cases the patient is likely to be even more confused.

Many patients who complain about bridges after they are fitted are unhappy with their appearance. Not only is it good planning to predict the final appearance of the bridge and seek the patient's acceptance before starting, but a record of the predicted appearance may also be useful from a dento-legal point of view should the patient eventually complain.

As well as the appearance of the final bridge, potential difficulties in preparing the teeth should be predicted when possible. These include problems with retention and path of insertion, and the possibility of endangering the pulps of the abutment teeth.

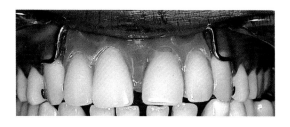

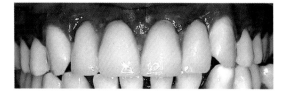

Figure 10.5

An intra-oral trial.

a A partial denture replacing four incisor teeth, which is to be replaced by a bridge. There is a buccal flange and a midline diastema.

b Denture teeth set on a wax baseplate being tried-in to ensure that the patient is happy about the appearance of pontics without a buccal flange or the midline diastema. Periodontal treatment will be provided before a bridge is made. The bridge will be six units, with the upper canines as the two abutment teeth.

Study casts

A second study cast should be poured of the arch in which the bridge is to be made. It is sufficient simply to cast the alginate impression a second time, if it can be removed from the initial cast intact. Alternatively, two impressions should be taken or the study cast duplicated in the laboratory.

The second study cast may be used for trial preparations to predict the problems outlined above as well as problems of the individual abutment preparation (see Figure 5.3c, d and e, page 91). The prepared study cast may be used to make a trial or diagnostic wax-up of the bridge to show to the patient. This is particularly useful when the shape of the abutment teeth will be altered by the retainer crowns or where orthodontic treatment is planned prior to bridge construction.

There are often alternative means of replacing missing teeth, and these change appearances in different ways. Figure 5.3 shows modified study casts illustrating two ways of changing the appearance that would be difficult to describe to the patient. Neither is ideal, and so the patient must be warned that compromise is necessary. The work should not be started until the patient understands and accepts this.

If the patient is to be shown the study cast, it is best to produce the wax-up in ivory-coloured wax, or to duplicate the waxed-up cast. The patient can thus look at a cast without the distraction of the contrast between the artificial stone and coloured wax. Most find it easier to compare the second, modified study cast with the first, rather than with themselves, partly because study casts look so artificial to them that they are better comparing two similarly artificial objects, but also of course because they have difficulty in relating a study cast, which is how others see them, to a reversed, mirror image of themselves. Other precautions are detailed in Chapter 5.

Intra-oral trials

Partial dentures   Many patients who are to have anterior bridges already have a partial denture. If the appearance of the artificial tooth on the denture is satisfactory and can be duplicated in a bridge, no further trial is necessary. However, if the denture carries a buccal flange, it is wise to try a denture tooth in the mouth without a buccal flange, usually attached to a simple wax or shellac base, to show the patient the effect (see Figure 10.5). The change can be dramatic. This form of intra-oral trial is suitable only when the shape of abutment teeth is not to be changed.

Other reversible intra-oral modifications

The size of potential abutment teeth can be increased by the addition of wax or composite attached by the acid-etch technique. In some cases a pontic can also be temporarily attached to adjacent teeth by means of composite. These modifications may be useful when predicting the final result, but are limited in that it is only possible to increase and not decrease the size of the teeth.

Temporary and provisional bridges

Once the preparations for a conventional bridge have been made in the mouth, it is possible to make a provisional bridge in the laboratory with acrylic, preferably incorporating acrylic denture teeth, or specially made facings. These provisional bridges are rather more permanent than temporary bridges (usually made at the chairside), which are only intended to last for two or three weeks while the permanent bridge is being made. One of the purposes of a provisional bridge is to allow further modifications to the shape of the bridge for aesthetic reasons or as modifications to the occlusion until both the dentist and patient are satisfied with the result. These modifications are then incorporated into the permanent bridge. The provisional bridge can also be removed and adjusted to allow periodontal or endodontic treatment as necessary.

An example of the value of a provisional bridge is in a patient who has had orthodontic treatment retracting the upper canines to make room for lateral incisors. The canines may relapse mesially, but this is not inevitable, and so it is unnecessarily destructive to make three-unit bridges as a matter of course, to prevent relapse: a two-unit cantilever bridge may be sufficient. The problem is to make the right prediction. Provisional two-unit cantilever bridges using the canines as abutments may be made in acrylic if the abutment teeth are to be prepared for a conventional bridge; alternatively a Rochette provisional may be made. The patient is then reviewed frequently with the aid of study casts taken when the bridges are first inserted to check for early signs of relapse. If relapse has not occurred within six months, the provisional bridges can be replaced with permanent ones. At the first sign of relapse, the provisional bridges are replaced by three-unit bridges.

Another example of the use of a provisional bridge is as an immediate insertion replacement of a tooth to be extracted. If the permanent bridge is to be a conventional design, the abutment teeth are prepared and the bridge made before the tooth is extracted – the preparation being protected by separate temporary crowns. If the permanent bridge is to be a minimal-preparation design, a Rochette type should be used to facilitate removal and modification as the extraction socket heals.

Practical steps in choosing a bridge design

So far, all the discussion of bridge design has been rather theoretical and somewhat inconclusive. This is inevitable, since designing bridges is still rather more of an art than a science. It is based partly on the clinical experience of the dentist, which will vary from person to person, and on the clinical condition of the patient, which again will vary. However, the design process has to start somewhere. Examples at the end of this chapter illustrate the logical steps in this process.

General approach

A list should be made of all the likely designs for a bridge in the case being considered. This should include the potential abutment teeth and their retainers, together with the basic design of bridge (fixed–fixed, fixed–movable, conventional, minimal-preparation and so on). In a simple case when the dentist is experienced, the list can be made mentally. For the less experienced and for more complex cases, it is helpful to write it down.

Every design is considered in turn and advantages and disadvantages listed.

In some cases, the optimum design will be obvious from this procedure. In others, further investigations with modified study casts, intra-oral trials or provisional bridges may be required.

Details of stages in the design process: Selecting abutment teeth

1 After the general examination of the patient and whole mouth, individual potential abutment teeth should be examined and a note made of

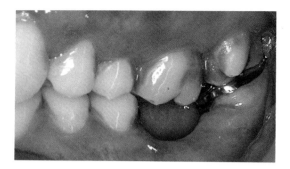

Figure 10.6

The upper first molar has over-erupted. It should be ground level to the occlusal plane prior to a lower bridge being made, in order to avoid occlusal interferences in lateral excursions. In some cases the tooth should be intruded to the original occlusal plane orthodontically.

the presence of caries or restorations and the extent and quality of any restoration present.

2 The periodontal state should be examined, including the presence of plaque and other deposits, gingival bleeding and periodontal pockets.

3 The vitality and mobility of the tooth should be tested and a periapical radiograph obtained.

4 Usually any major problems with the individual tooth should be dealt with first by appropriate treatment, but sometimes the more sensible solution is to extract the tooth and replace it as an additional pontic on the bridge, rather than retain a dubious tooth as an abutment when its presence may well jeopardize the future of the whole bridge. An example of this is where three lower incisor teeth are already missing and the fourth has very little bone support. The lower canines are sound and will make good abutment teeth. They will have to be used in any case to support the bridge. Including the remaining incisor will not add significantly to the support of the bridge and may detract from its long-term prognosis.

5 A judgement must be made as to the prognosis of all the teeth in the vicinity of the bridge to reduce the risk of another tooth having to be extracted shortly after the bridge is made

Selecting the retainers

The list of potential alternative retainers may include complete and partial crowns and minimal-preparation retainers. The choice of a complete crown is inevitable when the tooth is already heavily restored or the appearance of a partial crown would be unacceptable.

The choice between a crown and a minimal-preparation retainer will depend upon whether the abutment teeth have restorations in them, the occlusal clearance and the appearance of the abutment teeth. If the only difficulty with minimal-preparation retainers is the lack of occlusal clearance, it may be possible to create sufficient clearance by reducing the opposing teeth, partly preparing the enamel of the abutment teeth or moving them orthodontically. Sometimes a combination of these approaches is possible.

Selecting the pontics and connectors

The design of pontics and connectors is the responsibility of the dentist and not the technician. Detailed instructions should be given to the technician, particularly on the contour of the ridge surface of the pontic (see Chapter 9). When the technician is unfamiliar with the dentist's usual requirements, the details of the design should be drawn and sent to the technician as part of the prescription for the bridge. Where a metal–ceramic pontic is to be made, the dentist should indicate where the porcelain should be finished. In some cases an all-porcelain occlusal surface is required; in others the porcelain covers only the buccal surface and buccal cusp, leaving the remainder of the occlusal surface in metal. Again, this should be specified.

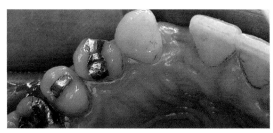

a

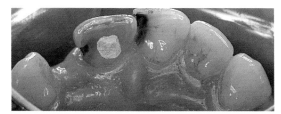

b

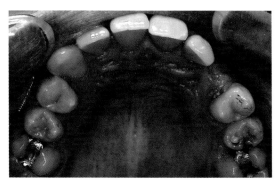

c

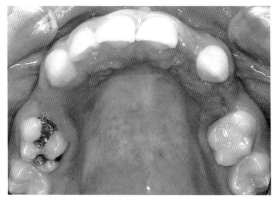

d

Figure 10.7

Bridge designs for single missing incisors.

a A missing upper lateral incisor with rotated canine and first premolar teeth. There is a Class 2 Division II incisor relationship with a deep overbite and minimal overjet. This means that no space is available for a minimal-preparation bridge, although orthodontic treatment might create some space. A fixed–fixed bridge using the central incisor and canine would be even more destructive of sound tooth tissue than usual, since they are not parallel. There would also be a risk of the central incisors not matching exactly. Splinting the rotated canine and first premolar together for a cantilever bridge would be possible, but would produce an awkward embrasure space that would be difficult to clean. Fortunately the occlusion is satisfactory for a simple cantilever bridge using just the canine tooth as the abutment, and its rotation can be corrected with a full crown. The first premolar has a failed amalgam restoration, which will be replaced separately with a porcelain inlay or composite restoration to improve the appearance.

b Another missing lateral incisor, this time with one discoloured, non-vital, root-filled central incisor and a large mesial carious lesion in the other. The central incisors are also misaligned. The canine is sound. Since the occlusion is not favourable for a cantilever bridge using only one abutment tooth, both central incisors will be crowned and connected to each other, and to a cantilevered lateral incisor pontic, once caries and periodontal disease elsewhere has been controlled.

c A missing upper canine tooth. These are difficult to replace by bridges when the occlusion will be guided by the pontic in lateral excursions, and in these cases several abutment teeth may be necessary. By grinding the lower canine slightly and leaving the pontic slightly short, it was possible to maintain group function in this patient rather than produce canine guidance by the pontic. The two premolar teeth were connected as abutments for a three-unit cantilever bridge. This design was chosen in preference to a fixed–fixed bridge so that preparing the sound, matching and well-aligned incisor teeth could be avoided.

A fixed–movable design with an inlay in the distal surface of the lateral incisor would not have been practicable, because the angulation of the lateral incisor would prevent a common path of insertion between the first premolar and a groove in an inlay in the incisor. This design would have been possible (although not desirable) if the lateral incisor had been more proclined.

A minimal-preparation bridge could be considered, but there is a greater risk of loss of retention with this occlusal relationship.

d A complicated case. If the only tooth missing was the upper lateral incisor then the ideal bridge design would probably be to cantilever a minimum-preparation bridge from the canine tooth. However this tooth is needed to help retain a bridge replacing the two premolar teeth. Therefore the design to replace the lateral incisor consisted of a minimum-preparation bridge cantilevered from the central incisor. The two premolar spaces were both restored by minimum-preparation, fixed–fixed bridges with the canine and first molar teeth as abutments.

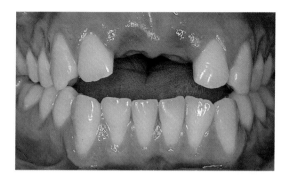

Figure 10.8

Replacing more than one tooth.

a With an anterior open bite and normal lateral incisors, a four-unit fixed–fixed minimal-preparation bridge with the lateral incisors as the abutment teeth would be satisfactory. There is no need to include the canine teeth.

This design is also acceptable in some cases where there is normal occlusion between the anterior teeth, but the left and right lateral excursions are canine-guided. In such cases the design may be minimal-preparation or conventional.

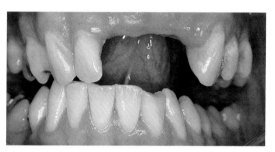

b Even with three incisors missing, with the occlusion being protected in right lateral excursion by a sound canine (shown here), the lateral incisor may be used as the only abutment on the right side for a five-unit fixed–fixed conventional bridge. The bridge could be extended to include the right canine, giving additional support and a more symmetrical appearance, but this would make the embrasure space between the lateral incisor and canine difficult to clean and would be unnecessarily destructive.

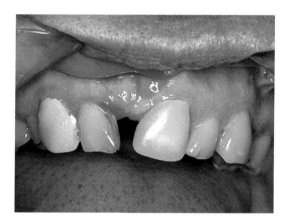

c and *d* The central incisor space is now reduced to approximately one-quarter of its proper width, although this is somewhat difficult to judge since the left central incisor has an acrylic jacket crown. The right canine also has an unsatisfactory acrylic crown. Trial wax-ups showed that a satisfactory appearance could be obtained by extracting the non-vital lateral incisor and making a four-unit fixed–fixed bridge. Both central incisors and the lateral incisor pontic would be small, but would give a better appearance than two large central incisors with the midline offset even further. The alternative of orthodontic treatment prior to bridgework was offered to the patient and declined. This is a similar problem to that of another patient, shown in Figure 7.7, page 160.

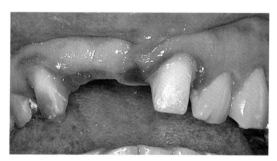

d The upper lateral incisor has been extracted and the two abutment teeth prepared. It is now clear that there will be sufficient space for the planned treatment. A provisional bridge will be fitted and periodontal treatment provided before impressions are taken for the permanent bridge.

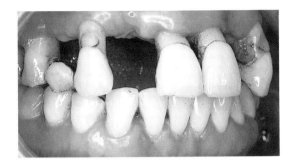

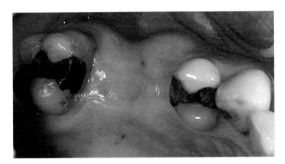

e Existing crowns and bridges following extensive, successful periodontal treatment and the extraction of the lateral incisors. None of the remaining teeth is a satisfactory abutment for a simple small bridge, and a partial denture replacing the lateral incisors and the totally unsatisfactory premolar pontic would be damaging to the periodontal tissues. A splint/bridge incorporating the principle of cross-arch splinting is indicated here.

f Sound restored abutment teeth and a span that will accommodate one premolar and one molar pontic. The buccal surface of the premolar is sound and of good appearance, and so one design could be a fixed–movable conventional bridge with a full crown on the molar tooth and an MOD inlay (without cuspal protection) in the premolar. The movable joint will be accommodated in the distal box of the inlay. A hybrid bridge would not be suitable, since the restoration in the molar tooth is too large for this tooth to have a minimal-preparation retainer.

Planning the occlusion

Details of this stage were given in Chapter 4. The first decision to be made is whether to articulate study casts and, if so, whether it is necessary to use a simple-hinge, semi-adjustable or fully adjustable articulator. With small bridges it is helpful to mount casts on a semi-adjustable articulator. With most large bridges a semi-adjustable or fully adjustable articulator should be used.

The second decision is whether any occlusal adjustment is necessary prior to tooth preparations for the bridge. With posterior bridgework it is often necessary to adjust an over-erupted opposing tooth (see Figure 10.6). The anticipated occlusal relationship of the pontic with the opposing teeth may influence the basic design of the bridge as well as the details of the occlusal surface of the pontic, and so, although this step is listed as the final one in the sequence, and it is usually considered last, if the bridge design is influenced by it, it will be necessary to introduce feedback loops to earlier stages.

Examples of the bridge-design process

See Figures 10.7 and 10.8 for practical examples, and the reasons for the choice; some alternative designs, and the reasons for rejecting them, are given.

Dentists will inevitably become biased in their selection of bridge designs by their own experience of clinical success and failure. Indeed, the author's own bias may be detected, for example, in the section on spring cantilever bridges and in Figures 10.7 and 10.8. Care should be taken to prevent this bias overriding more substantial clinical criteria.

As an additional example, the table on page 220 sets out over 30 different designs for the replacement of one upper lateral incisor. Some of the suggestions on this list are a little bizarre and would only be used under unusual circumstances. For example, it would not be common to splint together the central incisors as one of the abutments (No. 6 on the list), since in most cases

Alternative designs for a bridge to replace |2

	Basic design	Abutment teeth	Retainers	
*1	Fixed–fixed	|1 and |3	|1 FC	|3 FC
2			|1 PC	|3 PC
3			|1 FC	|3 PC
4			|1 PC	|3 FC
*5			|1 MP	|3 MP
6		1 |1 and |3	1 |1 FC	|3 FC
7			1 |1 MP	|3 MP
8	Fixed–movable	|1 and |3	|1 FC	|3 FC
9			|1 PC	|3 PC
10			|1 FC	|3 PC
11			|1 FC	|3 PC
12			|1 Cl III	|3 FC
13			|1 Cl III	|3 PC
*14	Cantilever	|3		|3 FC
15				|3 PC
*16				|3 MP
17		|3 and |4	|3 FC	|4 FC
18			|3 PC	|4 PC
19			|3 FC	|4 PC
20			|3 PC	|4 FC
21			|3 MP	|3 MP
*22		|1		|1 FC
23				|1 PC
*24				|1 MP
25		1 |1		1 |1 FC
26				1 |1 PC
*27				1 |1 MP
28	Spring cantilever	|4 and |5	|4 FC	|5 FC
29			|4 PC	|5 PC
30			|4 FC	|5 PC
31		|6		|6 FC
32				|6 PC
33		|7		|7 FC
34				|7 PC
35		|4		|4 FC
36				|4 PC
37		|5		|5 FC
38				|5 PC

Key: FC: full crown
PC: partial crown
MP: minimal-preparation
Cl III: Cl III inlay

Several of these designs would only be considered in unusual circumstances. The most common designs are indicated with an asterisk. In addition, when the adjacent teeth are sound, and in particular when the anterior teeth are spaced, a single-tooth implant may well be the treatment of choice.

just one central incisor would be sufficient. In other cases, however, the upper lateral incisor would be replaced almost incidentally as part of a much larger splint. In that case all the upper incisors and perhaps teeth further back in the arch would also be included.

So the list could be further extended to show an even greater variety of potential abutment teeth, and even further to show the choice of materials. The important point is to show the enormous variety of designs possible and the dangers inherent in becoming too reliant upon a limited number or an over-simplified 'cookery-book' approach to designing bridges.

Practical points

● Criteria for planning bridges are similar to those for crowns.

However:
● With bridges, a partial denture can first be tried and later replaced by a bridge if necessary.

● Teeth with active periodontal disease should be avoided as abutment teeth.

● The contour of the saddle area will be taken into consideration in deciding on whether a bridge, a bridge with removable buccal veneer or a partial denture should be made.

● It is best to predict the final appearance of the bridge using trial wax-ups on study casts and to ensure the patient's acceptance from the outset.

● The use of provisional bridges allows for further modification before final fitting of the permanent bridge.

11

Clinical techniques for bridge construction

This chapter should be read in conjunction with Chapter 6. Many of the techniques are identical, and so this chapter will deal only with those that are peculiar to bridges or where a different emphasis is necessary.

Pre-operative procedures

All the planning stages described in Chapters 5, 6 and 10 should be undertaken. In particular, the shade should be taken and an impression for the opposing cast made. The following additional pre-operative procedures may also be required.

Occlusal adjustment

It is more often necessary to carry out an occlusal adjustment in preparation for a bridge than for crowns. A new impression must be taken for the opposing cast, since the study cast will obviously no longer be accurate.

Additional space for anterior minimal-preparation retainers can be produced by using a Dahl appliance (see Chapter 6).

Preparations for a temporary bridge

It must be decided whether a temporary bridge will be made or whether the patient will be left with individual temporary restorations to protect the abutment teeth. When the patient has a satisfactory temporary denture and especially if the design is a cantilever or fixed–movable conventional bridge or any design of minimal-preparation bridge, it is often better to make separate temporary restorations rather than a temporary bridge. When the design is fixed–movable and the paths of insertion of the retainers will not be parallel to each other, it may be impractical to make a temporary bridge. Besides, when a minor retainer such as a distal–occlusal inlay is to be made for a fixed–movable bridge, the temporary bridge (which will be fixed–fixed) may loosen at the minor retainer.

However, in many cases, particularly for larger fixed–fixed conventional bridges, a temporary bridge is essential to protect the abutment teeth and to retain their relationship with each other and the opposing teeth. Temporary bridges may be made in one of two ways: either by one of the chairside techniques described in Chapter 6, or by making an acrylic temporary bridge on the study cast, using the trial preparations, and then relining and adjusting this at the chairside as necessary.

If a chairside technique is to be used, a trial wax-up on the study cast should be made and duplicated (by means of an alginate or elastomeric impression) to make a stone cast. A vacuum-formed PVC slip can then be produced (see Figure 6.17, page 124). Alternatively, a silicone impression of the waxed-up study cast may be used directly in the mouth to make the temporary bridge.

Figure 11.1 shows a laboratory-made temporary bridge, constructed before the teeth are prepared so that it can be adapted and cemented at the tooth preparation visit. Techniques for constructing chairside temporary bridges are described later.

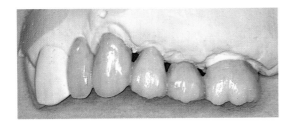

Figure 11.1

A laboratory-made temporary acrylic bridge (see also Figure 9.4d).

Preparing the abutment teeth

Paralleling techniques for conventional preparations

When the design of a conventional bridge requires two or more teeth to be prepared in a common path of insertion, special techniques are used to ensure that there are no undercuts and yet each individual preparation is as retentive as possible. These are listed in increasing order of complexity.

Paralleling by eye

Two or three teeth close together can be made parallel by eye. The clinician will become more adept at doing this with experience, and should concentrate on developing the skill. In the anterior part of the mouth it is possible to see along the long axis of the teeth by direct vision. Only one eye should be used, since binocular vision can 'see around' undercuts. Figure 11.2a shows a dentist assessing the path of insertion of the upper canine teeth, which are being prepared for a bridge replacing the four incisor teeth. It helps to look from as far away as possible. It may also be useful to make a small pencil mark on the two surfaces that may still be undercut. An assessment of parallelism or undercut can then be made by closing one eye and moving the head so that one of the pencil marks just disappears and then continuing to move the head until the other pencil mark appears.

In the lower jaw and in posterior parts of the mouth large mirrors are useful to show all the preparations in the same field. Parallelism cannot be assessed satisfactorily when two or more preparations can be seen only by moving the small mouth mirror. Many of the photographs in this book have been taken in larger, front-surface-reflecting mirrors (see Figure 11.2b).

It is also helpful to use a straight probe like a laboratory surveyor, but in the mouth. The probe is placed against one of the prepared tooth surfaces, and then, held rigidly, it is moved over to the other abutment tooth without its angulation being changed. This is not a completely reliable guide of course, and will detect only fairly gross undercuts or overtaper. But many clinicians do find it useful (see Figure 11.2c).

Extra-oral survey

With larger bridges and when teeth are prepared on both sides of the arch, the simplest and most reliable method of assessing parallelism is to take a simple impression (usually in alginate) once the basic reduction has been carried out on all the abutment teeth. The impression is cast at the chairside in a fast-setting plaster, usually with an accelerator such as alum added. The cast is then surveyed at the chairside and further preparation carried out as required (see Figure 11.3). The procedure may be repeated several times with more difficult cases or with large numbers of abutment teeth. When the abutments are satisfactory for the path of insertion, the final smoothing and finishing of the preparations is carried out.

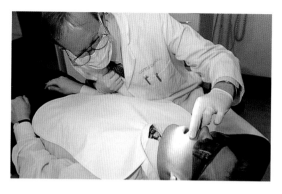

Figure 11.2

Clinical methods of assessing parallelism of bridge abutment preparations.

a Using direct vision, from a distance with one eye closed when, for example, upper canine teeth are being prepared for a fixed–fixed bridge.

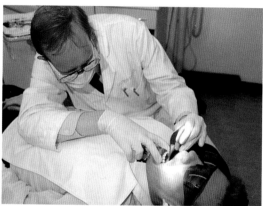

b Using a full arch mirror for the same purpose in the lower jaw. Full arch mirrors are used in clinical photography and many of the photographs in this book were taken with one of these large mirrors.

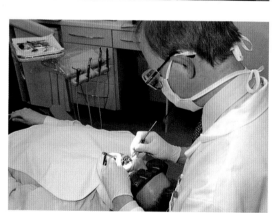

c Using a straight probe as an 'intra oral surveyor'. The operator must stay very still other than moving the probe round the abutment teeth in a controlled fashion. This, on its own, may not be enough but gives a guide to the presence of undercuts. Operators who make a significant number of bridges develop considerable skill in this technique.

Paralleling devices for crown preparations

Many of the devices available are cumbersome, unreliable or extremely expensive. One of the simpler ones consists of a stainless-steel mirror with vertical lines scribed on it. This is placed buccally or lingually and used to assess the mesiodistal parallelism of abutment preparations. It cannot be used for the buccal–lingual surfaces. Another device consists of a clear plastic disc with a pin passing through it. This is held against the occlusal surfaces and can be moved around,

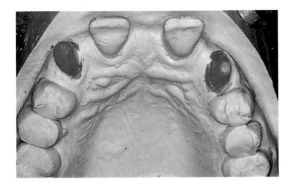

Figure 11.3

Surveying preparations.

a Initial preparations have been carried out on the upper canine teeth in the mouth and this cast has been made from an alginate impression. The two preparations have been varnished. The bridge will be a six-unit immediate insertion provisional bridge, and the two remaining incisors with extensive alveolar bone loss will be extracted.

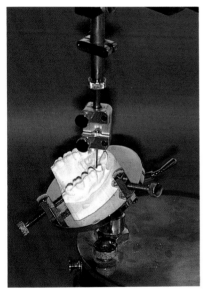

b The preparations are surveyed with a fine rod, and the cast is trimmed until they are parallel. Trimmed areas show up in contrast to the untouched varnished areas. Similar reduction is carried out in the mouth. The process may need to be repeated.

acting as a surveyor. These two devices may be useful, but the inexperienced dentist is better advised to master the basic techniques of surveying by eye and extra-oral surveying.

Preparations for minimal-preparation bridges

Since the introduction of minimal-preparation bridges, there have been fluctuations in fashion as to the degree of tooth preparation that should be carried out. Initially very little preparation was undertaken, and then over the next few years various authors recommended more and more extensive preparation with finishing lines, seating grooves at right angles to the path of insertion and location grooves in the line of the path of insertion all being advocated. Some dentists even went as far as using operating microscopes and complicated paralleling devices.

There is very little reliable evidence that any of these produce significant benefit, and so the fashion has swung back away from extensive preparation of the enamel. One danger of overpreparing teeth for these types of retainer is that if the retainer becomes debonded but the

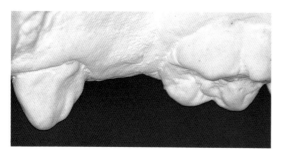

Figure 11.4

a The lingual view of an incompletely erupted upper canine tooth to be used as an abutment for a minimum-preparation bridge.

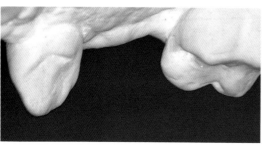

b Crown lengthening has been carried out to give a greater surface area and a horizontal seating ledge has been prepared at the cingulum. This is very small but sufficient for the purpose.

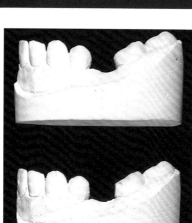

Figure 11.5

A fixed–fixed minimal-preparation bridge will require preparation of the proximal surfaces of the abutment teeth shown in the upper model to increase the surface area of enamel. In the lower model this has been done. However, this could be avoided by using a fixed–movable design.

bridge is held in place by other retainers, features such as grooves tend to become carious more rapidly than unprepared enamel surfaces, and, because the dentine is closer to the base of the groove, it too becomes carious with the result that a further minimal-preparation retainer is not possible.

The three principles that should guide the operator in deciding how much preparation is necessary are as follows:

- The maximum surface area of enamel should be used for retention of major retainers.

- The bridge should seat positively so that it can be held firmly in place without movement against the resistance of rubber dam while the cement is setting.
- Preparation may be necessary to allow an adequate thickness of retainer when the occlusion is unfavourable.

The maximum enamel surface area can often be achieved with anterior bridges without any tooth preparation other than a seating ledge (see Figure 11.4). However, with posterior fixed–fixed bridges, the abutment teeth have commonly tilted

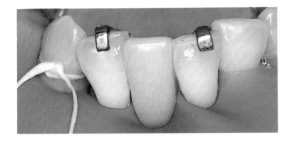

Figure 11.6

Temporary incisal hooks to allow firm stable pressure to be applied while the bridge is cemented. Once the cement has set, they will be cut off.

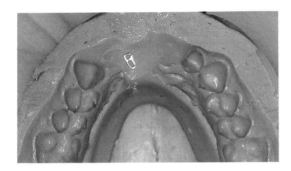

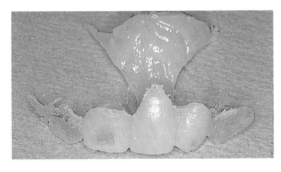

Figure 11.7

Chairside temporary-bridge construction.

a An alginate impression is taken before the preparations are started, with the temporary denture in place. The alginate is removed from the buccal sulcus area to facilitate reseating in the mouth before the temporary crown and bridge material is put into the impression.

b The plastic temporary bridge removed from the mouth. The material has flowed palatially into the space left by the plate of the denture. This can now be removed together with the thin flash over the adjacent unprepared teeth. The almost-transparent buccal–incisal surface of the upper right central incisor retainer shows that more preparation of the abutment tooth is needed here or the retainer will be too thick. To a lesser extent the same is true at the tip of the upper left lateral incisor. These modifications should be made to the preparations before the impression is taken.

towards the space and there is an undercut between their proximal surfaces. Slight reduction on one or both of the abutment teeth will allow not only a greater surface area of enamel but also more 'wrap around' of the retainer to the buccal surface (see Figure 11.5). An alternative and better solution if the occlusion permits is to make a fixed–movable bridge (see Figure 8.3, page 175).

With posterior bridges, occlusal rest seats are used to provide a firm stop against which the bridge can be seated. A shallow preparation is made in the enamel of the marginal ridge much like a rest seat for a partial denture, although it can be shallower. With retainers on anterior teeth, horizontal seating ledges or dimples are prepared. An alternative is to make the casting with an incisal hook that is cut part way through from the fit surface before cementation and is then cut off after cementation once it has done its job (see Figure 11.6).

Although some preparation of the axial walls of posterior abutment teeth is occasionally necessary, it should be avoided where possible and in any case kept to a minimum. Great care must be taken not to penetrate through to dentine, and this is sometimes difficult, particularly near to the gingival margin. Figure 11.8 shows a section of an unprepared molar tooth (a), together with a pattern for a minimum preparation retainer without preparing the tooth (b) and after preparing the tooth (c). In both Figures 11.8b and c there is inevitably a change of contour at the margin of the retainer, which must be kept clean by the patient. In this and many cases, there would be no advantage in preparing this axial surface. It has been suggested that a finishing line indicates to the technician where the retainer is to finish. This is a completely unjustifiable reason, because the same indication could be given by the dentist drawing the retainer outline on the study cast.

Making temporary and provisional bridges

Choice of material

Temporary bridges are nearly always made of one of the plastic materials. If made at the chairside, one of the higher acrylics, with or without reinforcing filler particles will be used; if made in the laboratory, they will usually be conventional acrylic or one of the higher acrylics, although laboratory light-cured composites may also be used. Metal castings or other metal components may be incorporated into longer-term provisional bridges, particularly those with long spans. However, the occlusal surface should usually be acrylic so that occlusal adjustments can be made readily if necessary. Modern plastics are sufficiently resistant to wear for this to be possible.

Choice of technique

Chairside construction

The majority of temporary bridges can readily be made at the chairside, often in less time than it takes to modify a laboratory-made temporary bridge, and of course avoiding the additional laboratory cost.

The chairside technique illustrated in Figure 11.7 is similar to the temporary crown techniques

shown in Figures 6.17, pages 124–5 and 6.18, page 126. The mould may be an impression of a study cast with the pontic made from a denture tooth, or it may be a vacuum-formed PVC slip. In many anterior bridges, though, the patient is already wearing a temporary denture, and it is sufficient to take an alginate or silicone putty impression of the arch with the denture in place and use this to make the temporary bridge. This is the technique illustrated in Figure 11.7. The excess material flowing into the areas of the impression previously occupied by the denture can be removed with an acrylic bur in a straight handpiece, once the plastic has set and the temporary bridge has been removed from the mouth.

For posterior bridges, where there is often no temporary denture, but where the appearance of the pontic is not important, an alginate impression may be taken (with nothing in the saddle area) before the teeth are prepared, and used to make individual temporary crowns for the abutment teeth.

Laboratory-made provisional bridges

If the provisional bridge is to last for more than a week or two, if it is large or if its appearance is particularly important then a laboratory-made provisional bridge is preferable to a bridge made at the chairside.

One technique is to make preparations of the abutment teeth on a study cast so that when the full-scale preparation is done in the mouth the temporary bridge will be a loose fit. If the preparations on the study cast are completed to full depth, it will be impossible to duplicate them exactly in the mouth, and the provisional bridge will not seat.

If full-scale trial preparations have been made to assess parallelism, this cast may still be used to make a provisional bridge, the prepared teeth on the study cast must be covered with a spacer of tin foil, or the fit surfaces of the bridge enlarged with a bur in the laboratory before the bridge is returned to the chairside. The bridge is waxed up and processed in the laboratory using conventional acrylic techniques, or acrylic denture teeth or special acrylic facings are ground to shape and incorporated as the facings for the bridge (see Figure 11.1).

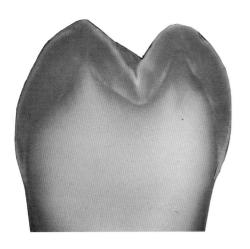

Figure 11.8

Alternative minimum-preparation retainer designs.

a A section through an extracted molar tooth.

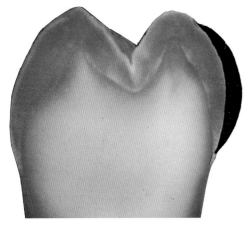

b The tooth has not been prepared and the retainer will be bonded directly to the enamel surface.

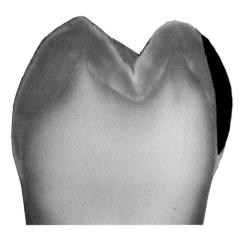

c There has been some preparation, entirely within enamel, and so the retainer is partly within and partly outside the original tooth contour.

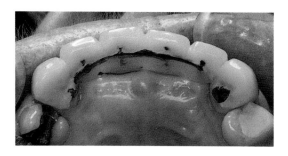

Figure 11.9

A long-term, immediate-insertion, provisional bridge in heat-cured acrylic incorporating a metal casting. The bridge has been in place six months while extraction sockets have healed. Note the space beneath the pontics that has resulted from the healing.

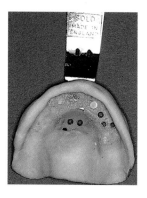

Figure 11.10

A plastic stock impression tray, stiffened with a higher acrylic and providing a soft tissue stop on the palate. A large amount of clearance is available for the impression of the anterior teeth.

Once the abutment teeth have been prepared in the mouth, the provisional bridge is tried-in and will usually need to be relined with a higher acrylic.

The technique using an accurate working impression of the prepared teeth to make a provisional bridge is more reliable, and often produces a better marginal fit but takes an extra appointment. This is necessary, however, if a metal casting is to be incorporated for extra strength (Figure 11.8).

Cementing temporary and provisional bridges

Temporary bridges should be sufficiently retentive not to cause trouble between appointments, but it should be possible to remove them without excessive force or damage. The temporary crown and bridge cementing materials are supplied with a modifying paste that may be combined in varying proportions with the base and catalyst pastes to weaken the final mix. Modified cement is recommended with large or very retentive bridges. Experience will guide the operator as to the correct proportions for the particular bridge and the particular patient. Fifty percent or more of the total mix may consist of the modifying paste.

Provisional bridges may also be cemented with temporary crown and bridge cement, but usually without modifying paste. If more retention is needed, a zinc oxide/eugenol cement may be used; in some cases zinc phosphate cement is necessary.

The working impression

Any of the impression materials or techniques described in Chapter 6 are suitable for bridgework. With fixed–fixed bridges it is often an advantage to have two working casts, one with removable dies for making the individual retainers and one that is not sectioned and therefore preserves the full contour of the saddle area together with the relationship of the abutment teeth. With good die location and a small bridge, an unsectioned model is not necessary, but with larger reconstructions where the dies have to be removed and replaced often, die location systems tend to wear, allowing movement of the dies. Then a solid model may be necessary.

All bridges should be made with full arch working impressions for maximum stability of occlusion. When all the teeth in one quadrant are missing or prepared, it is necessary to provide adequate stops on the impression tray to prevent it from seating onto the prepared teeth. In some cases these will be soft-tissue stops. Figure 11.10 shows an acrylic stock tray modified with a higher acrylic at the chairside to give a palatal soft-tissue stop. There are also improvements to the peripheral adaptation and rigidity. This tray would be suitable for use with a polyether impression material or an addition-curing silicone.

Figure 6.4 shows the construction of special trays.

Occlusal records

For the choice of appropriate occlusal records, see Chapter 4. The larger the bridge, the more time-consuming is any occlusal adjustment at the chairside, so it is likely that a semi-adjustable or fully adjustable articulator will be chosen (together with the appropriate occlusal records) to minimize this adjustment time.

Trying-in the metal framework or separate units

Metal–ceramic conventional bridges should be tried-in at the metal stage. Experienced operators making small bridges, who are familiar with their technician's work, sometimes omit this stage, but this is inadvisable under other conditions.

Metal–ceramic bridges of up to six units are often cast in one piece. When they are tried in,

all the checks listed in Chapter 6 should be made, and if the framework is acceptable, it may be returned to the laboratory for the porcelain to be added.

If the framework does not seat, and once obvious causes have been eliminated, such as tight contact points or air blows on the fit surface of the casting, it must be assumed that the relationship between the abutment teeth is the problem. This may be wrong either because the abutment teeth have moved since the impression was taken (perhaps because a temporary bridge was not provided) or because the die location is at fault. If this is suspected, the bridge should be divided and the separate components tried in. It is better to saw through the bridge with a fine fretsaw cutting diagonally through one of the pontics rather than through a connector (see Figure 11.11a). This gives a larger surface area for the bridge to be resoldered, and the solder joint will be covered by porcelain, which will further strengthen it. If the separate units fit, the bridge is relocated (see below) and soldered with a high-temperature solder before the porcelain is added. It is advisable to retry the bridge now.

If, once the bridge is sectioned, some of the retainers fit and others do not, a further impression is needed. This will be of the unsatisfactory abutments, with the satisfactory retainers and the attached parts of the pontic left in situ. They will be a guide to the technician in waxing-up the repeated sections. A further retry and localization in the mouth is necessary before soldering.

With larger bridges not cast in one piece, the separate sections should be tried-in before localization and soldering.

Bridges made in other materials are usually completed and not tried-in as separate units. Posterior all-metal bridges are necessarily relatively small, as are anterior all-porcelain bridges. Where metal units are to be soldered to metal–ceramic units, it is possible to try-in the separate retainers before the connectors are soldered.

Localization techniques

Now that full arch impressions are taken almost universally for bridgework, there is less need for localization of individual retainers than when individual impressions were taken of each

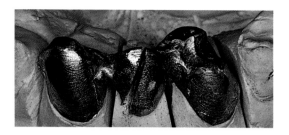

Figure 11.11

Localization

a The metal framework for a three-unit metal–ceramic bridge. This has been tried in the mouth and found not to fit. When sectioned diagonally through the pontic, the separate retainers fitted, and so it was relocalized in the mouth and soldered before the porcelain was added.

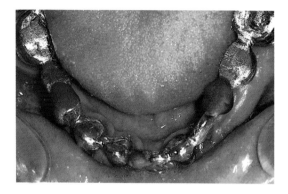

b A large bridge, cast in four sections, being localized in the mouth with fast-setting acrylic. To stabilize it, a bar will be attached across the back with more acrylic.

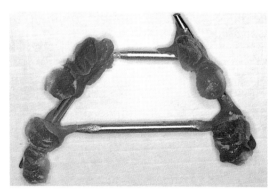

c Multiple separate bridge retainers connected with acrylic and old bur shanks. The castings have been removed from the acrylic. This assembly can now be reseated in the mouth and a new impression taken over it to record the saddle areas. The pontics are then made and soldered to the retainers.

abutment tooth. However, problems still arise, as outlined in the previous section, with the fit of one-piece castings. It may also be difficult to get a single impression of all the teeth at once, especially when large bridges are made in the lower arch. The tongue makes it difficult to obtain a dry field on both sides of the arch at the same time. In these cases separate impressions of groups of abutment teeth have to be taken and related to each other with a localization technique.

An overall impression of the castings in place may be used for localization. A rigid elastomeric material such as polyether must be used, since softer materials distort when the casting and dies are seated in the impression. An alternative is to use acrylic with a paint-on technique. When adjacent retainers are to be located or a cut pontic resoldered, it is sufficient simply to clean the surfaces, paint a fast-setting cold-cure acrylic over the surface and allow it to harden before withdrawing the bridge (see Figure 11.11b).

When the pontics are not yet made or where the bridge is large, the localization is stiffened and supported with metal bars or a metal framework.

The bars may be old bur shanks cut to suitable length (see Figure 11.11c).

Try-in and trial cementation of finished bridges

The checking procedure is as described in Chapter 6. In some cases the bridge does not fully seat and the operator may suspect that the teeth have moved, particularly if a metal stage try-in was satisfactory. Rather than sectioning the bridge again, it may be left in the mouth for a few hours, preferably with no cement, or with petroleum jelly and zinc oxide powder (which does not set) to prevent oral fluids from irritating the exposed dentine. If after a few hours the bridge has not seated, the next stage is to cement it with a very weak temporary crown and bridge cement with a large proportion of modifier. Bridges cemented in this way may be left for days or even weeks to settle before being finally cemented. This should be done routinely with larger bridges.

The advantages of trial cementation are that, as well as possible improvements in marginal fit, the patient has a chance to become accustomed to the appearance and feel of the bridge, which can still be modified out of the mouth if necessary. Any problems with the occlusion are likely to show themselves and can be dealt with before the bridge is permanently cemented.

Trial cementation should not be attempted with all-porcelain bridges or the minor retainers of fixed–movable bridges. Trial cementation is not possible with minimal-preparation bridges.

Permanent cementation

The cementation of conventional bridges differs from that of crowns only in that with fixed–fixed bridges the surface area of the combined abutment preparations is larger than an individual crown and so the hydrostatic pressure of the unset cement is much greater. Greater force therefore has to be applied to seat the bridge fully.

Because of the difficulty of cementing large bridges and the need for a long working time before the cement starts to set, zinc phosphate cement is still the most popular for large bridges. Its working time can be extended considerably: the mixing slab is cooled, very small increments of powder are added at a time, and mixed for a long period (approximately 90 seconds). Ready proportioned cement in a plastic syringe is also available and is mixed in a mechanical vibrator. If the syringe is used straight from the refrigerator, a consistent, slow-setting, air-bubble-free mix is obtained.

For preparations with nearly parallel walls the technician may use an additional layer of die-relief varnish on the axial walls. This increases the cement-film thickness in this area without increasing it at the margins, and so reduces hydrostatic pressure during cementation.

Glass ionomer luting cement is preferred for small conventional bridges for the reasons described in Chapter 6.

The cementation of minimum-preparation bridges depends on the technique used to make the bridge and the luting cement. The commonest types are now those with sand-blasted fit surfaces luted with an adhesive resin, or Rochette (macro-mechanically retentive) bridges or splints cemented with a conventional, chemically cured composite material. These are used when it is likely that they will have to be removed atraumatically. In addition, etched metal surfaces luted with chemically cured, low-viscosity luting cements are also still used.

Figure 11.12 shows the luting process for an etched bridge with a chemically cured composite cement. The process is very similar with adhesive resin cements except that the margins must be protected with a gel material to avoid air contamination while the cement sets.

Summary of clinical technique for minimal-preparation bridges

Minimal-preparation bridges are constructed as follows (see Figure 11.12).

● Thoroughly scale and polish the abutment teeth
  – and the remainder of the mouth, of course

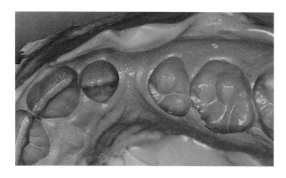

Figure 11.12

Clinical technique for a minimum-preparation bridge.

a The working impression.

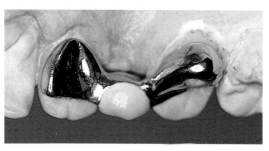

b The metal framework and pontic on the model. This is tried in the mouth and adjusted before etching or sandblasting. It should not be retried after etching, or the delicate etched surface will be damaged. The design is fixed–fixed because the tooth being replaced is an upper canine that will be in occlusion in lateral excursions. A cantilever bridge from the premolar would not have been adequate with this occlusion, and there was insufficient space to make a movable connector in the lateral incisor without excessive tooth preparation.

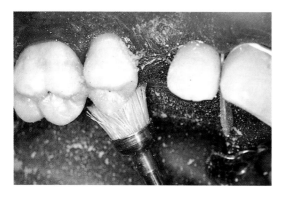

c Polishing the abutment teeth with pumice and water after applying rubber dam.

- Carry out any necessary tooth preparation
- Take an accurate working impression in elastomeric material
- Prepare the metal framework and pontic in the laboratory; the pontic is usually metal–ceramic
- Try-in the bridge; if it is a Maryland bridge, etch the metal fitting surface after trying it, and then do not touch the etched surface or retry the bridge, otherwise the delicate etched surface will be damaged
- Repolish the enamel surfaces to which the bridge is to be cemented, apply rubber dam and acid-etch the enamel surfaces
- Cement the bridge with a chemically cured composite resin (one made specially for the purpose), and remove excess composite from the margins
- If the bridge is to be cemented with a chemically adhesive cement, the metal should be sandblasted as late as possible before cementation. The bridge should be cemented under rubber dam and the gel material supplied with

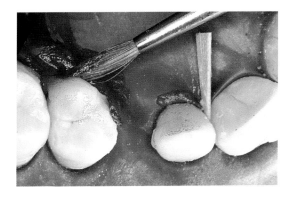

d Phosphoric acid gel applied carefully with a paint-brush or with a syringe to the areas to be covered by the retainers.

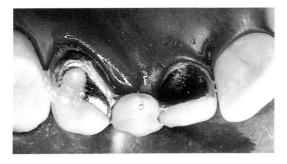

e Luting the etched bridge with a chemically cured composite specially made for the purpose. It would have been a good idea to place some floss between the abutment and the adjacent teeth before cementing the bridge. Pulling this through the contact points before the cement set would have helped to remove excess cement. If the bridge had been sandblasted and luted with an adhesive resin, the margins would be coated with gel to exclude air while the cement set.

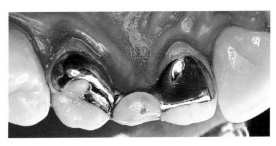

f Immediately after removing the rubber dam.

the cement applied to the margins of the retainer to exclude air since the setting of the cement is inhibited by air.

Oral hygiene instructions and maintenance

This is particularly important with bridges, and in some cases the techniques will be entirely different from those the patient has been taught to date or for crowns. The areas where different cleaning techniques may be needed are between the pontic and the ridge and the gingival margins of the abutment teeth beneath the connectors. The technique will depend upon the design of the ridge surface of the pontic, the part of the mouth where the bridge is situated and the patient's manual dexterity. With ridge-lap and saddle pontics, dental floss or tape may be threaded through an embrasure space and then passed under the pontic to clean it and the ridge. Even

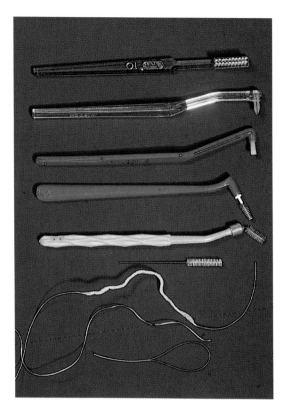

Figure 11.13

a Cleaning aids for use with bridges.

From the top: a soft toothbrush with two rows of bristles that can be used around dome and ridge-lap pontics;

two single tuft interspace brushes – these are often too stiff except in very large open embrasure spaces;

two 'bottle' brushes with multiple small lateral tufts that are useful for medium-sized embrasure spaces;

a 'bottle' brush with a simple wire handle;

superfloss, the most useful of the bridge cleaning aids – this has a stiffened end, right, and a furry section that is very useful for cleaning under pontics, and especially under smooth saddle pontics;

regular floss, which can sometimes be passed through embrasure spaces to clean under pontics; but when this is difficult it is used in conjunction with

a floss threader, a flexible nylon loop with a stiff end that passes easily between tight embrasure spaces.

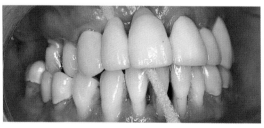

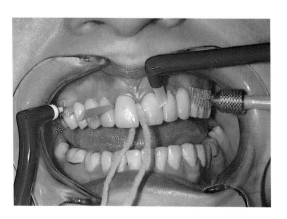

b Superfloss being used to clean beneath the pontic

c The clinical use of some of the cleaning aids shown in *a* and *b* – they would not normally all be used at once!

better is superfloss. Its furry section makes cleaning under pontics much easier (see Figures 9.5, page 199 and 11.13).

Wash-through and dome-shaped pontics are usually cleansable entirely with the toothbrush, although in some cases an interspace brush or other special brush may be an advantage.

Oral hygiene instruction should be given at the same appointment as the bridge is cemented. The patient should be seen again in one or two weeks to ensure that the new cleaning techniques are successful. At this stage it may be helpful to use disclosing tablets or solutions. At the same appointment the occlusion and the retainers should be checked.

It is advisable to see the patient at regular intervals, usually six-monthly, when the full range of checks of margins, gingival health, cleaning, occlusion and the mechanical integrity of the bridge are made. Chapter 13 deals with repairs and modifications to bridges where these checks reveal any problems.

Practical points

● Teeth should be prepared parallel to each other by eye, and if in doubt, and for larger bridges, a model of the initial preparations surveyed in the laboratory.

● Most temporary bridges can be made at the chairside.

● All bridges should be made with maximum stability of occlusion.

● Localization techniques may be needed when one-piece castings have to be cut and individual retainers are not satisfactory.

● Trial cementation will allow for possible improvements and will give the patient time to become accustomed to the feel and appearance of the bridge.

● Good homecare by the patient is essential if bridges are to succeed.

Part 3   Splints

12   Fixed splints

Many of the techniques used in constructing fixed splints are similar to those used to make crowns and bridges. Large splints often contain one or more pontics, and are therefore combination bridge/splints. There is no attempt here to describe removeable splints in detail, since the techniques for constructing them are more akin to partial denture construction. There is, however, a section of this chapter comparing fixed and removable splints.

Different types of splint are used depending on the time for which they will be needed. Short-term splints are made as an emergency measure, intermediate splints are made to last for a few months, usually while other forms of treatment are being carried out, and permanent splints are intended to last for the lifetime of the dentition or the patient.

Indications for fixed splints

Trauma

A blow may result in an incisor tooth being partially or completely subluxated. If the tooth is repositioned correctly in its socket very shortly after the accident, particularly with young patients, it has a good chance of surviving for a useful period, providing it is kept clean and other conditions are favourable. It will normally need to be stabilized by being attached to adjacent teeth while the periodontal ligament heals and the alveolar bone remodels. It is not usually necessary to provide intermediate or permanent splinting for traumatized teeth.

Periodontal disease

At one time splints were prescribed as a way of treating periodontal disease and preventing the loss of teeth through progressive loosening. This is no longer accepted as a reasonable form of treatment; and the proper treatment of periodontal disease itself is beyond the scope of this book.

However, once the disease has been successfully treated, there may be two conditions when a fixed splint is indicated:

● When the residual mobility of the teeth is such that the patient finds them uncomfortable and normal masticatory function is impractical.
● When teeth are missing and must be replaced for one of the reasons listed in Chapter 7. In many cases the remaining teeth are not satisfactory as denture abutments in view of their mobility or because it is considered that a partial denture will make oral hygiene procedures more difficult and will be likely to shorten the life expectancy of the remaining teeth. Individual teeth may also be unsuitable as bridge abutments, but a number of teeth splinted together may form a satisfactory abutment for a bridge or perhaps a precision-attachment retained partial denture.

Orthodontic retention

In the great majority of courses of orthodontic treatment the teeth are moved into new positions where, following a period of settling in, they are stable. There is sometimes a persistent tendency to relapse, and for fuller explanations for this the reader is referred to textbooks of orthodontics. Orthodontic relapse is more likely, and may indeed be anticipated, if the tooth movement is to realign teeth that have drifted following periodontal disease. Figures 4.5c and d, page 70 illustrate a case where, if orthodontic treatment is to be provided, fixed splint retention is very likely to be necessary.

Congenital defects

Cleft palate

One method of treating cleft-palate cases is to expand the palate rapidly by orthodontic means

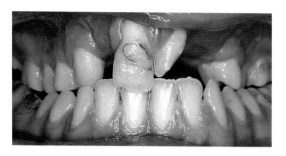

Figure 12.1

A bridge to stabilize a mobile premaxilla resulting from a bilateral cleft palate.

a The preoperative condition following surgical treatment.

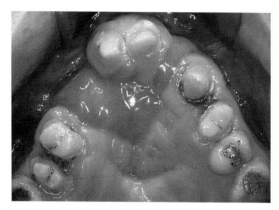

b The prepared teeth. Two abutments in each buccal segment are used together with the two teeth in the premaxilla.

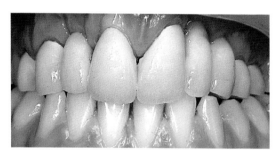

c The completed bridge stabilizing the premaxilla.

and to insert a bone graft. In some cases the result is not completely stable, and if there are missing anterior teeth (which is common), a bridge replacement may be made and a number of teeth on each side of the cleft splinted to form the abutments. These splinted abutments will also stabilize the two halves of the upper arch.

Occasionally the premaxilla is separated from the remainder of the upper arch, and, together with any teeth carried in it, it will be mobile. This can be splinted by means of a fixed splint/bridge (see Figure 12.1).

Dental defects

Acquired or congenital dental abnormalities can result in teeth of an unsual shape or consistency.

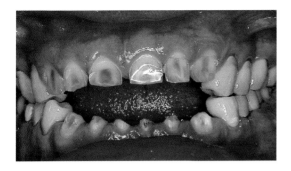

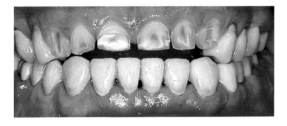

Figure 12.2

a and *b* Pin-retained splinted crowns to restore vital but badly worn lower incisor teeth. The upper incisor teeth were also crowned, but sufficient dentine remained for these crowns to be separate.

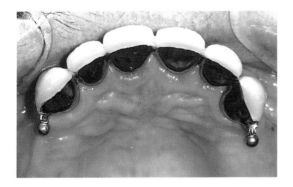

Figure 12.3

Splinted abutment teeth for a precision-attachment retained-free-end saddle denture. The six anterior teeth have reduced alveolar support and have been successfully treated periodontally. They were also heavily restored. Splinted crowns provide support for extra-coronal precision attachments that retain and stabilize a denture and avoid visible clasps.

If crowns are necessary, retention may be unusually difficult, but can be improved by splinting a number together. Figure 12.2 shows a case of gross tooth wear where the lower incisors are too small for adequate retention of conventional restorations and where radiographs showed pulp calcification so that post crowns were not possible. Splinted pin-retained crowns were made, each one gaining support from its neighbours.

Additional retention

With precision-attachment retained partial dentures, the abutment teeth carrying the attachment may need to be splinted together. This provides extra retention to resist the additional force during removal of the appliance (see Figures 7.3a, page 151 and 12.3).

Short-term, intermediate and permanent splints and diodontic implants

Short-term splints

When a tooth is loosened by a blow or is completely lost and replanted, an immediate temporary splint is necessary. The usual method of splinting is to attach the tooth involved to adjacent teeth with acid-etch retained composite (see Figure 8.9 page 184). Various other techniques are used for temporary splints, such as wiring the teeth together or cementing a cap splint made of acrylic, some other vacuum-formed material or cast metal. However, if sufficient enamel is present for acid etching, these other techniques are less satisfactory than composite splints because they are less hygienic and interfere with the occlusion.

Intermediate-term splints

These are used when teeth need to be immobilized for periods of between a few weeks and a few months, for example while periodontal treatment is carried out, before permanent restorations are made. They are usually one of the less permanent minimal-preparation types (see opposite), but may be intra-coronal. Cemented cap splints are not suitable, since they interfere with the occlusion and create great difficulty in cleaning.

Permanent splints

Conventional permanent splints for restored teeth are either partial or complete crowns, connected, or one of the proprietary splints. However, with unrestored teeth a minimal-preparation type of splint is now the treatment of choice.

Diodontic implants

An entirely different approach to permanently splinting an individual tooth is to stabilize it with a diodontic implant (see page 249). These are used when the root of the tooth is short, as a result of horizontal fracture in the middle third of the root, apical resorption or repeated unsuccessful apicectomies.

Fixed splints compared with removable splints

Advantages of fixed splints

● The most reliable splints for mobile teeth or those with a tendency to drift
● Can be kept entirely clear of the gingival tissues
● Occupy minimal or no additional space
● Cannot be left out by the patient.

Disadvantages of fixed splints

● Conventional splints are expensive and destructive to tooth tissue
● Minimal-preparation splints may be plaque-retentive and unreliable. The consequence of loosening and rapid caries development may be the loss of teeth.

Advantages of removable splints (e.g. cast cobalt–chromium)

● Can be removed for cleaning
● May be less expensive than fixed conventional splints and may be less destructive to sound tooth tissue.

Disadvantages of removable splints

● Removal and insertion inevitably causes movement of the teeth that are meant to be stabilized, and this may increase mobility
● With long-term orthodontic retention and cleft-palate cases, a removable splint has to be worn for 24 hours a day (except for cleaning), and this has harmful effects on the periodontium

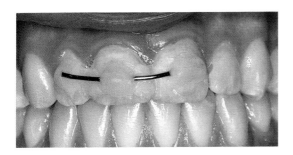

Figure 12.4

The right central incisor was partly displaced by a blow. It was mobile and uncomfortable. This wire-and-composite splint is rigid, allows the tooth to be positioned correctly in the occlusion while the splint is being attached, allows the tooth to be tested for vitality, does not interfere with the occlusion, and is accessible for cleaning. It was removed after three weeks, by which time the injured tooth was firm.

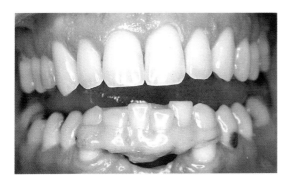

Figure 12.5

A wire-and-acrylic splint. This splint served a useful purpose during initial periodontal therapy, after which the roots of the four incisors were resected. The splint has remained effective until complete alveolar healing has occurred, and now the patient is ready to have a bridge – a temporary partial denture having been avoided.

● If the splint is broken or lost or has to be returned to the laboratory for repair, there is a risk of teeth moving while the appliance is out, so that the appliance will not fit when it is returned to the mouth.

Types of short-term intermediate and permanent fixed splint

Minimal-preparation (resin-bonded) splints

This group can be used either as short-term, intermediate or, in some cases, permanent splints. They have the advantage that they can be removed, and since the teeth have often not been prepared, they do not have to be restored. However, because these splints are applied to the surface of the teeth, they inevitably add to their bulk and make oral hygiene more difficult. There is also the problem of them interfering with the occlusion; and in some cases the ideal design for retention and splinting cannot be used because of the occlusion.

Acid-etch retained composite splints (see Figure 12.4)

A simple short-term splinting technique is to acid-etch the approximal surfaces of adjacent teeth and attach them with acid-etch retained composite. The technique is not sufficiently rigid to function as a permanent splint. To strengthen the splint, it is usually necessary to add stainless-steel wire or one of the proprietary splints that are similar to orthodontic brackets (see later).

Wire-and-acrylic or wire-and-composite splint (see Figure 12.5)

A satisfactory form of intermediate splinting, particularly for lower incisors, is the wire-and-

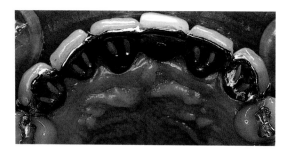

Figure 12.6

A minimal-preparation splint/bridge of the Rochette type. These large retention holes are no longer used (see Figure 8.9a). One central incisor has also been replaced.

acrylic splint. The technique can be used when some of the teeth are crowned and so cannot be etched for the retention of composite.

Briefly, the technique is to pass a wire loop around all the teeth to be splinted. Further loops, in thinner wire, are passed around the contact points, taking in the first loop buccally and lingually. The secondary loops are twisted and tightened in turn a little at a time, allowing adjustment of the position of the mobile teeth. When all is firm, the wire ends are cut off, tucked into the embrasures and the whole painted over with acrylic or composite without etching any enamel that is present. This type of splint is easier to remove than etch-retained splints.

Cast-metal minimal-preparation (Rochette and Maryland) splints

These have become the most common type of intermediate and permanent splints. They have the advantage that they do not require much or any preparation of the tooth and yet are thin and unobtrusive and do not significantly affect the patient's appearance. Figure 12.6 shows a Rochette splint. These splints have the advantage that it is possible to remove them fairly atraumatically by cutting the cement out of the retentive holes. Minimal-preparation-type splints of the micro-mechanical or chemical-adhesive types are more difficult to remove, and if removal is necessary, they usually have to be cut off, otherwise there is a risk of extracting any teeth with reduced alveolar support with the force necessary to remove them. However, for permanent

retention of orthodontically treated teeth with sound periodontal health, a minimal-preparation type of splint is preferred since it is more retentive and smoother lingually.

These splints are made and cemented in the same way as the minimal-preparation bridges described in Chapter 11. It is essential to use rubber dam while cementing them.

Intra-coronal splints

A variety of techniques have been suggested for splinting adjacent teeth with intra-coronal restorations using either amalgam or composite, with the teeth linked by wire or a proprietary device. Figure 12.7 (centre) shows a typical example of such a splint.

The major problems with this type of splint are first that forces applied to the unprotected part of the tooth surface tend to break down the seal between the restoration and tooth, with marginal leakage occurring followed by secondary caries. Second, mechanical failure at the connectors is fairly common. Third, because they are difficult to finish and polish, it is often harder to clean around this type of splint than around partial or complete crown splints with polished connectors.

Proprietary splints

A variety of splint systems involving anchoring a cast framework to the teeth with threaded pins

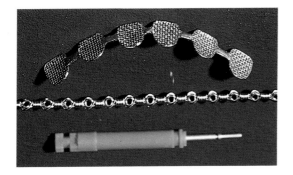

Figure 12.7

Two forms of composite retained proprietary splint. *Top:* a preformed splint, available in a variety of forms, is retentive for composite and is attached by the acid-etch technique to the lingual surfaces of the teeth to be splinted. It is commonly used as a permanent or semi-permanent orthodontic retainer. *Centre:* the chain is embedded in cavities prepared in the teeth from the lingual or occlusal surface and held in place with threaded pins. A self-shearing pin on a contra-angle shank is shown. Once the chain has been anchored in place, the cavities are filled with composite. This method is only used in cases where there are already multiple, large approximal restorations in the anterior teeth and therefore insufficient palatal or lingual enamel to retain one of the other systems. A full-crown splint is an alternative, but is often too expensive in view of the probable prognosis of the teeth to be splinted.

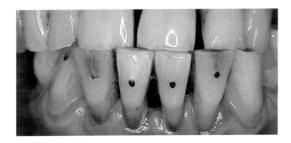

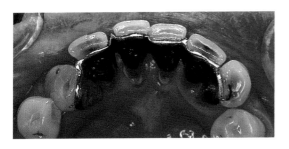

Figure 12.8

a and *b* A horizontal non-parallel-pin splint. This has been present for several years, but failed through caries developing around the pins in two of the lower incisors. With the splint removed, the pinholes filled and periodontal treatment provided, the teeth became sufficiently firm not to require further splinting.

were used at one time. These have been superseded by the acid-etch retained systems, but many patients were treated with them. Dentists still need to be able to recognize these splints so that at least they can provide suitable maintenance.

The type that has survived more than others is the non-parallel horizontal-pin splint. This was used for anterior teeth (see Figure 12.8). The lingual surface was prepared and horizontal holes drilled right through the tooth bucco-lingually. An impression was taken in a special tray with

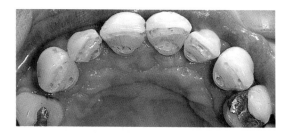

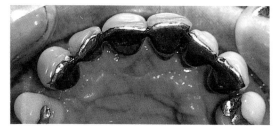

Figure 12.9

A partial-crown splint made before minimal-preparation techniques were available. Splints are now rarely or never made this way, but some patients still have partial-crown splints that need to be maintained.

a Teeth prepared with ledges and with three parallel-sided pins each. The pinholes were prepared using an intra-oral paralleling device. (See Figure 6.21e for the impression stage and Figure 7.8 for the buccal appearance.)

b The cemented casting.

impression pins provided as part of the kit and a cast-metal backing corresponding to the pinholes in the teeth. The backing was then cemented, and, before the cement set, pins were passed through the tooth and screwed through the backing. The heads of the pins fitted into countersinks on the buccal surface of the tooth. When the cement was set, the excess pin was removed, both buccally and lingually. The heads of the pins were reduced below the level of the buccal surface, and the teeth were restored with composite.

Partial-crown splints

As with proprietary splints, these have been superseded by minimum-preparation splints. However, again, maintenance is sometimes necessary, and it is easy for the inexperienced dentist to confuse a partial-crown retained splint (see Figure 12.9c) with a minimal-preparation splint.

Figure 12.9 shows a partial-crown splint retained by vertical parallel pins. Most partial-crown splints were retained in this way.

Complete-crown splints

Despite the advantage of minimal-preparation splints, complete-crown splints are still common. This is because the natural crowns of the teeth being splinted often already have large restorations or crowns, and some teeth may have been extracted, so that the appliance becomes a splint/bridge. Figure 12.10 shows a typical 12-unit splint/bridge where six teeth are missing and where the remaining teeth were uncomfortably mobile. A partial denture to replace the missing teeth would probably have increased the mobility of the remaining teeth; and the patient was most unhappy about wearing a removable appliance. The radiographs of this patient are shown in Figure 7.5.

The disadvantages of this technique are that it is very time-consuming, both at the chairside and in the laboratory, and therefore very expensive; and if failure occurs, it may be necessary to remove the entire splint and maybe extract several other teeth. This type of appliance should therefore only be provided for very highly motivated patients.

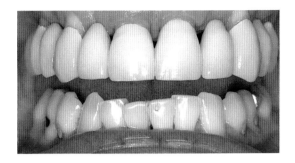

Figure 12.10

A 12-unit fixed splint/bridge. There are six abutment teeth and six pontics. Note the supragingival margins which have helped to maintain a good level of gingival health. Note also the opaque appearance of the retainer margins. This is because in order to make the six preparations parallel to each other it was not possible to prepare sufficiently wide shoulders without over-preparing the whole tooth and risking exposure. This was anticipated from the trial preparations and the patient was fully informed about this before the preparations were undertaken so that her consent to the procedure included understanding that the appearance would be compromised in this way.

Diodontic splints

A diodontic splint consists of a metal post that passes through the root canal and into bone apical to the root. It may extend a little beyond the position of the original apex of the tooth, but not so far that there is a risk of other structures being perforated, such as the floor of the nose or the maxillary sinus. Figure 12.11 shows a case where the roots of both upper lateral incisors had been partly resorbed by unerupted canine teeth in the palate. Following the removal of the canines, the roots of the lateral incisors continued to resorb. Before the diodontic implants were placed, both lateral incisors were very mobile.

With diodontic implants the tooth should be firm from the moment the implant is placed, and no further splinting is required. The technique will work only if there is sufficient healthy periodontal attachment at the gingival end of the root. The minimum is 2–3 mm of undisturbed periodontal attachment around the entire circumference of the tooth.

Diodontic splints are placed less often these days, but are still useful in some cases. For example, in young people who are still growing and when, although the long-term treatment may well be extraction and a single-tooth implant, a diodontic splint will tide them over their late teenage years without involving the adjacent teeth.

The appearance of anterior splints

A patient who has had extensive periodontal disease and treatment (particularly surgical treatment) often has upper anterior teeth that appear very long. When the lipline is high this is an aesthetic problem (see Figure 7.8c). If the incisor teeth are extracted and a partial denture made, artificial teeth, fitted to the ridge, will also appear to be too long; otherwise a flange may be used, and the edges will have an extremely artificial appearance. In any case, if the patient has been cooperative during periodontal treatment and this has been successful, he or she will obviously not want the teeth extracted.

If a full-crown splint is made, it will be necessary to prepare crown margins at the cement–enamel junction and try to disguise the crown margin as the CEJ, or at the gingival margin, producing very long thin preparations that endanger the pulp. The first alternative is often unsatisfactory, since the opacity of the metal–ceramic retainer is greater than that of the root surface. Neither makes any improvement in the appearance of the length of the teeth (see Figure 12.10).

With all these aesthetic problems, some patients and dentists would elect to extract the upper incisor teeth, re-contour the ridge by bone augmentation and replace the teeth with implants.

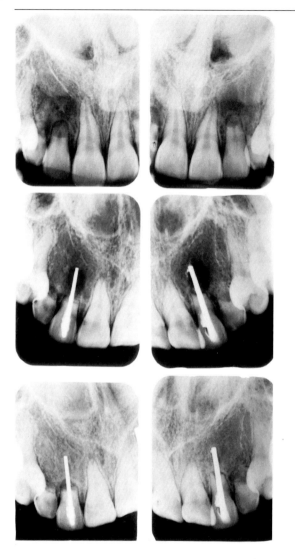

Figure 12.11

Diodontic implants.

a Unerupted canines have been removed from the palate in this young teenage patient, but resorption of the roots of the lateral incisors is continuing. This has been demonstrated by a series of radiographs taken over a number of months.

b Diodontic implants have been placed by an open approach. The apical part of the root surface has been removed to reduce the likelihood of the resorption continuing. The lateral incisors were firm immediately following the surgery.

c Six months later, with bone reformation almost complete. These implants remained in place for more than ten years and were replaced by single tooth osseointegrated implants when the patient was in her mid-twenties.

Selecting an anterior splint

It is important to make sure the patient understands how the splint will look, and what compromises are necessary. In a typical case the patient has:

- Mobile uncomfortable upper anterior teeth that have been successfully treated periodontally
- A high lipline with unattractive appearance of the upper incisor teeth

- An extreme reluctance to wear a removable appliance.

There is no ideal solution to these problems; the options are as follows, in increasing order of cost:

a Offer no treatment; the result will be a patient who continues to complain about mobility, the lack of comfort, the appearance and possible further drifting of the upper incisors

b Provide a minimal-preparation splint with or without a removable gingival prosthesis; the compromise here is the 'metal shine-through', but on the plus side are the conservative nature of the preparations and the relatively low cost compared with the alternatives. Sometimes this option is not possible because some of the teeth are heavily restored or crowned or the occlusion is unfavourable

c Extract the upper incisor teeth and provide a partial denture; some patients will refuse, and in any case it will provide only partial improvement in appearance

d Extract the upper incisors and provide a bridge; there is still the problem of the length of the pontics, but this may be the preferred treatment in some cases – there is little point in keeping teeth with a very poor prognosis if the same number of additional abutment teeth would be necessary to support them as would be prepared for a bridge; a removable gingival prosthesis may also be provided

e Provide a complete-crown splint with or without a removable gingival prosthesis; this has the disadvantages of time, cost and appearance described above, but may still be the preferred treatment in some cases

f Extract the teeth and provide ridge augmentation and implants.

Clinical techniques for permanent splints

The reader is referred to the literature on the treatment of traumatized teeth and the periodontal literature for full descriptions of temporary and intra-coronal splinting techniques. Similarly, the surgical procedures for placing diodontic implants are described in textbooks on surgical endodontics. The clinical techniques for minimal-preparation splints are the same as for bridges (see Chapter 11). Therefore clinical techniques will be described only for complete-crown splints.

Tooth preparation for complete-crown splints

One of the techniques described in Chapter 11 should be used to ensure that the preparations

are parallel. In the case of multiple-unit complete-crown splints, it may be necessary to take several intermediate impressions to check the parallelism of the preparations with a surveyor before the final impression is taken. Figure 12.10 shows a 12-unit splint/bridge with six abutment teeth. Six intermediate impressions were taken. This sounds very time-consuming, but with fast-setting plaster and a surveyor at the chairside, only two appointments were needed.

It is highly advisable to carry out trial preparations on a study cast to ensure that the ideal path of insertion is selected. This may not be in the long axis of all the teeth.

Temporary splints

With complete-crown splints it is possible to make a temporary splint at the chairside or in the laboratory using one of the techniques described in Chapter 11.

Impressions

When teeth are mobile, they should be splinted so as to be in an unstrained position within their remaining periodontal support, and preserving optimum occlusal relationships. There is a danger of them being moved away from this position by the force of the impression being inserted, so that the finished splint, although it may fit, will distort the alignment of the teeth. This risk is greater if a viscous material is used, particularly in a close-fitting special tray. This means that the putty-wash techniques and polysulphide impression materials are not ideal for these impressions.

There are two ways around this problem. One is to use an impression technique in which the teeth can 'float' into their natural positions before the material sets, the ideal material being reversible hydrocolloid. The second way is to take an impression in any material and have separate transfer copings made for each tooth. These are located in the mouth using a gentle technique that does not disturb the alignment of the teeth, for example painting on a self-curing acrylic material (see Chapter 11).

Cementation

Some teeth being splinted are likely to be more mobile than others, and this produces a cementation problem. Although the splint may fit well at the margins when it is tried-in, if some teeth can be moved apically in their sockets and others cannot, when the splint is being cemented the mobile teeth may be depressed by the hydrostatic pressure in the unset cement. The marginal fit of the retainers of these teeth is therefore unsatisfactory. Precautions should be taken to avoid this happening. In some cases the retainers are vented to allow free escape of cement, in others the splint should be pressed firmly home onto the stable abutments and then an instrument such as a Mitchell's trimmer hooked onto the abutment tooth, preferably at the amelo-cemental junction, and the tooth drawn down into its retainer. Because this takes time, zinc phosphate cement, mixed to produce an extended working time, is preferred to glass ionomer cement. Alternatively, floss is tied round each of the mobile teeth between the preparation margin and the gingival margins. After fully seating on the stable abutments, the mobile teeth can be pulled down into their retainers with the floss.

Practical points

● Permanent splints are not used in the treatment of periodontal disease, but may be necessary to stabilize mobile teeth and replace missing teeth after successful periodontal treatment.

● Permanent splints are also used in some cases of congenital defect and occasionally following orthodontic treatment.

● Short- and intermediate-term splints may be useful after injury or during a course of periodontal treatment.

● Minimal-preparation splints may be successfully used as permanent splints as alternatives to crowns.

● Overall, fixed splints have greater advantages than removable ones.

● Where anterior teeth need splinting and appear long as a result of periodontal disease, the final appearance will need careful consideration.

Part 4   Failures and repairs

13

Crown and bridge failures and repairs

The difficulties of estimating the risk of failure before a bridge is started and dangers of misinterpreting failure statistics were discussed in Chapter 7. A reasonable method of recording failures is as a percentage per year. Recent large surveys of bridges made in practice and elsewhere in different countries show that about 90% of bridges last at least 10 years.

Dealing with failures of implant fixtures and/or the prosthetic elements is a specialist subject beyond the scope of this book. If a dentist finds evidence of failure in an implant, the patient should be referred unless the dentist has had specialist training.

There are two major problems with these surveys of bridges. First, they are usually of selected and therefore biased samples – restorations made in dental schools, or specific practices – and second, there are difficulties in defining failure.

Looking at any crown or bridge, it is always possible to find some minor fault with the fit or the appearance of some other aspect. In many cases it is a matter of degree. There is nothing seriously wrong with the restoration, only that one dentist, looking at another's work, would have applied his or her skills in different ways – would have introduced a little more incisal translucence or placed the margin a little more subgingivally or supragingivally, or finished it better. These variations in judgement are to be expected and need to be encouraged. If every crown or bridge were standardized, there would be no room for development and improvement.

At the other extreme there are undisputed failures, for example, the fractured PJC or the loose bridge where extensive caries has developed. Between these extremes lies a large grey area of partial failures and partial successes. With these it is better to speak of levels of acceptability to patient and dentist (which may be different) and to consider what needs to be done to improve matters. This chapter first describes the causes of failure and some solutions, and then gives the techniques for adjustment or repair.

Causes of failure and some solutions

Loss of retention

With the exceptions of post crowns, where failure is usually due to inadequate post design or construction (see Figure 13.1), loss of retention is not a common cause of failure of individual crowns. But because of the leverage forces on bridges, one of the more common ways in which they fail is by one of the retainers becoming loose from the abutment tooth.

Fixed–fixed bridges and splinted retainers

When only one retainer becomes loose, this can be disastrous. Without a cement seal, plaque forms in the space between the retainer and the abutment tooth, and caries develops rapidly across the whole of the dentine surface of the preparation (see Figure 13.2). The same problems arise with loss of retention of one part of a minimal-preparation bridge, but, although caries does sometimes develop rapidly, because the surface of the tooth is enamel rather than dentine, the development of caries is usually slower.

Sometimes the patient is aware of movement developing in the bridge or experiences a bad taste from debris being pumped in and out of the space with intermittent pressure on the bridge. A good diagnostic test for a loose retainer is to examine the bridge carefully without drying the teeth, pressing the bridge up and down and looking for small bubbles in the saliva at the margins of the retainers.

If one retainer does become loose, it is a matter of urgency to remove at least that retainer, and usually the whole bridge. If a fixed–fixed minimal-preparation bridge becomes loose at one end but seems firmly attached at the

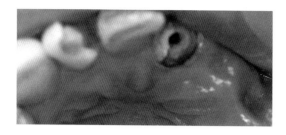

Figure 13.1

The upper central incisor had a post-retained crown but no diaphragm covering the root face. The tooth has split longitudinally and must now be extracted.

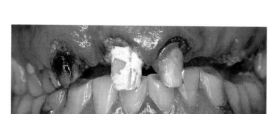

Figure 13.2

Carious abutment teeth revealed by removing a bridge that was still firmly attached to the sound abutment teeth.

other, one option is to cut off the loose retainer, leaving the bridge as a cantilever.

Other bridges

In the case of simple cantilever bridges with one abutment tooth, or the major retainer of a three-unit fixed–movable bridge, the loss of retention will result in the bridge falling out. The same is true if both ends of a fixed–fixed bridge become loose. There is usually less permanent damage in these cases, since plaque is not retained against the surface of the preparation, and the patient is obviously aware of the problem and seeks treatment quickly.

Minimal-preparation bridges

Partial or complete loss of retention is the commonest cause of failure of these bridges. It is argued by some that if the bridge can be cleaned and re-cemented without further treatment, it is not a true failure but only a partial failure. This is

a reasonable point of view, and when minimal-preparation bridges are made, the patient should be warned that re-cementation may be necessary as part of normal maintenance and should not be regarded as a disaster.

There is some evidence that minimal-preparation bridges are retained for longer periods when they have been re-cemented. It is difficult to imagine why this should be, other than perhaps the operator taking greater care the second time around.

There is now good evidence that fixed–fixed minimal-preparation bridges fail through loss of retention more readily than cantilever (with one abutment tooth) and fixed–movable designs. This is why these designs have been advocated earlier in this book. It is very unusual for a minor retainer for a fixed–movable minimal-preparation bridge to lose its retention, because there are no significant forces to dislodge it.

Solutions

If there is no extensive damage to the preparation, it may be possible to re-cement the crown or bridge, provided that the cause can be identified and eliminated. It may be that a bridge was dislodged by a blow or that some problem during cementation was the cause. However, if the underlying reason is that the preparation is not adequately retentive, it may be possible to provide additional retention by cross-pinning the preparation (see Figure 13.3), although ideally it should be made more retentive and the crown or bridge (or at least the unsatisfactory retainer) remade.

Alternatively it may be necessary to include additional abutment teeth in a bridge to increase the overall retention or to change the design in some other way.

Mechanical failure of crowns or bridge components

Typical mechanical failures are:

● Porcelain fracture
● Failure of solder joints
● Distortion
● Occlusal wear and perforation
● Lost facings.

Porcelain fracture

At one time pieces of porcelain fracturing off metal–ceramic crowns, or the loss of the entire facing due to failure of the metal–ceramic bond, were relatively commonplace. With modern materials and techniques this is much less common; but when it does occur it is particularly frustrating since, even though the damage may be slight, there is often little that can be done to repair it satisfactorily without remaking the crown or the whole bridge.

To prevent this type of damage to metal–ceramic bridges, the framework must be properly designed with an adequate thickness of metal to avoid distortion, particularly with long-span bridges. If there is any risk of the pontic area flexing, the porcelain should be carried on to the lingual side of pontics to stiffen them further.

An all-porcelain crown or bridge that is fractured must be replaced. Sometimes the cause is a blow, and then the choice of material can be

regarded as fortunate: had a metal–ceramic material been used it is more likely that the root of the tooth would have fractured. If the fracture is due to trauma, and particularly if the crown or bridge had served successfully for some time, it should be replaced by means of another all-ceramic restoration. However, if the failure occurs during normal function, shortly after the crown or bridge is fitted, the implication is that the conditions are not suitable for an all-ceramic restoration, and the replacement should be metal–ceramic.

Failure of solder joints

Occasionally a solder joint that appears to be sound fails under occlusal loading. This may be due to:

● A flaw or inclusion in the solder itself
● Failure to bond to the surface of the metal
● The solder joint not being sufficiently large for the conditions in which it is placed.

A problem, particularly with metal–ceramic bridgework, is that soldered connectors should be restricted from encroaching on the buccal side too much to avoid metal showing, restricted gingivally in order to provide access for cleaning, and restricted incisally to create the impression of separate teeth. Too much restriction can lead to an inadequate area of solder and to failure.

It is better whenever possible to join multiple-unit bridges by solder joints in the middle of pontics before the porcelain is added. This gives a much larger surface area for the solder joint, and it is also strengthened by the porcelain covering. A failed solder joint is a disaster in a large metal–ceramic bridge, and often means that the whole bridge has to be removed and remade. Figure 9.4f, page 197, shows a failed solder joint. There are no satisfactory intra-oral repair methods, and it is not usually possible to remove the bridge to resolder the joint without doing further damage.

Distortion

Distortion of all-metal bridges may occur, for example, when wash-through pontics are made

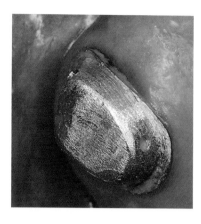

Figure 13.3

Cross-pinning for additional retention.

a A telescopic crown that has been in place for many years but is overtapered. The bridge cemented to this has become loose and been removed.

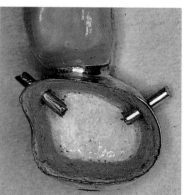

b The retainer (which fits over the telescopic crown) is drilled to receive gold-wire pins.

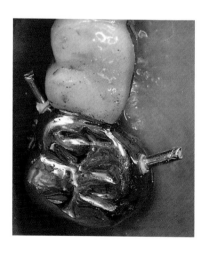

c The bridge is replaced and short holes cut through the telescopic crown (these can be seen in *a*), with the holes in the retainer being used as guides. A 0.7-mm-diameter twist drill that matches the gold wire is used. The retainer has now been cemented, and the gold pins cemented through it into the telescopic crown and the dentine beneath. When set, the excess gold wire will be removed and the surface polished.

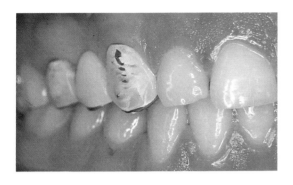

Figure 13.4

Badly worn acrylic bridge facings.

too thin or if a bridge is removed using too much force. When this happens the bridge has to be remade.

In metal–ceramic bridges distortion of the framework can occur during function or as a result of trauma. This is likely if the framework is too small in cross-section for the length of span and the material used. Distortion of a metal–ceramic framework invariably results in the loss of porcelain.

Occlusal wear and perforation

Even with normal attrition, the occlusal surfaces of posterior teeth wear down substantially over a lifetime. Gold crowns made with 0.5 mm or so of gold occlusally may wear through over a period of two or three decades. If perforation has been the result of normal wear and it is spotted before caries has developed, it may be repaired with an appropriate restoration. Occasionally, particularly if the perforation is over an amalgam core, it is satisfactory simply to leave the perforation untreated and check it periodically (see Figures 8.1b, page 174 and Figure 13.11h, page 269).

Occlusal perforations may also be made deliberately for endodontic treatment or vitality testing (see Figure 10.2c, page 209).

Lost facings

Materials are available to repair porcelain in the mouth (see Figure 13.10, page 266). Even if they last only a few years before discolouring or wearing, they can be replaced and are a reasonably satisfactory and less costly alternative to replacing the whole restoration.

Laboratory-made ceramic or acrylic facings may be entirely lost, and with acrylic facings, wear and discoloration are also common (see Figure 13.4). Although very few crowns or bridges are made nowadays with proprietary facings, it is not uncommon to find patients with old bridges missing long-pin, Steele's or other proprietary facings.

Changes in the abutment tooth

Periodontal disease

Periodontal disease may be generalized, or in a poorly designed, made or maintained restoration its progress may be accelerated locally. If the loss of periodontal attachment is diagnosed early enough and the cause removed, no further treatment is usually necessary. However, if the disease has progressed to the point where the prognosis of the tooth is significantly reduced then the crown or bridge, or the tooth itself, may have to be removed.

With a bridge the original indication will still be present, and so something will have to be done to replace the missing teeth. It may be possible to make a larger bridge, or the abutment teeth may be reduced and used as abutments for an over-denture. Teeth that have lost so much support that they are not suitable as bridge abutments are not suitable either as abutments for conventional partial dentures.

Problems with the pulp

Unfortunately, despite taking the usual precautions during tooth preparation, abutment teeth may become non-vital after a crown or bridge has been cemented. It is usually reasonable to attempt endodontic treatment by making an access cavity through the crown. There are of course problems in the application of a rubber dam, although these can usually be overcome by punching a large hole and applying the rubber dam only to one tooth, stretching the rubber over the connectors.

It is often difficult to gain access to the pulp chamber and remove the coronal pulp completely without enlarging the access cavity to a point where the remaining tooth preparation becomes too thin and weak to support the crown satisfactorily, or where the pin retention of a core is damaged. The crown may have been made with rather different anatomy from the natural crown of the tooth for aesthetic or occlusal reasons, so that the angulation of the root is not immediately apparent. Provided these problems can be overcome and a satisfactory root filling placed, the prognosis of the crown or bridge is only marginally reduced.

Teeth that were already satisfactorily root-filled when the crown or bridge was made may later give trouble. Occasionally it may be possible to root-fill the tooth again through the crown, but more commonly apicectomy is the solution. Care must be taken not to shorten the root of an abutment tooth more than is absolutely necessary so that the maximum support for the bridge can be maintained.

Caries

Secondary caries occurring at the margins of crowns or bridge retainers usually means that the patient has changed his or her diet, the standard of oral hygiene has lapsed or there is some inadequacy in the restoration that is encouraging the formation of plaque. The cause of the problem should be identified and dealt with before repair or replacement is started.

Fracture of the prepared natural crown or root

Fractures of the tooth occasionally occur as a result of trauma, and sometimes even during normal function, although the crown or bridge has been present for some time. With a bridge abutment it is usually necessary to remove the bridge, but occasionally the abutment tooth can be dispensed with and the root removed surgically, the tissue surface of the retainer being repaired and converted into a pontic.

Movement of the tooth

Occlusal trauma, periodontal disease or relapsing orthodontic treatment may result in the crowned tooth or bridge abutment becoming loose, drifting, or both. When the cause is periodontal disease or relapsing orthodontic treatment, this must be remedied before the crown or bridge is remade.

Design failures

Abutment preparation design

The pitfalls of inadequate crown preparation design were described in Chapter 3, and are the underlying cause of many of the problems listed so far in this chapter.

Inadequate bridge design

Designing bridges is difficult. It is neither a precise science nor a creative art. It needs knowledge, experience and judgement, which take years to accumulate.

So it is not surprising that some designs of bridge, even though well intentioned and conscientiously executed, fail. A simple classification of these failures is as 'under-prescribed' and 'over-prescribed' bridges.

Under-prescribed bridges These include designs that are unstable or have too few abutment teeth – for example a cantilever bridge carrying pontics that cover too long a span or a fixed–movable bridge where again the span is too

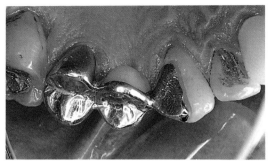

Figure 13.5

A bad design. The bridge is fixed–fixed and is firmly held by the premolar retainer. The inlay in the canine is, however, loose and caries has developed beneath it. Either the design should have been fixed–movable with a mesial movable connector or, if fixed–fixed, the retainer on the canine should have covered all occluding surfaces of the tooth and have been more retentive.

long, or where abutment teeth with too little support have been selected.

Another 'under-design' fault is to be too conservative in selecting retainers, for example intracoronal inlays for fixed–fixed bridges. With these design faults little can be done other than to remove the bridge and use another type of replacement (see Figure 13.5).

Over-prescribed bridges Cautious dentists will sometimes include more abutment teeth than are necessary, and fate usually dictates that it is the unnecessary retainer that fails. The first lower premolar might be included as well as the second premolar and second molar in a bridge to replace the lower first molar, no doubt so that there will be equal numbers of roots each end of the bridge. This is not necessary. Another example would be to use the upper canines and both premolars on each side in replacing the four incisor teeth. As well as being destructive, this gives rise to unnecessary practical difficulties in making the bridge. This, in turn, reduces the chances of the bridge being successful.

When an unnecessarily large number of abutment teeth have been included in a bridge and one of the retainers fails, it is sometimes possible to section the bridge in the mouth and remove the failed unit, leaving the remainder of the bridge to continue in function. The failed unit is remade as an individual restoration (see Figure 13.6).

The retainers themselves may be over-prescribed, with complete crowns being used where partial crowns or intra-coronal retainers would have been quite adequate; or metal–ceramic crowns might be used where all-metal crowns would have been sufficient. When the pulp dies in such a case, it is interesting to speculate whether this might not have occurred with a less drastic reduction of the crown of the natural tooth.

Inadequate clinical or laboratory technique

It is helpful to allocate problems in the construction of crowns and bridges to one of three groups:

- Minor problems to be noted and monitored but where no other action is needed
- The type of inadequacies that can be corrected in situ, and
- Those that cannot.

This is often a matter of degree, and many of the following faults can fall into any of these groups.

Marginal deficiencies

Positive ledge (overhang) A positive ledge is an excess of crown material protruding beyond the margin of the preparation. These are more common with porcelain than with any other margins. Considering that this is a fairly easy fault

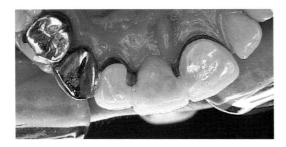

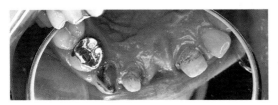

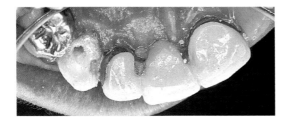

Figure 13.6

Overprescribed design.

a This four-unit bridge replaces only one central incisor. The partial-crown retainer on the canine has become loose. When the bridge was removed, the central and lateral incisors were found to be sound and adequate abutments, without the inclusion of the canine. Caries has spread across the canine, and the pulp has died.

b and *c* Fortunately it was possible to remove the bridge intact, and, after removing the canine retainer, the remaining three units could be re-cemented. A separate post crown was made for the canine tooth following endodontic treatment.

to recognize and correct before the crown or bridge is fitted, it is surprising how frequently overhangs are encountered (see Figure 6.27a, page 141). However, it is often possible to correct them without otherwise disturbing the restoration.

Negative ledge This is a deficiency of crown material that leaves the margin of the preparation exposed but with no major gaps between the crown and the tooth. Again it is a fairly common fault, particularly with metal margins, but one that is difficult or impossible to correct at the try-in stage (see Figure 6.27b). It often arises because the impression did not give a clear enough indication of the margin of the preparation and the die was over-trimmed, resulting in under-extension of the retainer (see Figure 6.28, page 142).

Provided that the crown margin is supragingival or just at the gingival margin, it is sometimes possible to adjust and polish the tooth surface. When the ledge is subgingival, and particularly when there is localized gingival inflammation associated with it, it may still be possible to adjust the ledge with a pointed stone or bur, although this will cause gingival damage. However, it is usually necessary to remove the crown or bridge.

Defect A defect is a gap between the crown and preparation margins. There are four possible causes:

● The crown or retainer did not fit and the gap was present at try-in
● The crown or retainer fitted at try-in, but at the time of cementation the hydrostatic pressure of the cement (particularly if the cement was beginning to set) produced incomplete seating
● With a mobile bridge or splint abutment, the

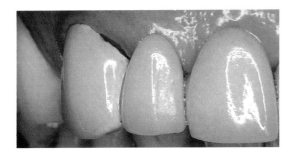

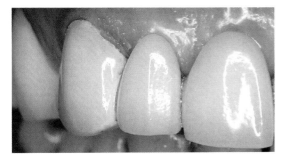

Figure 13.7

a A small gap at the mesial margin of the upper canine retainer on an otherwise very satisfactory bridge that has been in place for several years. The gap was not noticed at previous recall appointments, and although it may now have become apparent through gingival recession, it is more likely that the gap has been enlarged by over-vigorous use of dental floss. The patient demonstrated a faulty and damaging sawing action, with floss running into the gap.

b The defect repaired with glass ionomer cement. The patient has been shown gentler oral hygiene techniques.

cement depressed the mobile tooth in its socket more than the other abutment teeth, thus leaving the gap
● No gap was present at the time of cementation, but one developed following the loss of cement at the margin, and a crevice has been created by a combination of erosion/abrasion and possibly caries.

In any of these cases, the choice is to remove the bridge, restore the gap with a suitable restoration, or leave it alone and observe it periodically.

Purists may say that all defective retainers should be removed and replaced. But this is not always in the patient's best interest, and the skilful application of marginal repairs may extend the life of the restoration for many years (see Figure 13.7).

Poor shape or colour

More can be done to adjust the shape of a crown or bridge in situ than to modify its colour, although occasionally surface stain on porcelain can be removed and the porcelain polished. The shape of metal–ceramic crowns or bridges can be adjusted if they are too bulky (and this is usually the problem), provided that it is done slowly. At the first sign of the opaque layer of porcelain, the adjustment is stopped.

Successful modifications can often be made to open cramped embrasure spaces, reduce excessive cervical bulbosity, shorten retainers and pontics, and of course adjust the occluding surface. In all cases the adjusted surface, whether it is metal or porcelain, should be polished.

Occlusal problems

As well as producing abutment tooth mobility, faults in the occlusion involve damage to the retainers and pontics by wear and fracture.

The occlusion can change as a result of the extraction of other teeth, or their restoration, or through wear on the occlusal surface.

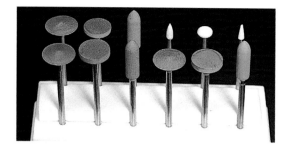

Figure 13.8

a A set of instruments for polishing porcelain.

b Scanning electron micrographs, at the same magnification, of three areas of the same porcelain surface. *Left*: the glazed surface showing some undulation and occasional defects. *Centre*: the surface ground with a fine porcelain grindstone. *Right*: the same surface repolished, after grinding, with the instruments shown in *a*. The surface is smooth, without undulations, but with some fine scratch marks and occasional defects.

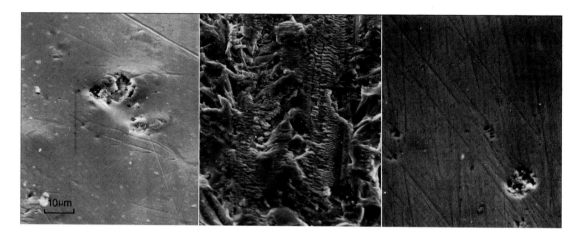

Techniques for adjustments, adaptations and repairs to crowns and bridges

Assessing the seriousness of the problem

In existing restorations there is not infrequently one or other of the faults listed above. A decision has to be made between:

- Leaving it alone, if it is not causing any serious harm
- Adjusting or repairing the fault
- Replacing the crown or bridge.

When action is necessary, it is clearly better to extend the life of an otherwise-successful crown or bridge with the second option than replace restorations too frequently. If there is any doubt, or when adjustment or repair must be carried out, the restoration must be kept under frequent and careful review.

Adjustments by grinding and polishing in situ

In some situations the margins of crowns with positive ledges can be satisfactorily adjusted. If the margin is porcelain, specially designed porcelain finishing instruments should be used. Alternatively, a heatless stone or diamond point can be used, followed by polishing with successive grades of composite finishing burs and discs. These are capable of giving a very good finish to non-porous porcelain, which the patient can keep

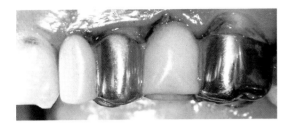

Figure 13.9

a A bridge with defective margins and extensive gingival inflammation.

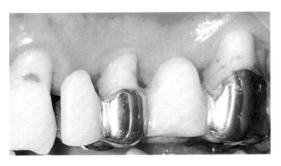

b The same bridge after a periodontal flap has been raised, the retainer margins adjusted by grinding and polishing, and the flap then apically repositioned. The gingival condition is now healthy.

as clean as glazed porcelain (see Figure 13.8). The contour of porcelain restorations can be modified in situ using the same instruments.

In the case of metal margins, a diamond stone followed by green stones, tungsten carbide stones or metal and linen strips may be used. Interdentally, a triangular-shaped diamond and an abrasive rubber instrument in a special reciprocating handpiece designed specifically for removing overhangs may be used. The margin should be polished with prophylactic paste and a brush or rubber cup, and interdentally with finishing strips.

Repairs by restoring in situ

Occlusal repairs

Occlusal defects in metal retainers can be repaired with amalgam, which usually gives quite a satisfactory result. However, a small gold inlay may be preferred. In porcelain or metal–ceramic restorations composite material can be used, but the repair may need to be redone periodically.

Repairs at the margins

Although repairs are justified to extend the life of an established crown or bridge, they should never be used to adapt the margins of a poorly fitting bridge on insertion.

Secondary caries that is identified at an early stage or early abrasion/erosion lesions at crown margins can be repaired using composite or glass ionomer cement. The cause should be investigated and preventive measures applied.

The cavity preparation at the margin must not be so deep that it endangers the strength of the preparation, although of course all caries must be removed. If there is poor access it may be better to remove part of the crown margin rather than an excessive amount of tooth tissue.

In some cases raising a full gingival flap may be justified. Retainer margins can be adjusted and restored under conditions of optimum access and visibility, and any necessary periodontal work or endodontic surgery carried out at the same time (see Figure 13.9).

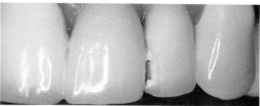

Figure 13.10

Repairing porcelain facings.

a The lateral incisor facing has chipped. The bridge is more than 10 years old.

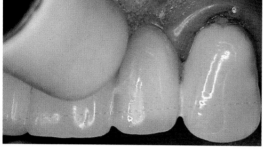

b After being polished with pumice and water, a silane coupling agent is painted over the surface, followed by a resin bonding agent and light-cured composite.

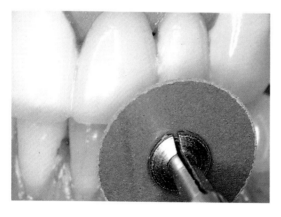

c Polishing the composite.

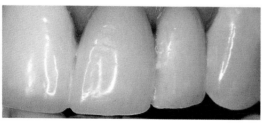

d The finished result. This is unsatisfactory, since the metal shows through. An opaquer should have been used over the metal.

Repairs to porcelain

Materials are available to repair or modify the shape of ceramic restorations in the mouth. These are basically composite materials with a separate silane coupling agent that allows optimum bonding. It is not an acid-etch bond like the bond to enamel and is not strong, so the use of the material is limited to sites not exposed to large occlusal forces (see Figure 13.10).

Repairs by removing or replacing parts of a bridge

Replacing lost facings

It is sometimes possible to replace a failed facing on a bridge, usefully extending its life. But this is not worth attempting on individual crowns – it is better to replace the whole crown.

Preformed or proprietary facings Some of the older proprietary facings were designed specifically so that they could be replaced in situ, for example the long-pin facing. When these are lost, provided the remainder of the bridge is sound, it is possible to take an impression of the backing and make a new porcelain facing, a metal–ceramic facing, or an acrylic or composite facing retained by pins (see Figure 13.11a, b).

Ceramic facings When the porcelain is lost from a metal–ceramic unit and a composite repair is not possible, there is often little choice but to remove the whole crown or bridge. However, with a pontic it is sometimes possible to drill holes through the backing and take an impression with suitable pins so that a new pin-retained metal–ceramic facing can be constructed rather like the proprietary long-pin facing. Almost inevitably, this will be bulky and will not perfectly match the appearance of the original (see Figure 13.11c, d).

Alternatively, it is sometimes possible with retainers or pontics to remove all the porcelain and re-prepare the metal part, producing enough clearance without damaging the strength of the metal. A new complete crown covering the skeleton of the old retainer or pontic can then be accommodated. These are sometimes made in heat-cured acrylic or laboratory light-cured composite. They are known as 'sleeve crowns'. A metal–ceramic sleeve crown is shown in Figures 13.11e,f and g).

'Unit-construction' bridge facings Before the routine use of metal–ceramic materials, bridges were often made with a metal framework and separate PJCs cemented to it. This design was known as 'unit-construction'. The individual PJCs often broke, since they were considerably reduced approximally to accommodate the connector. However, a new PJC could easily be made, and some patients were even provided with a second, spare set when the bridge was cemented (see Figure 13.11h and i).

Removing and/or replacing entire sections of a bridge

Bridges are sometimes so designed that if a doubtful abutment tooth becomes unsaveable, it can be removed with its associated section of the bridge, leaving the remainder undisturbed. This is one of the purposes of removable, telescopic crown-retained bridges and of dividing multiple-unit bridges into smaller sections. When part of a bridge is removed, the remainder can sometimes be modified, perhaps by cutting a slot for a movable joint and then replacing the lost section.

Extending bridges

Provision is sometimes made to extend a bridge if further teeth are lost. Figure 13.12 shows a large bridge with a slot in the distal surface of the premolar retainer on the left of the picture so that a further fixed–movable section can be added if the second premolar (which has a questionable prognosis) is lost. The slot is filled in the meantime by a small gold inlay.

Removing crowns and bridges

In removing any crown or bridge, and in particular posts and caries, it is often helpful to break up the cement by vibrating the restoration with an ultrasonic scaler. This works best with zinc phosphate cement.

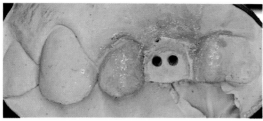

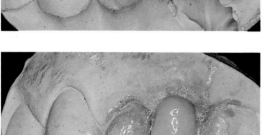

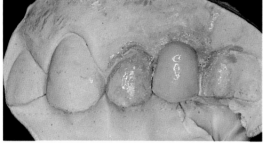

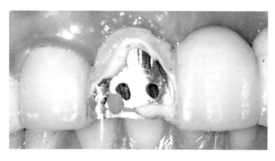

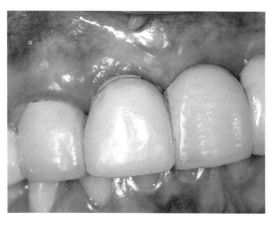

Figure 13.11

Techniques for repairing bridges.

a The cast of a bridge pontic that had lost its long-pin facing. The impressions of the pinholes were taken with stainless-steel wire of matching diameter.

b A metal–ceramic laboratory-made replacement long-pin facing.

c Most of the porcelain facing has been lost from this metal–ceramic pontic. Pinholes are drilled through the metal framework, the margins shaped and an impression taken.

d A new facing made in metal–ceramic material. This is inevitably bulky, but if the alternative is to remove the entire bridge and remake it at very high cost, this compromise may be preferable. In any case, further periodontal treatment is needed before a replacement bridge is made.

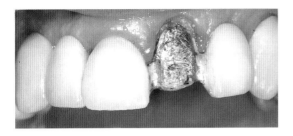

e The porcelain on this bridge retainer has fractured. It has all been removed and the tooth prepared for a 'sleeve-crown'.

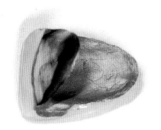

f The sleeve-crown with a metal lingual surface replacing the original lingual porcelain.

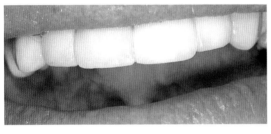

g The sleeve-crown in place.

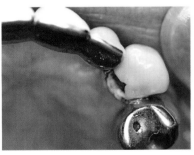

h A fractured PJC, which has been made over a gold coping as the canine retainer for a bridge. Apart from this, and the hole worn in the occlusal surface of the premolar partial crown retainer, the bridge is still serving satisfactorily after more than 20 years. The pontics have long-pin facings.

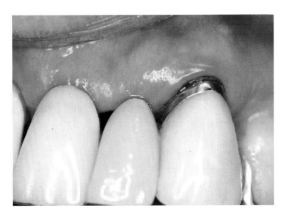

i The replacement PJC cemented

(*Note:* This figure (*h* and *i*), with the same caption, was published in the first edition of this book in 1986. In 1996 the bridge with its replacement PJC is still in place – showing that repairs of this sort are well worthwhile.)

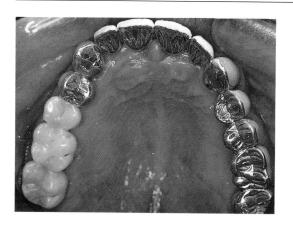

Figure 13.12

Provision for the extension of a bridge (see text for details).

Crowns

Removing metal crowns

Complete and partial metal crowns can sometimes be removed intact by levering at the margins with a heavy-duty scaler such as Cumine or Mitchell's trimmer. Alternatively, a slide-hammer type of crown- or bridge-remover may be used, or one of the other devices specially designed to remove crowns; Figure 13.13 shows a selection. If these techniques do not work, the crown will have to be cut off (see under 'Removing metal–ceramic crowns').

Removing posts and cores

Unretentive posts can often be removed by gripping the core in extraction forceps and giving it a series of sharp twists. This should not be attempted by the inexperienced!

There are several devices designed to remove posts and cores intact and to remove broken posts (see Figure 13.13).

Removing PJCs

These cannot usually be removed intact, and should be cut off. A vertical groove is made with a diamond bur in the buccal surface, just through

to the cement, and then the crown is split with a suitable heavy-duty instrument (see Figure 13.14a).

Removing metal–ceramic crowns

It is sometimes possible to remove metal–ceramic crowns intact by using one of the devices shown in Figure 13.13, but they are more rigid than gold crowns and the porcelain is liable to break, and so they usually have to be cut off.

A groove is cut vertically from the gingival margin to the occlusal surface, preferably on the buccal side just through to the cement, and then the crown is sprung open with a heavy instrument such as a Cumine scaler, Mitchell's trimmer or a heavy chisel, breaking the cement lute. Sometimes the cut will need to extend across the occlusal surface (see Figure 13.14b–d).

Cast metal is best cut with a special solid tungsten carbide bur with very fine cross-cuts (beaver bur). This is capable of cutting metal without juddering or jamming, and there is less risk of the bur itself breaking than with a conventional tungsten carbide bur. Eye protection should always be worn by the patient, the dental nurse and dentist, particularly when cutting metal.

Diamond burs cut cast metal slowly, but are ideal for rapidly cutting porcelain, and so metal–ceramic units are best sectioned using different burs for the two materials. Since it is

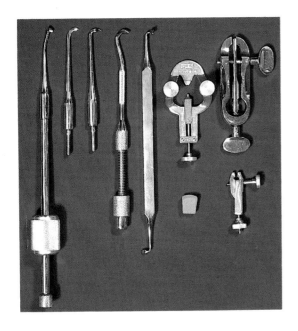

Figure 13.13

A selection of instruments for removing crowns and bridges. *From the left:*

a slide-hammer remover with two alternative screw-in tips: the tip is hooked into a crown margin or under a bridge connector, and the weight slid down the handle and tapped against the stop at the end;

a spring-loaded slide hammer, also with replaceable tips;

a special heavy-duty instrument that is hooked under crown margins and twisted to remove them;

below: a turquoise-coloured polymer that is softened in hot water and bitten upon by the patient. The material is cooled with water and the patient asked to jerk the jaw open;

above: this instrument is clamped beneath the crown and the two screws (the heads visible here) are screwed down on to the occlusal surfaces of adjacent teeth, lifting the crown;

two clamps that fit on to posts and cores, with a screw that presses on to the shoulder of a post-crown preparation and draws the post and core out of the tooth.

possible to cut porcelain much more quickly than metal, the metal on the buccal surface is usually thinner than that on the palatal or lingual surface, and visibility and access are far better buccally, the groove is easier to make on the buccal side.

Removing bridges

There are three sets of circumstances:

● When the abutment teeth are to be extracted and so it does not matter if the preparations are damaged, the bridge will be removed in the most convenient way, often with a crown- and bridge-remover. In some cases it may not be necessary to remove the bridge at all, for example with simple cantilever bridges with one abutment tooth. In others it is quicker to divide the bridge through a pontic or connec-

tor and extract the abutment teeth individually with their retainers in place.
● When it is the intention to retain the abutment teeth – either to make a new bridge or to use them to support a partial denture or an over-denture – it does not matter whether the bridge is damaged during its removal, but the preparations should be protected. The retainers should be cut and the bridge carefully removed with the bridge-remover.
● There are occasions when it would be helpful to remove the bridge intact, modify or repair it and then replace it, if only as a temporary measure. In this case neither the bridge nor the preparations should be damaged.

Removing bridges intact

The slightly more flexible structure of all-metal bridges and of minimal-preparation bridges allows

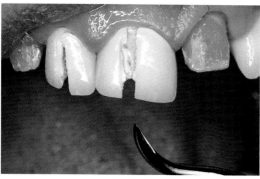

Figure 13.14

Removing crowns and bridges.

a Removing PJCs. A cut is made with a diamond bur down the buccal surface and across the incisal edge. The crown can then be split with a suitable heavy-duty instrument.

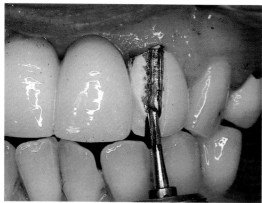

b Removing a metal–ceramic bridge by cutting through the buccal porcelain with a diamond bur.

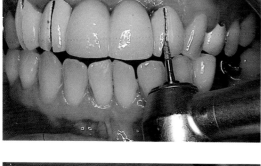

c Then changing to a special metal-cutting (beaver) bur to cut through the metal until the cement just shows.

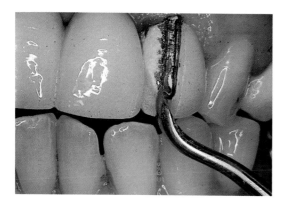

d Springing open the retainer with a heavy-duty instrument. It is sometimes necessary to continue the cut round to the lingual surface.

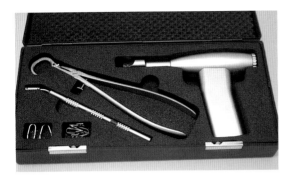

Figure 13.15

a Specialized equipment for removing crowns. The pistol-shaped instrument is supplied with compressed air and vibrates one or other of the attachments against the crown or bridge. The equipment is expensive and only available in specialist centres.

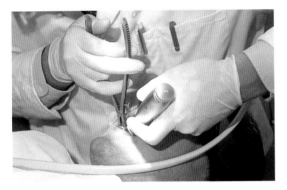

b The equipment shown in *a* being used clinically.

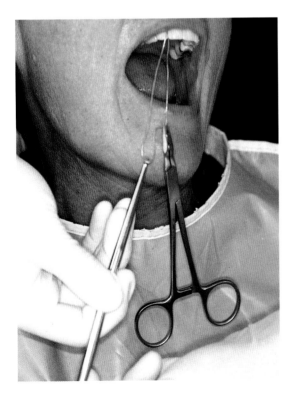

Figure 13.16

Removing a bridge with a soft brass wire loop. The locking forceps are clipping the twisted ends of the wire together to prevent the sharp ends damaging the chin. The slide-hammer (see Figure 13.13) is being used in the wire loop rather than under the bridge pontic. This is more controllable and effective and less dangerous.

them to be removed intact rather more readily than metal–ceramic conventional bridges. However, all types can sometimes be removed by sharp tapping, which fractures the cement lute without too much risk to the periodontal membrane of the abutment teeth. The nature of the force is quite different to the slow tearing applied in extracting teeth.

Slide hammers are specially designed for the purpose with replaceable tips to fit under retainer margins, under pontics or into embrasure spaces (see Figure 13.13). Sometimes it is necessary to drill a hole in the palatal surface of the retainer or pontic and fit an attachment from the slide hammer into it.

Various other techniques can be used. Figure 13.15 shows an air-driven appliance and ultrasonic vibration with a scaler can loosen crowns and bridges.

A more common technique is to make loops of soft wire beneath the contact points of the bridge and use a slide hammer in the wire loop (see Figure 13.16). Alternatively, if a slide hammer is not available, a heavy metal object is passed through the loops well outside the mouth, and sharp blows applied to it with a mallet or other heavy instrument. This is a rather dramatic approach, and the patient needs to have a phlegmatic personality and to be properly informed of what is proposed beforehand.

Practical points

● A large proportion of 'failures' are partial, and a level of acceptability needs to be established between patient and dentist. This is particularly true for minimal-preparation bridges.

● Changes in the abutment teeth due, for example, to periodontal disease can frequently be treated so that the prognosis for the crown or bridge is not significantly affected.

● Although repairs are justified to extend the life of an established crown or bridge, they should never be used to cover-up poor design, for example to adapt the margins of a poorly fitting bridge on insertion.

● Bridges can be made with 'fail-safe' features – for example so that one section can be removed if necessary, leaving the remainder undisturbed.

Further reading

Chapter 1

Treatment of traumatized teeth
Andreasen JO, *Traumatic injuries of the teeth* (1981) Saunders, Philadelphia.

Tooth wear
Smith BGN, Knight JK, A comparison of patterns of tooth wear with aetiological factors, *Brit Dent J* (1984) **157**: 16–19.

Smith B G N. Some facets of tooth wear. *Ann R Aust Coll Dent Surg* (1991) **11**: 37–51.

Bleaching
Warren K, Bleaching discoloured endodontically treated teeth, *Restorative Dent* (1985) **1**: 132–8.

Fisher N L and Radford J R. Internal bleaching of discoloured teeth. *Dental Update* (1990) **17**: 110–114.

Anterior composites
Lutz F, Philips RW, A classification and evaluation of composite resin systems, *J Prosth Dent* (1983) **50**: 480–8.

Facings in composite
Jordan RE et al, Labial resin veneer restorations using visible cured composite materials, *Alpha Omega Scientific Issue* (1981) **74**: 31–9.

Porcelain veneers
McConnell RJ et al, Etched porcelain veneers, *Restorative Dent* (1986) **2**: 124–31.

Dunne S M and Millar B J. A longitudinal study of the clinical performance of porcelain veneers. *Brit Dent J* (1994) **175**: 317–321.

Restoration of root-filled teeth
Martin DM, Glyn Jones JC, The relationship of endodontic procedures to the coronal restoration, *Restorative Dent* (1986) **1**: 10–16.

Chapter 2

Porcelain and metal-ceramic restorations
McLean JW, *The science and art of dental ceramics,*

Vol. I (1979), Vol II (1980), Quintessence, Chicago.

Alternatives to precious metal alloys
Council on dental materials, instruments and equipment, Statutory report on low-gold-content alloys for fixed prostheses, *J Am Dent Assn* (1980) **100**: 237–40.

Retention
Lorey RE, Myers GE, The retentive qualities of bridge retainers, *J Am Dent Assn* (1968) **76**: 568–72.

Chapter 3

Crown preparation taper
Jorgensen KD, The relationship between retention and convergence angles in cemented veneer crowns, *Acta Odont Scand* (1955) **13**: 35.

Mack PJ, A theoretical and clinical investigation into the taper achieved on crown and inlay preparations, *J Oral Rehab* (1980) **7**: 255–65.

Crowns margins and gingival health
Silness J, Periodontal treatment of patients with dental bridges, 3 The relationship between the location of the crown margin and the periodontal condition, *J Periodontal Res* (1970) **5**: 225–9.

Chapter 4

Occlusion, general
Ash MM, Ramfjord SP, *An introduction to functional occlusion* (1982) Saunders, Philadelphia.

Mohl N D, Zarb G A, Carlsson G, Rugh J D Eds. A textbook of occlusion. Quintessence, Chicago (1988).

Gross MD, Mathews JD, *Occlusion in restorative dentistry* (1982) Churchill Livingstone, Edinburgh.

Occlusal records
Simpson JW et al, Arbitary mandibular hing axis locations, *J Prosth dent* (1984) **51**: 819–22.

Mandibular dysfunction
Zarb G A, Carlsson G E, Sessle B J, Mohl N D Eds. Temporomandibular joint and masticatory muscle disorders. Munksgaard, Copenhagen (1994).

Robinson P D. A review of temporomandibular joint pain. *Pain Reviews* (1995) **2**: 138–151.

Chapter 5

Examining the whole patient
Tyldesley WR, *Oral diagnosis* (1978) Pergamon Press, Oxford.

Planning crowns for endodontically treated teeth
Nicholls E, *Endodontics* (1984) John Wright, Bristol.

Appearance
McLean JW, *The science and art of dental ceramics.* Vol. 1 (1979), Vol. 2 (1980) Quintessence, Chicago.

Chapter 6

Shade selection
Scharer P et al, *Esthetic guidelines for restorative dentistry* (1982) Quintessence, Chicago.

Tooth preparation
Shillingburg HT et al, *Fundamentals of fixed prosthodontics* (1997) Quintessence, Chicago.

General
McLean JW, *Dental ceramics. Proceedings of the first international symposium on dental ceramics* (1983) Quintessence, Chicago.

Chapter 7

Choice between fixed and removable prostheses
Zarb GA et al, *Prosthodontic treatment for partially edentulous patients* (1978) Mosby, St Louis.

Embouchure: musicians
Corcorcon DF, Dental problems in musicians, *J Irish dent Assn* (1985) **31**: 4–7.

Precision attachments
Preiskel HW, *Precision attachments in prosthodontics,* Vol. 1 (1984) Quintessence, Chicago.

Implants
Hobkirk J A and Watson R M. Dental and maxillofacial implantology. Mosby-Wolfe, London (1995).

Chapter 8

Minimal-preparation bridges
Rochette AL, Attachment of a splint to enamel of lower anterior teeth, *J Prosth Dent* (1973) **30**: 418.

Livaditis GL, Thompson, VP, Etched castings: an improved retention mechanism for resin bonded retainere, *J Prosth Dent* (1982) **47**: 52.

Chapter 9

Pontics
Stein RS, Pontic-residual ridge relationships: a research report, *J Prosth Dent* (1966) **16**: 251–85.

Clayton JA, Green E, Roughness of pontic materiald and dental plaque, *J Prosth Dent* (1970) **23**: 407–11.

Chapter 10

Abutment support for bridges:
'Engineering' evidence
Reynolds JM, Abutment selection for fixed prosthodontics, *J Prosth Dent* (1968) **19**: 483–7.

Wright KWJ, Yettram AL, Reactive force distributions for teeth when loaded singly and when used as fixed partial denture abutments, *J Prosth Dent* (1979) **42**: 411–16.

Clinical evidence
Nyman S, Lindhe J, Prosthetic rehabilitation of patients with advanced periodontal disease, *J Clin Periodont* (1976) **3**: 135–47.

Nyman S, Ericsson I, The capacity of reduced periodontal tissues to support fixed bridgework, *J Clin Periodont* (1992) **9**: 409–14.

Chapter 11

Provisional and temporary bridges
Capp NJ, The diagnostic use of provisional restorations, *Restorative Dent* (1985) **1**: 92–8.

Technique for minimal-preparation bridges
Gratton DR et al, The resin bonded cast metal bridge: a review, *Restorative Dent* (1985) **1**: 68–76.

Chapter 12

Splints and periodontal disease
Lindhe J, *Textbook of clinical periodontology* (1983) Munksgaard, Copenhagen.

Cleft palate and splints
Kantorowicz GF, Bridge prostheses for cleft palate patients: an analysis, *Brit Dent J* (1975) **139**: 91–7.

Dental defects and splints
Mars M, Smith BGN, dentinogenesis imperfecta: and integrated conservative approach to treatment, *Brit Dent J* (1982) **152**: 15–18.

Chapter 13

Failures in general
Wise MD Failure in the restored dentition (1994) Quintessence, London.

Surveys of bridge failures
Roberts DH, The failure of retainers in bridge prostheses, *Brit Dent J* (1970) **128**: 117–24.

Reuter JE, Brose MO, Failures in full crown retained dental bridges, *Brit Dent J* (1984) **157**: 61–3.

Dunne S M and Millar B J. A longitudinal study of the clinical performance of resin bonded bridges and splints. *Br Dent J* (1993) **174**: 405–411.

Removal of bridges
Kantorowicz, GF, The repair and removal of bridges, *Dent Practitioner* (1971) **21**: 341–6.

Index

Note. Main headings for appliances used in bridgework are in UK terminology, with cross-references provided from the US terms.

Abutment teeth
  alignment of, retention and, 192–3
  changes causing problems, 259–60
  condition of, retention and, 194
  definition, 173
  examination, 211–12
  healing, in ridge augmentation, 164, 165
  occlusal load on, 207–8
  preparing, 223–9
  removal of bridge and extraction or retention of, 271
  selecting, 207–10, 215–16
  splinting with precision-attachment partial denture, 243
  support by, 207–10
  transmucosal, see Transmucosal abutment
Acid-etch retained composite splints, 245
Acrylic(s), see also Wire-and-acrylic splint
  biteplane, 74
  buccal prosthesis, 161
  cast-metal crown facings, 29
  pouring with temporary crowns, 122, 124
  provisional bridge, 197
  special trays, 103, 104–5
  veneers, 11, 13
Adaptations, see Adjustments and adaptations
Adhesive bridge, see Minimal preparation bridge
Adhesive cements, 47, 144
Adjustments and adaptations, 264–5
  with bridges, 264–5
    occlusion, 222
  with crowns, 264–5
    axial contours during trying-in, 143
    intercuspal position, 83
    in mouth, 83–4, 146
    shade, 143
Aesthetics, see Appearance
Age
  and crowns, 85–7
  and replacement of missing teeth, 159
Air, compressed, gingival retraction, 135, 136
Alginate impressions in bridgework
  for assessing parallelism, 223, 225
  for chairside temporary and provisional bridge
    construction, 228, 229, 230, 231
Aluminium temporary crowns, 122

Alveolus
  bone loss, and replacement of missing teeth, 162, 164
  ridge, see Ridge
Amalgam (for restorations)
  choosing, 23
  copper ring and, temporary crowns of, 125
  cores of, 36
  mercury toxicity, 19
  pin-retained, 17–19, 36
Amelogenesis imperfecta, crowns, 4
Anterior crowns, 8–9, 24–34, 54, 114–15
  alternatives, 9–16
  complete, 24–33, 109, 114–15
    vital teeth, 24–9
  designing, 53, 54, 58–9
  indications, 8–9
  partial, see Partial crowns
  preparation of teeth, 109, 114–15, 116–22
  root-filled teeth, 29–33
Anterior splints, 249–51
  appearance, 249–50
  selecting, 251
Ante's rule/law, 207, 209
Appearance/aesthetics
  crowns, 6–8, 43–4, 89–90, 92–5
    after fitting/cementation, 146
    metal–ceramic, 29
    planning, 89–90, 92–5, 101–5
    porcelain, 25
  replacements for missing teeth (bridges etc.), 154, 161–2, 210–11
    pontics, 195
    retainers, 192–3
  splints, 249–50
Appointments, 98
Approximal surfaces, see Proximal surfaces
Arcon-type articulator, 80, 81
Articulating paper, 75
Articulators, 77–82
  casts mounted on, 82
    study, 76, 78–9
  fully-adjustable, 81–2
  semi-adjustable, 80–1
  simple-hinge, 77–80

Attitude of patients
  crowns, 85
  replacements of missing teeth, 158–9
Autogenous grafts for ridge augmentation, 162, 164
Automix gun for delivering polymers, occlusal records, 139
Axial surfaces/contours (with bridges), 228–9
Axial surfaces/contours (with crowns)
  checking/adjusting, during trying-in, 143
  reduction
      partial crowns, 115
      posterior crowns, 112–14

Biteplane
  acrylic, 74
  fixed anterior (Dahl appliance), 71, 72, 73, 108–9
Bleaching, 9, 12
Bone loss, alveolar, and replacement of missing teeth, 162, 164
Boxes, 116
Bridge(s) (US term = fixed partial denture), 149–237,
      255–74
  children, *see* Children
  components, 173, 191–206, *see also specific components*
      mechanical failure, 258–9
  construction, 222–37
  designs, *see* Designs
  extending, 267, 270
  failure, 157–8, 255–74
      causes, 255–63
      solutions (repair/replacement etc.), 256–8, 267, 271–4
  impression materials, 130–1
  indications (compared with partial dentures and implant-
      retained prostheses), 149–72
  materials used for, *see* Materials
  occlusal objectives, 76–7
  over-prescribed, 261
  planning, 210–15
  predicting final result, 212–14
  removing bridge and parts of, *see* Removal
  replacing part of, 267
  temporary and provisional, differences between, 128–9
  terminology/definitions, 149–52, 173
  trial preparations, 95, 214–15
  types, 149, 150, 173–90, *see also specific types*
  under-prescribed, 260–1
Bridge splint (splint/bridge), 248–9
Brittleness, porcelain jacket crowns, 25
Broken-down teeth
  amalgam restoration, 18
  assessing structure and environment, 98
  crowns, 4, 5
      posterior, 16
  veneers, 13
Buccal prosthesis, acrylic, 161
Buccal surfaces
  crowns, reduction, 43
      anterior crowns, 114–15
      posterior crowns, 112

pontics, 202–3
Build up techniques
  cores, 106–9
  temporary partial crowns, 125
Bur(s), 109
  for mesial and distal surface preparation, 114
Burnishing crown margins, 145

Canines, retainers, 193
Cantilever bridge, 153, 174, 176
  advantages/disadvantages, 181, 182
  approximal surface, pontics and, 202
  combined with fixed–fixed design, 178–9
  practical examples, 217
  retainers, failure, 256
  span length, 212
  spring, *see* Spring cantilever bridge
Caries
  crowns for
      anterior, 8
      fillings vs., 3
  secondary, 265
      with bridges, 157, 260
      with crowns, 260
Cast(s)
  articulating, 82
  opposing, 100
  study, *see* Study casts
  trimming, 82
Cast ceramic crown, 26
Cast cobalt–chromium removable splints, 244
Cast connectors, 204
Cast-mesh bridge, 184, 186
Cast-metal bridges, 180, 186, 187
Cast-metal crown
  acrylic-faced, 29
  anterior, 29
  posterior, 34
Cast-metal minimal preparation splints, 246
Cast post and cores, 60
  making, clinical and laboratory stages, 96, 97
Cast posterior cores, 39
Casting, crowns, difficulties, 53–4
Casting alloys, bridges, 183
Cements (and cementation), 143–5, 230
  with bridges, 233, 234–5
      permanent cementation, 233
      with temporary and provisional bridges, 230
      trial cementation, 233
  with crowns
      choice, 143–4
      glass ionomer, *see* Glass ionomer cement
      luting, 47
      root filling, removal, 116
      technique, 144–5
      with temporary and provisional crowns, 129
  with splints, 252

Centric occlusion, 66
Centric relation, 66
Ceramic materials, *see also* Metal–ceramic; Porcelain
  bridges, 180
    fracture, 258
  crowns
    fracture, 258
    posterior, 34–5
  facings, 267
  inlays for posterior teeth, 21, 22
Cerec machine, 22
Cermets, 38–9
Chairside
  temporary bridge construction, 228, 229
  temporary crowns, 122–5
    construction, 122–5
    planning, 106
Checking procedure, crowns, 140–3
Children, crowns and bridges, 85–6
  oral hygiene and, 89
Choosing restorations, *see* Decision-making
Chroma, 102
Class IV gold inlays as alternative to anterior crowns,
    10–11, 12
Cleaning and cleansability with bridges, 210, 236, 237
  pontics, 194
Cleft palate
  bridgework, 156
  splints, 241–2
Clinical stages and techniques
  with crowns, 77–83, 96–7, 98–9, 100–46
  inadequate technique, 261–3
Cobalt–chromium removable splints, cast, 244
Colour of teeth (matching of crown restorations), 102
  poor match, 263
  posterior restorations, 19–21
Combination designs, bridges, 178–9
Composite materials (restorations made from), *see also*
    Wire-and-composite splint
  acid-etched retained, splints attached with, 245
  as alternative to anterior crowns, 10
  appearance, 7
  core, for posterior crowns, 38
  core and crown, for root-filled anterior teeth, 31
  for crown facing, 29
  inlays, 20, 21
  veneers, 11–16
Compressed air, gingival retraction, 135, 136
Confidence of patients, replacement of missing teeth and,
    159
Congenital defects, splints, 241–3
Connectors/joints, 204–6
  definition, 173
  fixed–fixed bridge, 176, 205, 206
  fixed–movable bridge, 176
  in hybrid designs, 179
  selecting, 216

Consent, informed, 85
Construction/manufacture
  bridges, 222–37
  crowns, 100–46
    clinical stages and techniques, 96–7, 98–9, 100–46
    laboratory stages, 96–7, 98–9
    occlusal objectives, 76–7
Contact(s), occlusal, 66, 67
  checking points of, during trying-in of crown, 143
  premature, 69
Copper ring and amalgam, 125
Cords, retraction, 135, 136
Cores, 36–9, 98, 106–9
  building up, 106–9
  and crown, 36–9
    for anterior teeth with root fillings, 31
    partial crown, for partial restoration, 18, 23
    for posterior teeth, 18, 23, 36–9
  need for, 98
  pins retaining, *see* Pin-retained cores
  posts and, *see* Posts
  removal, 270
Cost
  bridges, 158, 194
  crowns, 87
    porcelain jacket, 25
Cross-pinning, 257, 258
Crowns (restorations) and crown preparations, 1–146, 255–74
  alternatives to, 9–16
  anterior, *see* Anterior Crowns
  children, *see* Children
  contraindications, 3–23
  cores and, *see* Cores
  decision-making, 21–3, 92
  designing, 41–61, 76–7
  impression materials, 130–1
  indications, *see* Indications
  lengthening, 46, 106
  making, *see* Construction
  multiple, 6
  paralleling devices, 224–5
  partial, *see* Partial crowns
  planning, *see* Planning
  posterior, *see* Posterior crowns
  problems/failure, 8, 255–74
    avoiding, 47–54
    causes, 255–63
    repair, *see* Repair
  provisional, 128–9
  as retainers, 173, 191
  sleeve, 267, 269
  splints retained by
    by complete crowns, 248–9, 251
    by partial crowns, 248
  temporary, *see* Temporary crowns
  trying-in, 140–3
  types, 24–40, *see also specific types*

Crowns (teeth), condition when considering crown
    restoration, 90, see also entries under Intra-coronal
Cusp, functional, 112

Dahl appliance, 71, 72, 73, 108–9
Decision-making (selection/choices)
    anterior splints, 251
    bridges, 207–11, 215–19
        construction technique, 229–30
        materials, 229
        retainers, 192–4
    crowns, 21–3, 92
    fixed vs. removable prostheses, 158–67
    posterior restorations, 21–3
Dental floss, bridges, 235–7
Dentinogenesis imperfecta, 4, 86
Dentures, partial, see Partial dentures
Designs
    bridge, 173–80, 207–21
        advantages/disadvantages, 180, 181, 182
        combinations, 178–9
        example of design process, 219–21
        pitfalls, 260–1
        pontics, 194–5
        selection criteria, 207–11
        variations, 180
    crown, 41–61, 76–7, 261
        pitfalls, 47–54, 260
Diodontic splints, 244, 249, 250
Direct bridges, 184
Discomfort, bridges, 158
Displacing forces, retention against, see Retention
Distal surface preparation for crowns, 113–14
Distortion, all-metal bridges, 258–9
Dome-shaped pontic, 196, 199, 200

Eating ability, replacements for missing teeth, 155
Elastomeric materials
    impression recording, 130, 132, 134
    occlusal recording, 139
Electrosurgery, 135
Enamel
    hypoplasia, 5, 45
    surface area for bridge retention, 226–8
Equipment, see Instruments and equipment
Erosion, see Wear
Etched bridge, 233, 235, see also Acid-etch retained
    composite
Examination, patient
    with bridges, 211–12
        recall, 237
    with crowns, 85–92
        of occlusion, 74–6, 78–9
        recall, 145
Extension of bridge, 267, 270
Extra-coronal restorations, general indications, 3–8
Eye, paralleling by, 223

Facebow, 78
Facings
    lost, 259, 268
        replacing, 267, 268
    pontic, see Pontics
    preformed, 267
    proprietary, see Proprietary facings
    repair, 266
    'unit-construction', 267
Fillings
    crowns vs., 3, 92
    root, see Root-filled teeth
Finishing
    anterior teeth for crowns, 115
        for post crowns, 121–2
    porcelain in mouth, 84
    posterior teeth for crowns, 114
Fit of crown, checking, 141–2
Fixed anterior biteplane (Dahl appliance), 71, 72, 73,
    108–9
Fixed connectors, 204
Fixed–fixed bridge, 173–6
    advantages/disadvantages, 181, 182
    combination of
        with cantilever design, 178–9
        with fixed–movable design, 179
    connectors, 176, 205, 206
    hybrid designs, 179
    practical examples, 218
    preparation, 226, 226–8
    retainers, 173
        failure, 255–6, 256
    span length, 212
    unsatisfactory design, 174, 175
Fixed–movable bridge, 174, 175, 176
    advantages/disadvantages, 181, 182
    combined with fixed–fixed design, 179
    hybrid designs, 179
    practical examples, 219
    retainers, failure, 256
    span length, 212
Fixed partial dentures (US term), see Bridge
Fixed prostheses (in general), choice between removable
    and, 158–67
Fixture, 153
    definition, 151–3
Flossing, bridges, 235–7
Fracture
    bridges, 258
        retainer, 269
    crowns, 258
        porcelain jacket, see Porcelain (jacket) crowns
    tooth tissue
        in abutment teeth, 260
        with crowns, 52
Function (with crowns)
    design considerations, 42–3

occlusion and, 62–4
restoration, 8

Gap between crown and preparation margins, 262–3
Gender, *see* Sex
Gingiva (with crowns), 44
  retraction, 131–5, 136
Gingival–palatal reduction, 115
Glass ionomer cement (for restorations), 144
  as alternative to anterior crowns, 10
  appearance, 7
  bridges, 233
  core
      and crown, for root-filled anterior teeth, 31
      for posterior crowns, 38–9
Gold alloy, 34
Gold bridges, trying-in of retainers, 231
Gold crowns
  adjustment in mouth, 84
  making, clinical and laboratory stages, 97
  posterior, 34, 35
      designing, 55–6
  removal, 270
Gold inlays
  as anterior crown alternatives, 10–11, 12
  as posterior crown alternatives, 17, 18, 19
      choosing, 23
Grafts, bone, for ridge augmentation, 162, 164
Grinding in situ, 264–5
Grooves, 116
Gutta percha root filling, removal, 116

'Half' crown, 36
Hammers, slide, 271, 274
Hand-held models for occlusal records, 77
Health, general, and replacements for missing teeth,
      159–61
History, patient, crowns and, 85–7
Hue, 102
Hybrid bridge designs, 179
Hydrocolloid, reversible, 130–1, 132
Hygiene, *see* Oral hygiene
Hyperplasia, gingival, crowns and, 44
Hypodontia, partial dentures, 168
Hypoplastic conditions, crowns, 5, 45
  anterior, 9

Implant-retained prostheses (osseointegrated implants),
      151–3
  definition, 151–3
  indications for, 169–71
      compared with bridges, 149–72
Impregnated retraction cords, 135, 136
Impressions
  in bridgework
      for assessing parallelism, 223, 225
      in chairside temporary and provisional bridge

construction, 228, 229, 230, 231
      working, 230–1
  for crowns
      planning, 102–5
      working, 129–37
  materials, 130–1
  for permanent splints, 251–2
Incisal hooks, temporary, 228
Incisal–palatal reduction, 115
Incisal reduction, 43, 114
Incisors
  crowns for, 106, 108
      lateral peg-shaped incisors, 4, 46
      porcelain jacket, preparation, 112
  retainers, 193
  single missing, bridge designs, 217, 219–21
Inclination of teeth, crowns altering, 6
  anterior, 9
Indications
  bridges (compared with partial dentures and implant-
      retained prostheses, 149–72
  crowns, 3–23
      anterior, 8–9
      combined indications, 6
      posterior, 16
  splints, *see* Splints
Inflammation, alveolar ridge, pontics and, 200, 201
Informed consent, 85
Injury, *see* Trauma
Inlays
  as anterior crown alternatives, 10–11, 12
  as posterior crown alternatives, 17, 18, 19, 20, 21
      choosing, 23
Insertion of crowns
  after cementation, 145
  path, 44
Instruments and equipment
  for removing crowns and bridges, 271, 273, 274
  for tooth preparation, 109
Intercuspal position, 66
  adjusting, 83
Intermediate-term fixed splints, 244, 245–50
Interocclusal space, creation, 71, 72–3
Intra-coronal retainers, 191
Intra-coronal splints, 246
Intra-oral practices, *see* Mouth

Joints, *see* Connectors

Keratinization with pontics, 200, 201

Laboratory stages and techniques
  bridges, 261
  crowns, 77–83, 96–7, 98–9, 129
  inadequate technique, 261–3
Lateral excursions of mandible, left and right, 66–8
  adjustments with restoration in mouth, 84

Ledge
  negative, 262
  positive, 261–2
Length
  of crown preparations, 50
  root, 90–1
  of span, abutment support and, 209
Lengthening, crowns, 46, 106
Light-curing acrylic for impression trays, 103
Lingual surfaces
  pontics, 202–3
  posterior crowns, reduction, 112
Localization techniques, 231–3
Luting cements
  bridges, 233
  crowns, 47

Macro-mechanically retentive bridges, 184–8, 189–90
Making crowns and bridges, see Construction
Mandible
  dysfunction, 71–4
  movements, 64–8
    and occlusal adjustment in mouth, 84
Manufacture, see Construction
Margins
  crown, 43–4, 114, 146
    burnishing, 145
    deficiencies, 261–3
  gingival, retraction, 131–5, 136
  repairs at, 265
Marking materials, occlusal, 75–6, 83
Maryland bridge, see Minimal preparation bridge
Maryland splint, 246
Materials, see also specific materials
  bridges, 180–3
    pontics, 203–4
    retainers, 183, 192
    temporary/provisional, 229
  crowns, 41–2
  impression, 130–1
Mechanical problems
  bridge components, 258–9
  crowns, 8, 258–9
Medium-mechanically retentive systems, 184, 188
Mercury toxicity, 19
Mesial surface preparation for crowns, 113–14
Metal(s)
  distortion (in crowns), 43
  noble and base, 41
Metal bridges, 180
  distortion, 258–9
Metal–ceramic bridges, 180
  fracture of porcelain, 258
  soldering, 183
  strength of pontic, 195
  trying-in, 231

Metal–ceramic crowns, 25–9, 34
  anterior, 25–9
  designing, 42, 54, 57
  fracture of porcelain, 258
  making, clinical and laboratory stages, 96, 97
  posterior, 34, 36, 57
    pins, 36
    preparation for, 110, 111
  removal, 270–1, 272
Metal–ceramic pontics, 183
  loss of facing, 268
Metal–ceramic retainers, 183
Metal crowns
  design considerations, 41, 54
  making, clinical and laboratory stages, 96
Metal powder, glass ionomer cement containing, cores for
    posterior crowns, 38–9
Metal retainers, 183
Micro-mechanically retentive bridges, 188, 189
Minimal preparation (resin-bonded) bridges
    (Maryland/adhesive bridges), 149, 150, 173, 184–90,
    225–9, 227, 233–5
  advantages/disadvantages, 182
  cementation, 233
  definition, 149
  disadvantages, 190
  fixed–movable, 175
  practical examples, 218
    single missing incisor, 217
  preparations for and construction of, 225–9, 233–5
  retention systems, 184–8, 192
    failure, 256
    in hybrid designs, 179
  types, 184–90
Minimal preparation (resin-bonded) splints, 245
  cast-metal, 246
Moulding techniques, temporary crowns, 122–5, 127
Mouth
  adjustments in, 264–5
    crowns, 83–4, 146
  repairs to crowns and bridges in, 146, 265–7
  trials of bridge in, 214
  whole, crowns and consideration of, 87–9
Movable connectors, 204–6
Mucous membrane reactions with pontics, 200, 201
Multiple crowns, 6
Muscle hyperactivity disorder, 71–4
Myofascial pain dysfunction syndrome, 71–4

Nickel–chromium metal surface of bridge, 187
Non-vital teeth, crowns, 8

Occlusal contacts, see Contacts
Occlusal interferences, 68–9, 74
  absence (=occlusal harmony), 69
Occlusal load on bridge, 207–8
Occlusal perforations, 259

Occlusal relationships
  avoiding loss, 77
  with temporary restorations, maintaining, 77
Occlusal repairs, 265
Occlusal surfaces
  of crown, shaping, 82
  of pontics, 200
  reduction, 112–14
  of tooth, 90
Occlusal vertical dimension
  with bridges, 156
  with crowns, 69–71, 106
    planning changes to, 93, 95, 106
Occlusal wear with crowns, 43, 259
Occlusion
  with bridges, 194
    adjustment, 222
    assessment, 212, 213
    as indicator for bridge, 166, 167
    objectives, 76–7
    planning, 219
    recording, 231
  with crowns, 62–84, 90
    adjustment, 83–4, 143
    alteration, 6
    checking, 143
    design considerations and objectives, 42–3, 76–7
    examination and analysis, 74–6, 78–9
    functional approach, 62–4
    management, clinical and laboratory, 77–83
    recording, 77–83, 138–40
    reduction, partial crowns, 115
    reduction, posterior teeth, 43, 110–12
    stability, *see* Stability
  problems, 263
Occupation and replacement of missing teeth, 156, 159
Opposing casts, 100
Oral hygiene
  with bridges, instructions and maintenance, 235–7
  with crowns, 87–9
    instructions and maintenance, 145
Orthodontic treatment, 62–3
  bridges and, 156
  splints and, 241
Osseointegrated implants, *see* Implant-retained prostheses
Overhang, 261–2
Over-prescribed bridges, 261
Overtrimmed die, 142

Palatal reduction with metal–ceramic crowns, 28, *see also*
    Gingival-palatal reduction; Incisal–palatal reduction
Palate, cleft, *see* Cleft palate
Parallel pinholes, 116
Parallel plastic pins, 133, 135
Parallel-smooth or serrated posts, 31, 32, 33
Parallel-threaded posts, 32, 33

Paralleling techniques
  complete-crown splints, 251
  conventional bridges, 223–5
Partial crowns, 33–4, 35–6, 61, 115–16
  anterior, 33–4
    designing, 61
    distortion of metal, 53
  core and, 18, 23
  posterior, 35–6
    designing, 61
  preparing teeth for, 115–16
  as retainers, 191
  splints retained by, 248
  temporary, build-up, 125
Partial dentures, 151
  bridge replacing, intra-oral trial, 214
  definition, 151
  fixed (US term), *see* Bridge
  indications, 168
    compared with bridges, 149–72
  precision-attachment, 149–50
Patient
  crowns and consideration of whole, 85–7
  examination, *see* Examination
  removable prostheses (bridges) and consideration of
      whole, 211–12
    fixed prostheses vs., 158–62
Peg-shaped lateral incisors, 4, 46
Perforations, occlusal, 259
Periodontium/periodontal tissue
  bridges and, 158
  crown preparation design and, 44–6
  disease
    abutment teeth affected by, 259–60
    splints, 155, 241, 249–50
Permanent splints, 244, 245–50, 251–2
  clinical techniques, 251–2
  types, 245–50
Petroleum jelly–zinc oxide powder, cementing temporary
      crowns, 129
Photographs, 100
Pier, definition, 173
Pin(s), *see also* Cross-pinning
  broken-down teeth, 16
  parallel plastic, 133, 135
Pin-retained amalgam restorations, 17–19, 36
Pin-retained cores, 16, 18, 36, 37
  construction, 106, 107
Pinholes, 137
  impression, 135
  partial crowns, 116
Planning
  bridges, 210–15
  crowns, 85–99
    clinical stages, 98–9, 100–9
    laboratory stages, 98–9
Plaque resistance, porcelain jacket crowns, 25

Plastic pins, parallel, 133, 135
Plastic strips (for occlusal examination), 75–6
Plastic temporary bridges, 228
Polishing in situ, 264–5
Polyacrylics, *see* Acrylics
Polycarbonate temporary crowns, 122, 123
Polycarboxylate cements, 144
  temporary crowns, 129
Polyether impression materials, 130, 132, 133
Polymer materials
  for impressions, 131–5
  for occlusal records, 139–40
Polysulphide impression materials, 130
Polyvinylchloride (PVC) slip, 122, 124
Pontics, 194–204
  definition, 173
  design principles, 194–5
  facings, 203, 268
    loss and replacement, 268
  metal–ceramic, *see* Metal–ceramic pontic
  selecting, 216
  spring cantilever bridge, 176
  support, 207–10
  surfaces, 195–203
Porcelain (with restorations), *see also* Ceramic materials
  with crowns
    in crown preparation design, 41–2
    finishing in mouth, 84
    occlusal shaping with, 82
  fracture, 52–3, 258, 269
  repair/replacement, 258, 267
Porcelain cantilever bridge, 177
Porcelain connectors, 204
Porcelain facings
  pontic, 203
    loss and replacement, 268
  repair, 266
Porcelain-fused-to-metal (=metal–ceramic), *see*
  Metal–ceramic
Porcelain inlays
  as anterior crown alternatives, 11, 12
  as posterior crown alternatives, 21, 22
Porcelain (jacket) crowns (PJCs)
  for anterior teeth, 24–5, 58, 59
    strengthened, 27
  designing, 52–3, 54, 58, 59
  fracture, 52–3, 269
    replacement, 269
  making, clinical and laboratory stages, 96, 97
  for posterior teeth, 34–5
  preparation of incisors for, 112
  removal, 270, 272
Porcelain veneers, 11–16, 17
Post(s), 31–3, 60
  and cores, 18, 60
    cast, *see* Cast post and cores
    construction techniques, 106, 107

for posterior crowns, 39
  removal, 270
  and separate crowns, for root-filled anterior teeth, 31
  shapes, 31–3
Post crowns/post-retained crown, 54–61, 116–22
  designing, 54–61
  one-piece, 33
  temporary, 125
  tooth preparation, 116–22
Post hole, preparation, 116–21
Posterior crowns, 16, 34–9, 54, 110–14
  alternatives, 17–21
  complete (and in general), 16, 34–9, 54, 110–14
    designing, 54, 55–6
    indications, 16
    tooth preparation, 110–14
  partial, *see* Partial crowns
Posterior restorations (in general), 19–23
  choosing, 21–3
  tooth-coloured, 19–21
Posterior teeth, reduction for crowns, 43, 110–12
Pouring techniques, temporary crowns, 122, 124
Precision-attachment partial denture, 149–50
  splinting of abutment teeth, 243
Preformed facings, 267
Preformed temporary crowns
  construction, 122
  planning, 106
Premature contact, 69
Proprietary facings, 267
  pontics, 203
Proprietary splints, 246–8
Prosthesis
  acrylic buccal, 161
  choice between fixed and removable, 158–67
  definition, 154
  implant-retained, *see* Implant-retained prostheses
Protrusive excursions of mandible, 66
  adjustment with restoration in mouth, 84
Provisional bridges, 215, 229–30
  acrylic, 197
  cementation, 230
  construction, 229–30
  practical examples, 218
Provisional restorations (in general), 128–9
  crowns, 128–9
    cementation, 129
  differences between temporary and, 128–9
  laboratory made, 129
Proximal/approximal surfaces
  bridges, 200–2
  crowns, reduction, 43, 44
    anterior, 114
Pulp
  of abutment teeth, giving problems later, 260
  in crown preparation design, 46–7
  replacements for missing teeth damaging, 156–7

Putty and wash, 131
PVC slip, 122, 124

Recall examination
  bridges, 237
  crowns, 145
Recording occlusion
  bridgework, 231
  crowns, 77–83, 138–40
Reduction (of tooth surfaces for crowns), 110–14, 114–15
  anterior, 114–15
  palatal (with metal–ceramic crowns), 28
  posterior, 43, 110–14
Removable bridges, 149, 150, 180
  definition, 149
Removable prostheses (in general), choice between fixed
    and, 158–67
Removable splints compared with fixed splints, 244–5
Removal
  bridges, 271–4
    parts, 267
  crowns, 267, 270–1
  root filling cements, 116
Repairs to crowns and bridges, 256–8, 265–7
  in situ, 146, 265–7
Replacement
  bridge part, 267
  missing tooth/teeth, *see* Tooth
Resin(s), chemically retentive, 188
Resin-based cements, 144
Resin-bonded bridges and splints, *see* Minimal preparation
    bridges; Minimal preparation splints
Restorations, *see also specific types*
  crowns as part of another, 6
    anterior, 9
    posterior, 16
  decision-making, *see* Decision-making
  extra-coronal, general indications, 3–8
  materials, *see specific materials*
  provisional, *see* Provisional restorations
  temporary, *see* Temporary restorations
Retainers/retention systems (for bridges), 184–90, 191–4
  choosing, 192, 216
  definition, 173
  failure, 255–6, 269
  fixed–fixed bridges, *see* Fixed-fixed bridge
  gold bridges, trying-in, 231
  in hybrid designs, 179
  metal–ceramic retainers, 183
  metal retainers, 183
  minimal preparation retainers, *see* Minimal preparation
    bridges
  over-prescribed, 261
Retention
  bridges, *see* Retainers
  cores, *see* Cores
  crowns, 47–52

  checking, 142–3
  loss, 255
  by pins, *see* Pins
  by posts, *see* Posts
  in vertical loss prevention, 47–51
  orthodontics, 156, 241
Retraction, gingival, 131–5, 136
Retruded contact position (RCP), 66, 67
Retrusive movements of mandible, 66
  adjustment with restoration in mouth, 84
Ridge, alveolar
  augmentation, 162, 164
  pontics and the, 195–200
  shape, 212
Ridge-lap pontic, 197, 198, 199, 200
  modified, 197, 200
Rochette macro-mechanical retentive bridges, 184–8,
    189–90
Rochette splint, 246
Root
  of abutment teeth, fracture, 260
  length, 90–1
Root-filled teeth
  as abutments
    examination, 212
    giving trouble later, 260
  crowns, 16, 29–33, 90
    anterior, 29–33
    removing root filling, 116

Saddle-shaped pontics, 198, 199, 200
Safety precautions, trying-in of crown, 140
Sandblasting, 83
Selection of restoration, *see* Decision-making
Self-curing acrylic for impression trays, 103, 104–5
'Seven-eighths' crown, 36
Sex
  crowns and, 87
  replacement of missing teeth and, 159
Shade, 95, 101–2
  checking and adjusting, 143
  techniques for selecting, 101–2, 103
Shape
  crown, poor, 263
  ridge, bridges and, 212
  tooth, crowns altering, 6
    anterior, 9
Shaping
  occlusal surfaces of crown, 82
  post hole, 116–21
Short-term fixed splints, 244, 245–50
Silicone impression materials, 130, 132
Size of teeth, crowns altering, 6
  anterior, 9
'Sleeve crowns', 267, 269
Slide hammers, 271, 274
Social history and crowns, 87

Soldering
  connectors, 204
  failure of solder joint, 258
  metal–ceramics
    bridges, 183
    crowns, 29
Span
  definition, 173
  length of, 212
    abutment support and, 209
Speech quality, replacements for missing teeth, 155
Splint(s), fixed, 241–52
  diodontic, 244, 249, 250
  indications, 241–4
    periodontal disease, 155, 241, 249–50
  intermediate-term, 244, 245–50
  permanent, *see* Permanent splints
  removable splint compared with, 244–5
  short-term, 244, 245–50
  types, 245–50
Splint/bridge, 248–9
Splinted retainers, failure, 255–6
Sports players and replacement of missing teeth, 159
Spring cantilever bridge, 174, 176–8
  pontics, 203–4
Stability of occlusion
  crowns, 69, 70
    check with restoration in mouth, 84
  replacements for missing teeth, 154–5
Stainless-steel temporary crowns, 122
Strength
  metal–ceramic crowns, 28, 29
  pontics, 195
Strengthened porcelain crowns, 27
Study casts
  with bridges, 212, 214, 229
  with crowns, 75–6, 78–9, 100
    'cheating', 92, 94
    trial preparations on, 94, 98
Support, pontic, 207–10
Surveying in bridge preparation, 223, 225

Taper of crown preparations, 49–50, 50
Tapered-smooth or serrated posts, 31, 33
Tapered-threaded posts, 32–3, 33
Teeth, *see* Tooth
Temporary bridges, 215, 222, 229–30
  cementation, 230
  construction, 229–30
    preparations for, 222, 228
Temporary crowns, 122–9
  cementation, 129
  construction, clinical techniques, 122–7
  planning, 106
  post crowns, 125
Temporary restorations (in general)
  differences between provisional and, 128–9

maintaining occlusal relationships, 77
Temporary splints, 251
Temporomandibular joint dysfunction, 71–4
Tetracycline staining, 9, 10, 11
Threaded posts, 39
  parallel, 32, 33
  tapered, 32–3, 33
'Three-quarter' crown
  anterior, 34
  posterior, 35–6
Tooth/teeth
  abutment, *see* Abutment teeth
  adjacent
    in crown design, 44–6
    replacement of missing teeth considering, 168
  artificial, as part of bridge, *see* Pontic
  broken-down, *see* Broken-down teeth
  colour, *see* Colour
  defective/abnormal, splints, 242–3
  extraction
    bridge removal accompanied by, 271
    decision-making, 92
  inclination, *see* Inclination
  missing, replacement of
    adjacent teeth considered with, 168
    advantages/disadvantages, 154–8
    splints and, 241
  non-vital, crowns, 8
  preparation (for bridges), 223–9
  preparation (for complete-crown splints), 251
  preparation (for crowns), 109–22
    for cementation, 144
    reduction of surface, *see* Reduction
    stages in, 110–22
  remaining, assessing structure and environment, 98
  root-filled, *see* Root-filled teeth
  shape, *see* Shape
  size, *see* Size
  trauma, *see* Trauma
  value, 89
  vital, anterior crowns, 24–9
  wear, *see* Wear
Tooth tissue
  conservation of (with bridges), 210
    retention and, 194
  removal/destruction
    for metal–ceramic crown, 29
    for porcelain jacket crown, 25
  trauma, *see* Trauma
Transmucosal abutment (TMA), 152, 153
  definition, 154
  in ridge augmentation, 165
Trauma/damage, *see also* Fracture
  crowns causing, 52, 260
    to adjacent teeth, 44
  crowns with, 4, 5
    anterior, 8

replacements for missing teeth causing, 156–7, 260
splinting, 241
Trays, impression, special
  bridge construction, 230, 231
  crown construction, 102, 103–5
Trial cementation, bridges, 233
Trial preparations (bridges), 95, 214–15
  intra-oral, 214
Trial preparations (crowns)
  on study casts, 94, 98
  wax-ups, 91, 92, 93, 94–5, 101
Trimming casts, 82
Trying-in
  bridges, 231, 233, 234
  crown, 140–3

Undercuts, interlocking minor, 48
Under-prescribed bridges, 260–1
Unit, definition, 173
'Unit-construction' bridge facings, 267

Value
  as dimension of colour, 102
  of tooth, 89
Veneer restorations, 11–16
Vital teeth, anterior crowns, 24–9

Wash-through pontic, 196, 197, 198
Wax (for occlusal examination), 75, 150
Wax-added technique, 82

Wax carving, 82
Wax records, functionally generated, 82–3
Wax-ups
  with bridges, 214
  with crowns
    diagnostic, 91
    trial, 91, 92, 93, 94–5, 101
Wear/erosion (crowns), 43, 259
Wear/erosion (tooth), gross, 106–9
  crowns with, 4, 5, 106–9
    anterior, 8–9
  partial dentures with, 168
  veneers with, 13–14
Wind-instrument players, replacements for missing teeth,
  156, 159
Wire-and-acrylic splint, 245–6
Wire-and-composite splint, 245–6
Wire loop, bridge removal, 273, 274
Working impressions
  bridgework, 230–1
  crowns, 129–37
Worn teeth and crowns, *see* Wear

Zinc oxide–eugenol
  cementing temporary crowns, 129
  occlusal registration paste, 138, 140
Zinc oxide–petroleum jelly, cementing temporary crowns,
  129
Zinc phosphate cements, 144
  temporary crowns, 129